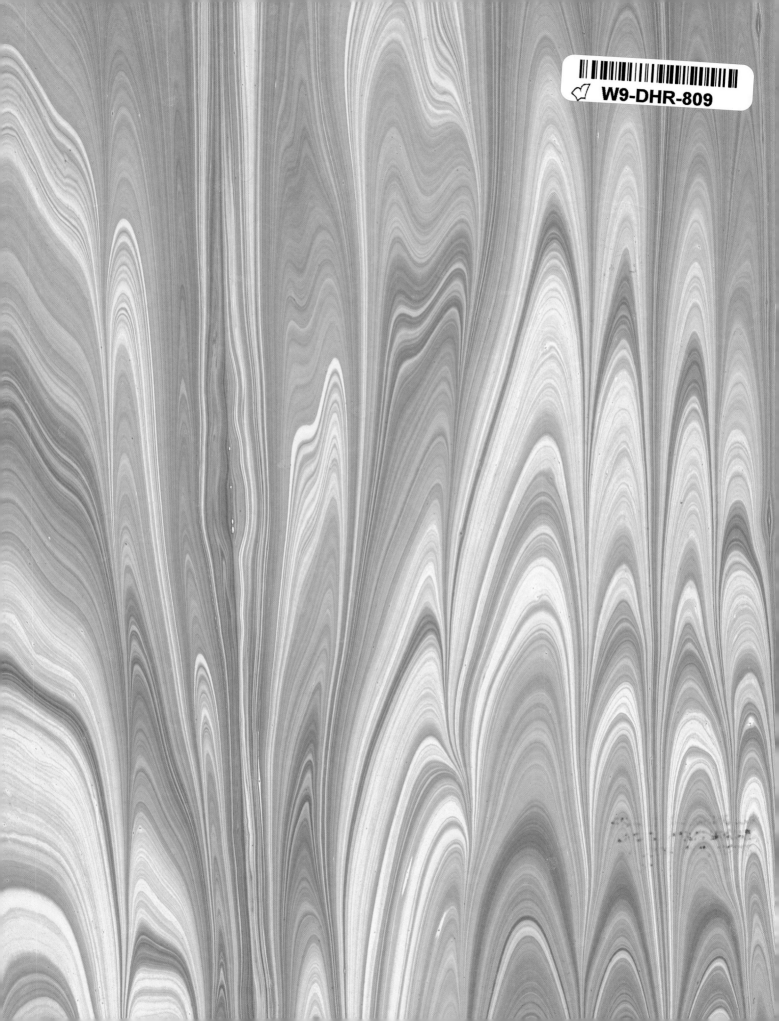

CANES
THROUGH THE AGES
With Value Guide

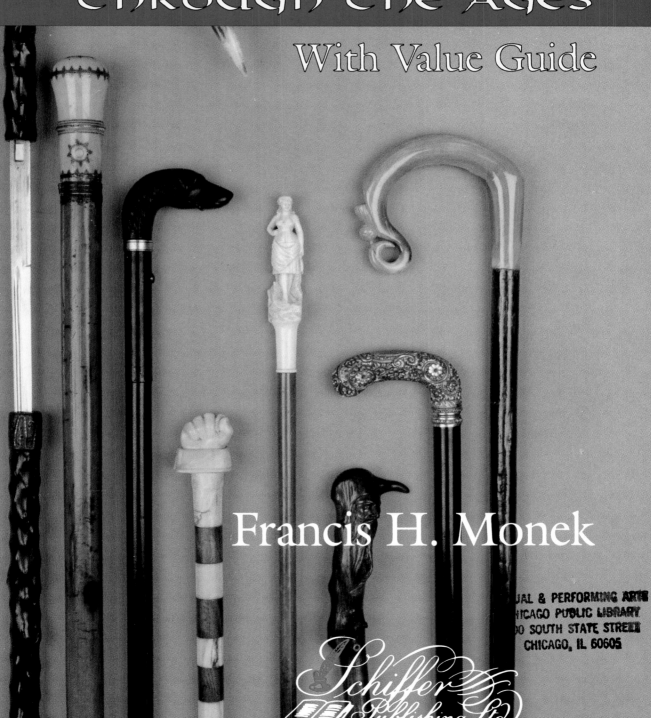

Francis H. Monek

Schiffer Publishing Ltd
77 Lower Valley Road, Atglen, PA 19310

Dedication

To Carol, my lovely and patient wife
of 55 years, the cheerful mother of my 10
children; the happy grandmother of 22;
the ecstatic great grandmother of one, and
the understanding and adoptive mother of
one dog, one cat and 5000 canes and
walking sticks.

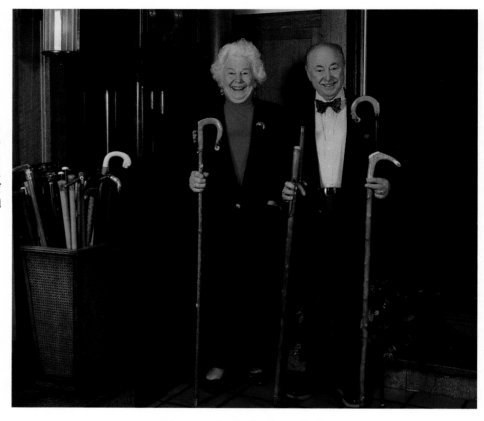

Photography by Barbara Collins

Library of Congress Cataloging-in-Publication Data

Monek, Francis H.
    Canes through the ages : with value guide / Francis H. Monek.
        p.   cm.
    Includes bibliographical references (p.   ) and index.
    ISBN 0-88740-862-1 (hardback)
    1. Staffs (Sticks, canes, etc.) I. Title.
GT2220.M66   1995
391'.44--dc20   95-31567
                CIP

Printed in Hong Kong
ISBN: 0-88740-862-1

Published by Schiffer Publishing Ltd.
77 Lower Valley Road
Atglen, PA 19310
Please write for a free catalog.
This book may be purchased from the publisher.
Please include $2.95 for shipping.
Try your bookstore first.

We are interested in hearing from authors
with book ideas on related subjects.

Contents

Acknowledgment and Appreciation

I wish to thank the following for their assistance in making this book possible:

The magazine *Antiques* for furnishing copies of old pictures and prints; Barbara Collins, professional photographer; Melissa Griswold, professional photographer; Youseff Kadri, editor of *Der Stocksammler* for copies of old prints. Frank J. Monek, my son, who not only continuously encouraged me but unstintedly allowed me use of his office facilities; Linda Redmann, who patiently typed and retyped numerous renditions of this text; Robert Sheldon, Curator of Musical Instruments of the Library of Congress; and most of all, Jeffrey B. Snyder, noted photographer and author of *Canes From the Seventeenth to the Twentieth Century* who provided needed publishing expertise in all departments and took over 1200 pictures and artistically portrayed my canes to their best advantage.

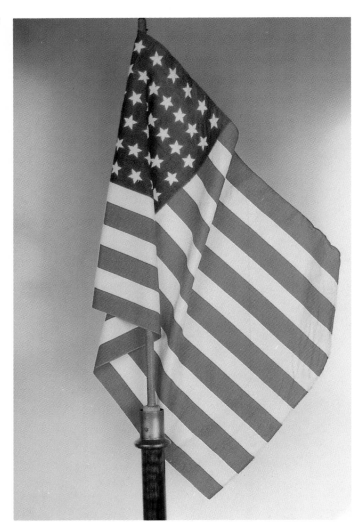

Introduction

This is a book on canes from the experience and viewpoint of a cane collector. It is a monologue by a collector of canes for collectors of canes and those who wish to be.

I have tried to answer all the questions most frequently asked of me in my lectures and conversations. How did I start collecting canes? What was my first cane? How many do I have? Where and how does one go about finding canes; how much does one pay, and how could one start collecting canes at this late date in the present renaissance of this abundant field?

Accordingly, this is not a catalogue of canes—there are enough books on this subject and some very good ones too that try to display every cane ever made, many of which are one-of-a-kind and will never be seen again. This is an eclectic history of one man's experience in hunting for these elusive sticks, were to go, what to look for, what to pay, how to make sure that the stick is all you are bargaining for, and what pleasures and surprises you can expect. As such, all of the canes depicted herein, except the Dayton C. Miller Flute Collection and those shown in the auction catalogues, are part of the collection of the author.

For those who want to know the kinds of canes that have been and still may be available for the persistent hunter, I have enclosed an exhaustive index of over 1580 canes patented in the United States, England, and Germany, giving the date of the invention, the name of the inventor, the number and description of the invention.

For those who are already bitten and thirst for more knowledge, I have appended the most exhaustive bibliography ever published on this subject.

For those who want to know the value of canes, I have not given my personal opinion or that of any alleged expert. I have, however, enclosed a guide compiled from an auctioneer's illustrated prospectus of his two most recent auctions, stating the estimated low and high sales prices before each auction and the actual sales prices received. These two auctions were run by the most reputable "canes only" auction house in America.

Cane collecting can be enjoyed by all as no one can ever garner them all. I've been at it 40 years and I don't have them all. There are enough canes out there for those who would specialize in glass canes, ivory canes, presidential and presentation canes, weapon canes, animal and figural canes, memorial canes - the list is unlimited and inexhaustible. There are rare antique canes and even fine modern canes that years from now will be antique.

You are now all set to expertly find and critically examine and purchase canes to start your own collection. So that you may experience the same joy and happiness this hobby has afforded me, I will answer any questions you find uncovered in this book. You can write me at the address below.

Best Wishes and Happy Hunting.

Francis H. Monek
950 E. Westminster
Lake Forest, IL 60045

October 1994

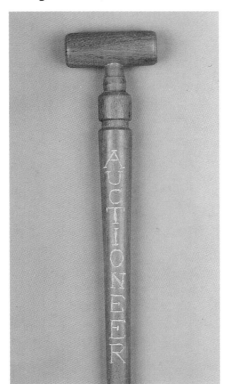

Auctioneer's gavel cane, all wood, 34" high.

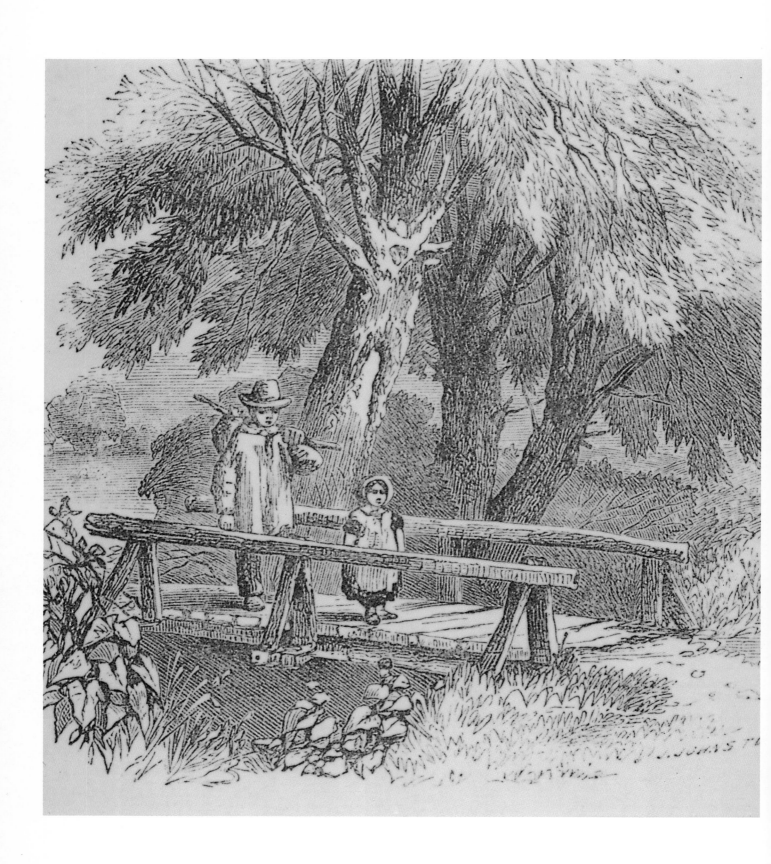

Chapter 1
A Collecting Hobby and Your Health

My profession as a trial lawyer was a very strenuous one. It was necessary that I be away from home for long periods of time as I had cases all over the United States. Tensions arose when a Federal Judge in Detroit notified me I was scheduled for trial in a week from Monday, and then suddenly his docket cleared and I was pushed up for trial on the day after tomorrow. Unfortunately, I was already assigned out before another judge in Philadelphia on the same day. I couldn't be on trial in both places, but this did not deter either judge.

Then there was the problem of getting witnesses, and especially doctors, to certain locations to testify. Then too, frequently the defendant would make a large settlement offer, but I would have to decline it as inadequate even though the judge recommended I accept it. To continue on with the trial was tension indeed. If I got less than the offer, the client could sue me for malpractice. All this was stress piled upon stress and naturally something had to give. I suffered a massive heart attack 30 years ago.

It was a ragged rat race, but for 50 years I enjoyed it. But I paid a price. To shorten my time away from home, I would work until very late at night to get the work done sooner. On top of that I had a growing family, ending up with ten children whom I saw infrequently.

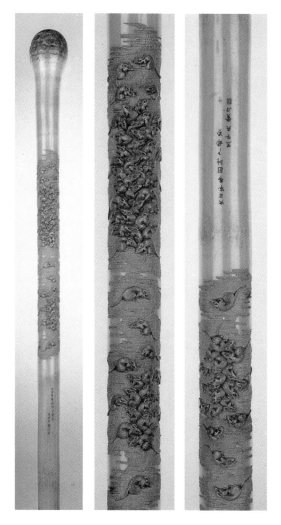

Chinese cane of bamboo with carved swarming rodents and Oriental signature and writing below, 36" high.

I was often away from home, frequently worked late, saw my ten children infrequently, and had a heart attack. Then my cane collecting hobby came to my rescue.

But then my hobby apparently came to the rescue. Just before the heart attack and my hospitalization, I had been negotiating with a man in the upper Northwest to buy his Remington gun cane that had an ivory dog-head handle. I had sent him the money he requested and was awaiting receipt of the cane. Now from the hospital, every day I called home to see if it had arrived. When my wife visited me daily, I asked her if the cane had come. She said no—maybe tomorrow. This went on for six weeks while I was in the hospital, and I stayed alive for each tomorrow because I would have received my finest cane. It never did come; the man was a fraud but in retrospect, he saved my life. I did however help the government to prepare a mail fraud case against him. He pled guilty and was given probation though I never got the cane or my money back.

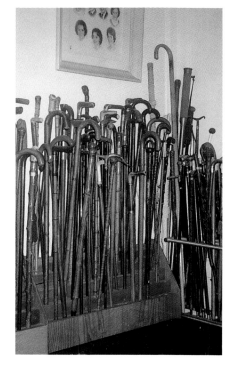

Having such an all controlling hobby as collecting canes gives one a reason to live for tomorrow as the mail might bring a treasured object. I had a running ad in a national collectors paper and received mail every week about canes for sale. At 82, I have now outlived all of my partners and many of my friends who had no real hobby to distract them from the stress of their occupations. Into my busy trial schedule, I somehow was able to lecture on canes, write articles on canes and avidly pursue new sticks in every town I had to be in for business. It was a relief from the stress of my occupation.

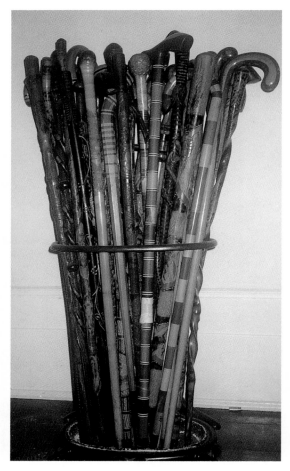

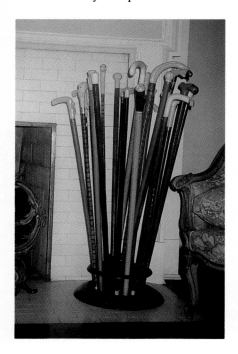

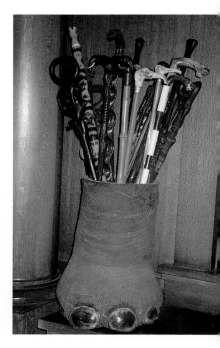

Having such an all controlling hobby as collecting canes gives one a reason to live for tomorrow.

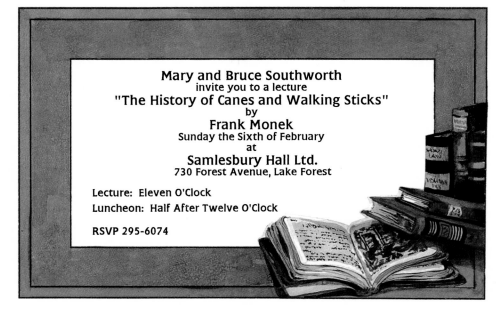

Mary and Bruce Southworth
invite you to a lecture
"The History of Canes and Walking Sticks"
by
Frank Monek
Sunday the Sixth of February
at
Samlesbury Hall Ltd.
730 Forest Avenue, Lake Forest

Lecture: Eleven O'Clock
Luncheon: Half After Twelve O'Clock

RSVP 295-6074

Collecting also was remunerative for my occupation. It was a delightful talking point with clients and broke the ice with reluctant witnesses.

On one occasion I had taken vital information from a witness who, however, refused to sign the statement though he admitted that everything was true. Though I persisted, he was adamant. I, therefore, arranged a meeting with him at my home and assured him if he took his day off work, I would reimburse him his lost day's pay for discussing the case further with me.

The day he came to my home, and walked into my den-office, he was somewhat surly until he saw about 100 canes standing one by one against the wall on the top of the oak wainscoting that circled the room above our heads. He remarked, "My, are all those canes?" I said, "No." He remarked, "Well, if they are not canes, what are they?" I said, "Each one is a gun." After a long silence he said, "Would you show me one?" I showed him one and explained the detail of its firing mechanism, and then I showed him another sample. Finally, he said, "Well, let's sit down and show me where to sign." He had suddenly become very friendly and if it hadn't been for the vital evidence he supplied, I may have lost the case.

The Pleasures of and Surprises in Collecting Canes and Walking Sticks

I have collected canes for about 45 years and now, though I already have over 5,000 sticks, I still continue searching for that unusual and elusive cane that I absolutely must have. This may be because it is made of unusual wood or other material or contains or does something not readily apparent.

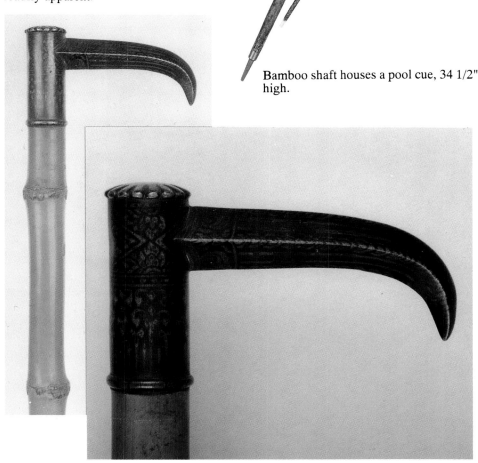

Bamboo shaft houses a pool cue, 34 1/2" high.

Bangkok elephant driver's cane, 1850, 33 1/2" high. A rare gadget cane.

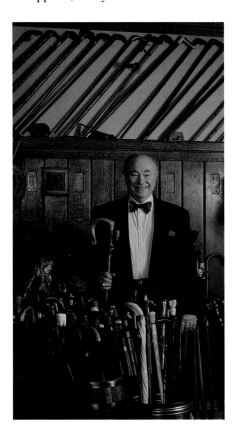

Roughly one hundred gun canes stand against the wall on the top of the oak wainscoating that circles the room. *Photography by Barbara Collins*

9

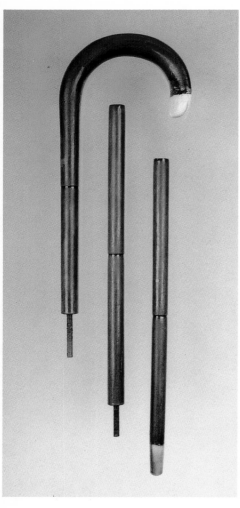

Traveling cane, crook handle with ivory tip, unscrews into three sections, partridge wood shaft, ivory tip with monogram JMK, 35" high.

My first cane was acquired in adulthood, after I was married, and had children. My profession as a lawyer required that I visit the city of Philadelphia, Pennsylvania, where I had to spend many weeks at a time living in the Bellevue Stratford Hotel. Weekends and evenings away from home were lonesome, so I would visit antique shops on Pine Street, in an area over 300 years old. Pine Street at that time had many antique shops. I would visit these shops as an observer, much like I toured museums, to take up my spare time.

One day while in an antique shop, I saw a fine ivory-headed and ivory-ferruled sword cane, made of malacca and with a snake carved on the ivory handle. I immediately remembered seeing an ad in an old monthly magazine called "Hobbies" wherein a Dr. B.W. Cooke advertised every month for canes and walking sticks. Hoping that I could buy this stick

and sell it to him at a profit, I purchased the cane for $12.00. There was an economic depression on at that time, the early 1940's, and though the amount seems trivial now, it was a large sum to a young lawyer with a young, growing family. I actually went without lunch for over a week to pay for this stick.

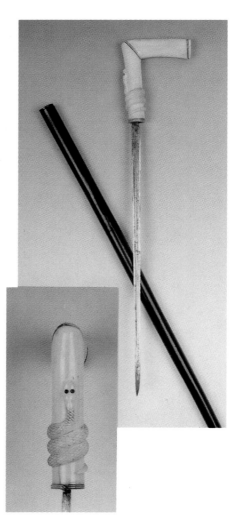

Physician's sword cane, ivory handle with snake, ebony shaft, c. 1840, 34 3/4" high.

When I arrived home in Chicago, I showed it to my wife, and as an excuse for the expenditure, I told her I was going to make a profit on its sale and I immediately called the doctor and told him about this beautiful sword cane. His comment was, "What, another sword cane? I already have over a hundred." He wasn't interested in my sword stick at any price. I apologized to my wife and she bravely said, "It won't break us and you better keep it as the children love it—but keep it out of reach as they might hurt one another."

A few weeks later I was back in Philadelphia. As I walked up Pine Street, I saw the dealer who sold me the cane sitting in a chair in front of his shop. When he saw me, his greeting was, "Here comes the cane man." I had bought only one stick in my life and already I was a cane man! The name seems to have stuck and wherever I go and am recognized, I am called the "cane man."

He invited me in and when I left, I had purchased two more canes. One was a fine cherry stick with a curved ivory handle, the end of which had a carved lion with jeweled eyes and a ferrule that was made of silver. With the cane came a silver and meerschaum pipe bowl in a leather case. To use it one would unscrew the ivory handle and an amber mouth piece was then seen at the top end of the stick. One now unscrewed the ferrule, and taking the pipe case out of one's pocket, inserted the shaft bottom of the cane into the meerschaum pipe bowl and smoked away.

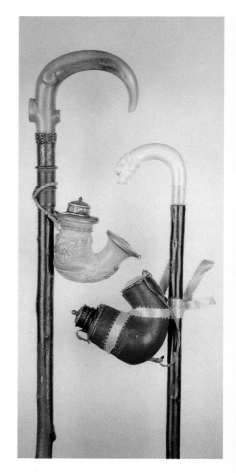

Two smoking canes, German, the full length of the shaft is a pipe. Left: horn handle, 36 1/4" high; right: ivory lion's head, 35" high.

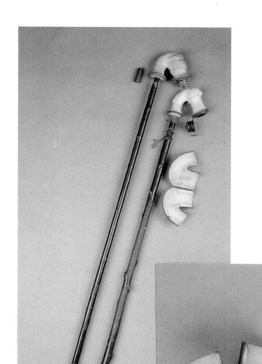

and told him I was a young lawyer from out of state and collected canes. He very graciously invited me to come visit him.

He was a friend and neighbor of the Ford family. He told me his daughters were friends of the Ford girls and we made similar small talk as at that time I had over four daughters (I now have eight, plus two sons). He then took me to his basement and showed me his canes - three fiber board barrels full of very rare and exquisite sticks. He said his deceased mother had collected them and he showed me her journal of each cane and when and

cherished fine canes to have them. He then asked me to make him an offer. I told him I bought one cane at a time considering my growing family, etc., but I loved all of his canes. He finally came to the conclusion that I fitted his description of a proper buyer and he quoted a price that I could afford. The aggregate was almost too high for me, but the individual price was about $1.35 a stick.

I was so excited at this deal. I wouldn't leave the canes out of my sight for fear he might change his mind, so I immediately phoned a car rental agency

I Find and Purchase My First Collection

As the history of the cane unfolded, sadly by the 1930s the cane was no longer either a fashionable article of wear nor even much of a collectible and with time and the depression conditions became worse. In the forties is when I started collecting canes, and I also had to travel the country and try cases in the larger cities of the nation.

Whenever I was in a town of any size, I would call up every antique shop in the Red Book and look for canes. I would do this in the recess and after court hours and between visits from clients. On one occasion in the later forties or early fifties I had done this in Detroit while I was at the Pontchatrain Hotel interviewing witnesses for an upcoming trial. I learned that one elderly man in Grosse Pointe had a fine collection, but he was reclusive and didn't show it to people. I learned his name, looked up his number, phoned him

where in the world she had obtained it. She sure had traveled the world and brought many stick mementos home. I was a very eager but novice collector he soon discovered, and he seemed pleased with my sincere enthusiasm and fondness for his sticks. Apparently no one except he and I treasured them. Hence they were relegated to an ignominious portion of the basement in three old barrels.

He then told me because of his own advanced years he would like to dispose of the canes, but he dreaded it because of what he had seen at a recent auction of the collection of a world famous founder and head of a pharmaceutical company. This latter man had chased canes all over the world in visiting his world-wide company. Now upon his death, his family had seen his immense, beloved and prized collection sold for as little as 10 cents a piece at auction. In some bids, two canes went for 10 cents - canes that had at one time cost hundreds of dollars.

Rather than face this humiliation with his deceased mother's collection, he wanted someone who dearly loved and

and ordered a car sent to me at his home. I then filled the trunk with the three large paper barrels containing the finest and most wonderful canes, plus his mother's journal of all her cane purchases - when and where - from 1907 to 1931. This journal is a real cane Odyssey. I then drove to the Pontchatrain Hotel, picked up my luggage and drove to Ann Arbor where I arrived just in time to give a scheduled lecture on law that evening. And all the time I worried about the safety of my newly found treasures sitting outside in those barrels.

Sadly, by the 1930s the cane was no longer either a fashionable article of wear nor even much of a collectible. With time and the depression, conditions became worse. The handle is a copy of a monument commemorative of the Swiss Guards that died in battle in Paris in 1792 defending the Tuileries. This monument is called the "Lion of Lucerne" and is designed by Thorwoldsen. It is hewn out of solid rock. It is in Lucerne, Switzerland, marked with the date MDCCXCII. Carved dead lion on shield with shattered spear in his side. 35 1/2" high.

Veteran Collection

These canes were part of that first collection I bought. In the cane diary kept by the mother of the man from whom I purchased the sticks, she wrote that they were made by Willard M. Chandler of the Soldier's home at Togus, Maine, 4 miles south-east of Augusta. She obtained them in 1918 from the estate of collector Walter L. Lauler of Brookline, Massachusetts through Mrs. Day of Kennebunkport.

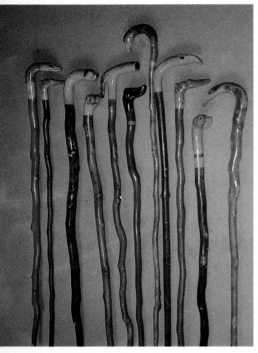

The Veteran's Canes. They were made by a veteran in an old veteran's home in Maine. These canes were part of the first collection I bought.

Many have a very attractive and knotty appearance - a few have natural blemishes which add to their attractiveness.

All of them were carved with a pocket knife into various shapes and figures:

	These all have a number on the ferrule from 407
78 dogs	to 560
58 eagles	
44 alligators	
12 frogs	
15 snakes	
5 ducks	
9 parrots	
2 horses	

2 deerfoot
1 monkey
1 boat
2 human hands
2 seals
52 miscellaneous

_____

299 Total

When I bought the collection only 11 of these canes were left and I appreciate these much more then the factory made canes as they are so natural and light to carry that they seem to be an extension of one's own arm. All are one piece - top to bottom - these were made from woods selected in the neighboring forest and carved by a war veteran using only a pocket knife and old fashioned black glass-topped straight pins for eyes.

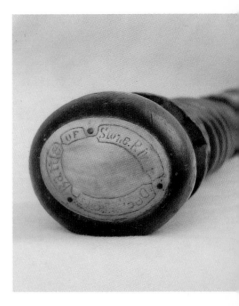

Top view, W.H. Baker's military cane, reading "Battle of Stone River."

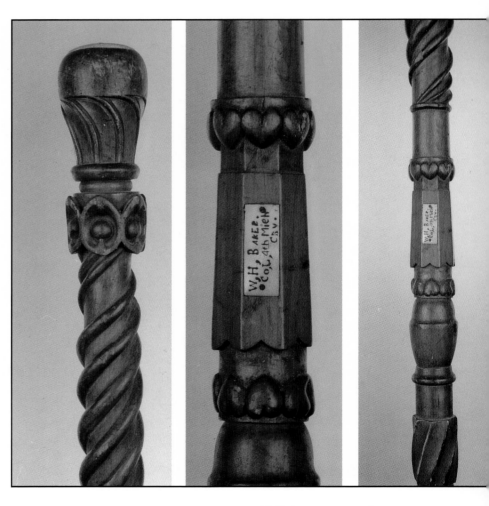

Other canes of war. Civil War cane, carved and signed in inlay "W,H, Baker. Co,L, 4th Mieh CRV." An odd feature, hearts carved below the signature join and then become two faces. On an inlay on top of the handle is carved "Battle of Stone River." 34 3/4" high.

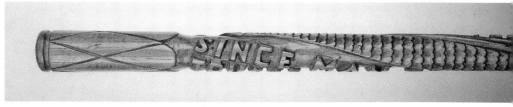

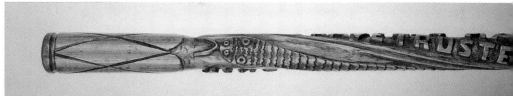

Prisoner of war captive's cane carved with a snake and completed with the phrase: "SINCE MAN TO MAN IS SO UNJUST. I HARDLY KNOW WHICH ONE TO TRUST. I HAVE TRUSTED. AND TO MY SORROW. PAY TODAY. I'LL TRUST TOMORROW." 35 1/2" high.

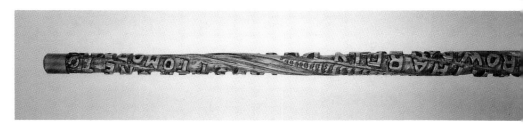

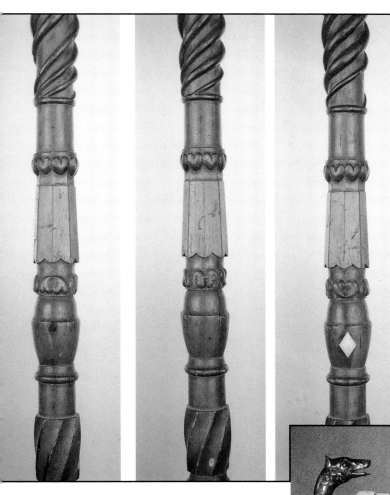

This is how I obtained my first collection which has now grown to over 5,000 sticks. Sadly at that time canes were cheap, but money was also scarce. Many antique dealers, having no customers for fine canes, cut off the beautiful ivory and precious metal handles of their finest sticks and attached them to large magnifying glasses where many can still be found.

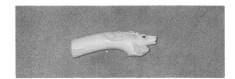

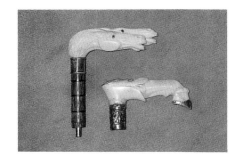

Fine ivory horses' heads handle and an ivory horse's hoof handle.

Handles featuring dogs' heads.

Hooked

I was now all enthusiastic and really hooked as a cane man. Thereafter I spent all my spare money on canes, particularly the gadget-types. A few months later I found my first Remington cap-and-ball, gutta-percha gun cane and I became a cane collector for life.

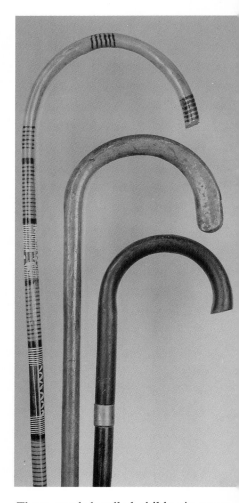

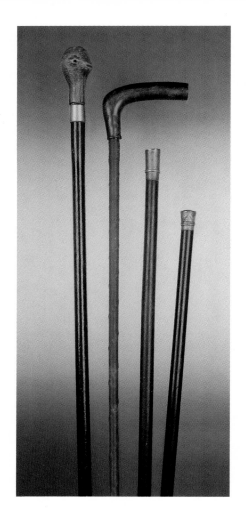

Four small canes for children. The left hand cane is a wooden duck's head, the L handle and the two knobs are all metal. These canes range from 21 to 28 1/2" high.

Three crook handled children's canes, ranging from 22-24" high.

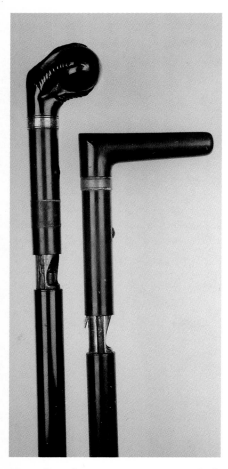

Two Remington gun canes. Left: Remington cap and ball gun cane with an eagle's claw and ball, 34 1/2" high; right: L handled Remington 32 caliber cartridge gun cane, 32 3/4" high.

I am always amazed at the things I find in canes, especially when this is unknown to the seller.

As time went by, my business and my fortunes increased ... and so did my family. Now I have ten children, 22 grandchildren, and over 5,000 canes. My children and their friends are fascinated with my canes and always want me to demonstrate the marvels within them.

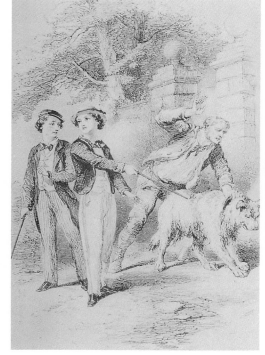

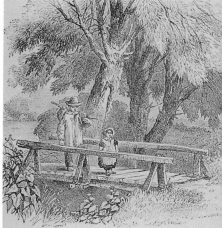

Children with canes.

14

As 20 years went by and I became known as a cane collector, I was contacted by a man who wanted to sell me a presidential cane, actually, the stick of the man who killed our famous president, Abraham Lincoln. His price was high, so I had him visit my house and we negotiated. During our conversation, I discovered he was the son of B.W. Cooke for whom I had purchased my first sword cane only to have him refuse it. His father was dead and his family had what was left of an immense collection, together with all his correspondence in purchasing these canes by mail in answer to his add in "Hobbies Magazine". You can already anticipate what happened. I now have all the canes he inherited; and then I met his brother and got all that he had too, including a violin cane. All this was made possible because they felt I knew their father and they knew I appreciated his collection and they wanted me to have it.

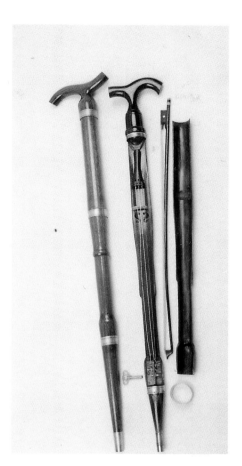

Two violin canes, left: 35 1/2" high; right: 34" high.

Subsequently I purchased other collections, as I was truly bitten by the cane-collecting bug, and in every collection, I have found gadgets that the owners never suspected. In one group of walking sticks, I obtained a very fine camera cane. These can be considered the perks of knowing all about canes and makes the collecting of them such an adventure.

Although in most sales transactions, the rule of *caveat emptor* (let the buyer beware!) prevails, the reverse fortunately may be true in the purchase of canes by a knowledgeable collector. Depending upon his experience, he may find treasures the dealer selling them may not even suspect.

Most antique dealers obtain individual canes or even whole collections because some avid and dedicated searcher who had accumulated them dies, and his wife (or husband), never appreciative of the hobby, immediately rids the house of these "dust collectors." Not knowing the rare container canes, or losing their identity in the sheer numbers of the sticks, she sells them en masse to a dealer who likewise has little experience with walking

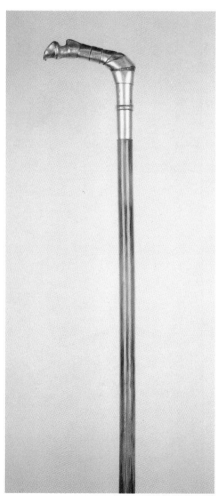

Very slim gold plated L handle in the shape of a horse's hoof, attributed to J. W. Boothe, 31 3/8" high.

sticks. As a consequence, the buyer suspects, and the dealer doesn't know, fine specimens can be purchased at a fraction of their value. This adds zest to the hobby (is the kill of the chase) and evens off the often exorbitant prices the collector has had to pay in his less experienced days.

It is a truism that many collections end in the sunnier climates preferred by the elderly when they retire. Therefore, for all collectors the happy hunting grounds are in Florida, California, Arizona, etc.

On one occasion my wife and I were in Boca Raton, Florida and I recalled having corresponded with a collector in Fort Lauderdale so I phoned him. I was advised by his wife that he was on his sailboat, but would be back in two to three hours so I eagerly drove down to his place and waited for him—but he never showed up. His wife sympathized with me. She was most considerate and suggested I come back the following day. The next day I made the 100 mile round trip again and after a long wait, his boat sailed into his slip at the end of his yard and we introduced ourselves to each other. He advised me that now sailing was his all-consuming hobby and consequently he was thinking of selling all his canes. He had about 25 canes he said but no container or gadget sticks. Would I be interested? This to a collector! Even if there were no gadget canes, I might buy them all, probably very reasonably because he was no longer interested. I could use them as traders for more desirable sticks with another collector. This could be a find—after all aren't oranges cheaper by the dozen?

I looked over his collection with well disguised cupidity, I thought. I soon learned in making small talk (actually sizing up an opponent) that this man was a real estate dealer and very experienced in the give and take of negotiations. He would not state a price but wanted me to make an offer. I hesitated lest I offer more than he would take. Our banter was leading us nowhere so he finally said off the bat that this was to be a one shot deal and no haggling; I would have to pay his price. He suggested I write my offer for all his canes on a piece of paper and he would likewise write his price on a piece of paper, and then both of us would throw our papers into the center of the rug in the middle of the room. I was to pick up his and he mine. If I was over his price, he'd still sell at his price, but if I was under, the whole deal was off. He was a real trader—what chance did I as a mere lawyer have against such a shrewd real estate dealer. He reiterated if we were anywhere close we could negotiate further. If we weren't close, the deal was off and I could go back to my hotel.

Well, I wanted the canes, but at the least expense. So I averaged about $10.00 apiece and wrote $300.00 (Remember this was in the days when the first-class U.S. postage stamp was 2 cents.) I was shocked when I opened his demand of $3,000.00. Didn't he know oranges were cheaper by the dozen?

We were nowhere close, so he said that ends the negotiations as he wanted about ten times what I was offering. In my law practice of settling and trying personal injury and other cases, my then employer and subsequent partner and my mentor always advised me—never, ever close a deal with finality, always leave the door open for further negotiations.

So I told my opponent that perhaps all his canes were too rich for my blood so how about half of them? He let me pick out the half I wanted but then insisted on the same charade, and when I picked up his paper and he mine, we were still the same distance apart. He still wanted ten times what I was offering. To shorten the telling, after more tries we were down to only one stick.

I had carefully looked over his canes and when he wasn't looking, I'd try to twist or pull a handle or strike the cane shaft against my leg to see if I could hear a rattle that would indicate something might be inside the cane. One—a very plain malacca with a stag-horn handle was somewhat suspicious to me. I thought I saw a slight line of demarcation near the bottom of the handle indicating two pieces of wood had been pieced together, but it was so well done that I was doubtful. Really of his whole collection, this was the only stick I coveted.

He then told me we apparently couldn't agree on any deal, but if I'd give him a good sword cane from my collection, he'd give me the choice of several of his canes. He said he walked his dog every night and would like the security of a weapon cane, especially when he traveled to and in New York City on his real estate deals. He said he was afraid in

New York City at dusk and nighttime when he regularly inspected large buildings. This was long before the metal detecting checks on the airlines that could have discovered a sword concealed in a cane.

I still wanted some of his canes, but as he was adamant I said I'd like to buy just one so I wouldn't go home empty handed. I picked out the one—the simple horn-handled stick. He said, "Why, that's the worst in the lot—it's a stick I use to walk my dog every day and is not nearly as valuable as any of the others." I said perhaps it is the only one I can afford. We talked awhile and he again asked if I had a sword cane. I said I had many. He expressed an interest in buying one as he said he had been collecting canes for years and could never find a decent sword cane. Then we talked about the matter at hand— the old malacca he used to walk his dog— but he still want ten times what I wished to pay. He asked $100.00 and I offered him $10.00. His wife finally intervened, as she had been watching the entire charade. She told her husband that I had come 100 miles round trip the day before when he didn't show up because he was out sailing and the wind had been adverse to his keeping our appointment. She also said I had nevertheless come back again and here he wouldn't even sell me the least of his canes by his own admission. After some more bargaining, she shamed him into selling me the stick for $15.00, and as I left, he said to remember him if I found an extra sword cane in my travels.

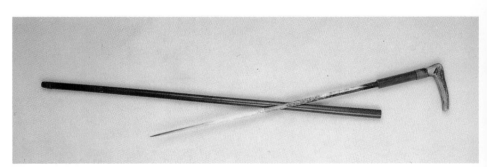

Sword cane with an antler handle, silver collar, malacca shaft, and a double edged blade decorated roughly half way down the blade. 35 1/4" high.

I could hardly wait to get back to the car and examine this cane more carefully. I had suspected that it was a container cane, but what kind I didn't know. I now worked harder on separating or opening

the cane without success and when I finally got to my hotel and entered our room, my wife, seeing I was carrying only one cane said, "Was it worth all that trouble for just one stick?" (She is not a collector, so she doesn't understand the mania). I said we would find out in a minute. As I held up the stick with my hands, one on each side of a slight line of demarcation I had seen on the stick, I started to bend the stick. She screamed, "You'll break it!" And with that there was a sudden pop as the stick separated and I pulled out a beautiful sword that hadn't been drawn out in about 100 years. Here, the man who so longed for a sword cane, was walking with one every day for many years entirely oblivious to its true nature. Whenever I tell this story, I am asked if I ever told the real estate dealer about this. My answer is always, "Would you?"

I have many, many similar stories to tell, but now I will tell about one cane that perhaps one of you readers can help me decipher.

About 20 years ago, I bought a beautiful thick mahogany cane with a silver handle and thick horn ferrule. It is a fine stick, but it has one drawback—it is very heavy, weighing about 3 1/2 pounds—too heavy for anyone to wear, carry or even use. This troubled me for a long time until one day I read about valuable objects being hidden in canes. Many handles unscrew to disclose secret compartments, and it has been reported when an old ivory-handled cane was cleaned, it was found to unscrew and in the opened hiding place was found a fine opal. Early miners out West had hollow shafted canes concealing gold dust; other shafts have concealed numerous coins and rods of precious metal. So, I checked my cane again. I balanced it from the center and felt that whatever made it heavy was in the entire length of the cane. I put a magnet to it along its entire length, but it was non-magnetic. I was now getting excited, as I thought it must be gold that was smuggled out from somewhere. Not wishing to destroy the cane or leave visible marks on it, I carefully worked off the heavy horn ferrule and then drilled upward in the bottom of the shaft. When yellow-like turnings came out, I was sure it was gold! I had an old acid gold tester and applied it to the turnings. It was gold! My wife and I were excited. We weighed the cane, multiplied it by the then present value of gold, and we were rich indeed. To be absolutely certain, the next day I took the turnings to a jeweler who was a client of mine. He tested it with a not-so-old tester—and it turned out to be nothing but brass! There the bubble burst, but the collector in me still wants to know who and why one would build such a very heavy cane, so finely made, when one couldn't use it except as a possible lure in a store where it would be alone in a container and no one could steal it and get away with it because of its weight. For years I was troubled about the use of this cane and then last year, in Maine, I found another walking stick exactly like this one—heavy as can be and yet beautifully made. It is over four pounds in weight.

There must have been a purpose for this cane. It's not an accident, as I have two alike. Can anyone tell me about it? But then, ever hopeful, maybe the brass rod is only at the bottom 3 inches of the cane—a decoy to conceal the gold rod above it. Some day I am going to remove the top handle and drill down from the top, or I may even drill crosswise at the middle of the cane. Strangely enough, that second cane from Maine is different in that it is magnetic from top to bottom.

Two mystery canes, very heavy. Left: 35 3/4" high; right: 35" high. These are too heavy to carry easily. What is their purpose?

Over the years I have frequently been asked if I'm ever going to write and publish a book on canes. Time went by and I frequently wrote articles for the Readers Digest, Der Stocksammler, and the Cane Collector's Chronicle and occasionally a few pages on the proposed book. In addition, I have allowed many authors to copy my source material and photograph my canes, all for their own books.

Once while giving a lecture on canes, a young lady commented that my talk was very interesting and informative and did I ever intend to write a book. Facetiously, I stated that at the rate I was progressing on the book, it would probably have to be published posthumously. The young lady said, "Wonderful, I hope we won't have to wait too long!!"

Many of my daughters were very helpful in assisting me with my collection. One in particular - our Mary, who is now a very prominent interior decorator, cleaned up my cane room while my wife and I were out of town at a legal convention. When I came home I noticed, not only had she cleaned my den very nicely, but she had tacked on the wall under a display of gun canes surrounding my den, a typewritten note that read, "The only difference between men and boys is the cost of their toys."

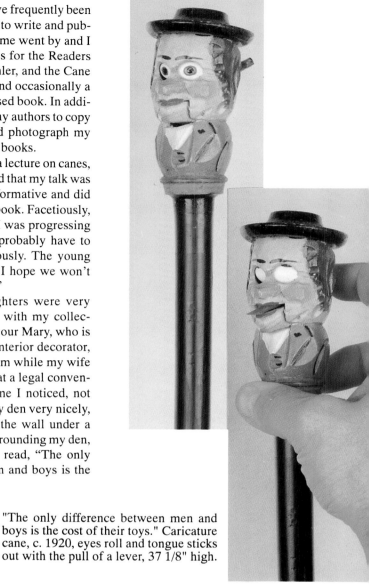

"The only difference between men and boys is the cost of their toys." Caricature cane, c. 1920, eyes roll and tongue sticks out with the pull of a lever, 37 1/8" high.

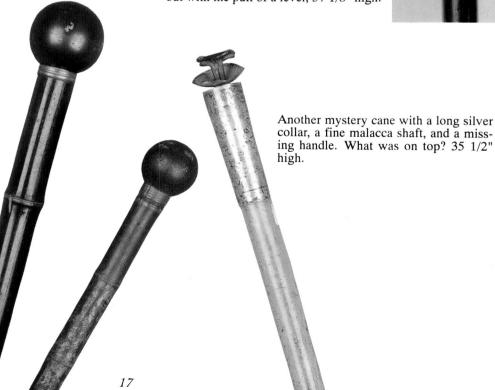

Another mystery cane with a long silver collar, a fine malacca shaft, and a missing handle. What was on top? 35 1/2" high.

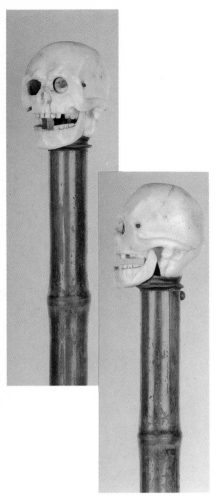

Skull handle that rolls its eyes and wags its jaw at the push of a button, c. 1890. 40" high.

I thought this pretty mature for a 12 year old and even a little brazen. Nevertheless, for the work she had done I wrote her a check for $12.00. This was her first check - she had never before had one made out to her and asked how she could cash it. I suggested she go to our local bank, which she did. She was gone a long time and when she returned, I asked her what took her so long. She was evasive at first and then said it was very complicated. When she went to the bank, the cashier, noting her youth, said she'd have to get the check approved by an "officer". Mary dutifully walked to the nearby police station and told the officer in charge that she required his approval on the check. He patiently explained her need was for a bank officer and not a police officer and she somewhat shamefully went back to the bank and got the proper endorsement. This story always stops her when she begins talking about Daddy and his toys.

As I have frequently written articles and lectured both on radio and television on canes and walking sticks, my name has often appeared in various newspapers and national magazines from the finest periodicals down to the sensational tabloid type.

One year while we were on vacation in Maine, my wife received a letter from one of our eight daughters who was in our home town of Lake Forest, Illinois. She was shopping in our finest food store called, "Don's Finest Foods," when Leslie, a clerk well known to and loved by all of us said to her, "Mrs. Davis, your father is pictured in the 'National Enquirer'." This is a newspaper-type magazine catering to sensational tattler news and is sold at the checkout counters in national food chains and other food stores.

Though as a trial lawyer, I had appeared frequently in print on national cases that I was trying and of which publicity my children evidenced a certain pride, none of these cases were of the sort that would appear in tabloids catering to notoriety.

She was appalled and wondered, what had daddy been up to now? She quickly went to the magazine rack and surreptitiously picked up the paper. There indeed was a picture of her father, all smiles, in the midst of hundreds of canes. Breathing a sigh of relief, she left the store and as she passed a nearby chain store, another friend called out, "You should see the 'Star', it has a big picture and write up about your father!" Hurrying into the store, she obtained a copy and fortunately it was on the same subject matter. Apparently that anyone had about 5,000 canes and walking sticks was sensational enough to merit inclusion in these tattler magazines. She wrote to her mother. "It was a shock to hear about Daddy in such magazines. Not only was he pictured in one, but two sensational tattlers in one week. But, thank God, nothing bad!"
A few weeks later I received a letter from Europe enclosing a clipping from the German version of these notorious magazines. Publicity of even such a mild sort prompts numerous letters and calls, some of interesting canes and others of pathetic or curious nature.

One evening, I received a call from a man who said he heard I had some gun canes. I admitted this and he said he wished to purchase one but a very good workable one. I told him I was a collector and all my canes were antique. Further, I never sold any gadget canes as they are hard to find and I use my duplicates as traders for canes I desire more. He begged for a cane and said he'd pay any price I demanded as he needed it for protection. I again reminded him I was a collector and wouldn't dare shoot one of my gun canes for fear that due to its age it might explode and injure me. He said he'd have any gun cane I sold him repaired and that it would be workable. I refused to sell and asked why he was so desperate to obtain such a weapon.

His story was pathetic. He said he was a witness for the government on a case against the Mafia. I told him the government had a protection program for such witnesses. He said that in his case he was guarded throughout the trial, and for long thereafter, through the appeals, but then when the felons were incarcerated, his protection became lax. One day as he got into his car and stepped on the starter, the car exploded. After many months in the hospital he said he left on two crutches. He is now a paraplegic and

Three rare pepper box gun canes with stilettos of Belgium manufacture.

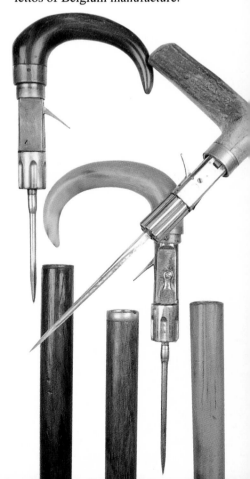

must use the two crutches the rest of his life. He fears "they" will try again and he needed a defense as he was in terror for his life. He felt he could walk with two canes and if one were a gun cane, he would feel more secure. I advised him to get a permit and carry a pistol. The police would not permit this he said.

I felt sorry for him but told him I could not sell him a gun cane, and under no circumstances would I, as they are just antiques and unsuitable for his purpose. Further, all gun canes using modern cartridges must be reported to and registered with the Federal Government under stiff penalties for any failures.

One year my wife and I attended a legal convention of the International Academy of Trial Lawyers in New Zealand and Australia. In New Zealand we had a seminar in the City of Christ Church with the local bar association. The President of our Academy and I, as its Dean, were invited with our spouses to be the dinner guests at the home of a prominent citizen of the town.

Other prominent townspeople were there too and our host had a beautiful home on the side of a mountain overlooking the city below. In the nighttime the houses of the city beneath us were lit up brightly and more and more sparsely up the hillside so that the vista was like one big Christmas tree with us as its top-notch at its pinnacle.

After the natural exclamation of the beauty of the vista, the evening started out stiffly with small talk about our respective origins, occupations, etc. as we groped for a mutually apolitical topic of conversation. Finally, our host inquired of me whether I engaged in any hobby or sport. When I advised him I was a cane collector, his face lit up and he said, "I recently read something really interesting that will appeal to you. It was in a magazine and it was about a great variety of canes. It is in my library and I'll go see if I can find it." He was gone awhile and then rejoined our group. As he was paging through the magazine, he stopped suddenly and said, "Oh my God, that's you!" as he read the title aloud and it's author.

It appeared he had an Australian or New Zealander edition of the Reader's Digest that ran an article of mine on canes. That year the Digest had printed this article in some seventeen languages, includ-

ing Chinese, Japanese, Arabic, French, German, Spanish, and Italian. This really broke the ice and I became the center of attention. Immediately the conversation of everyone turned to canes and continued so throughout the meal which was, of all things, mutton. But then New Zealand had a population of two million inhabitants and 90 million sheep. Had it not been for the canes, it would indeed have been a stiff and formal evening.

About thirty years ago, while in Hong Kong with my lawyers academy, I skipped some lectures and seminars and hunted for some oriental canes. An opium pipe would be a real find—but no one knew where I could find one. I was wandering through a local village on the Chinese side making signs that I wanted a pipe. One man understood and took me to a small place—I can't say it was a shop as it had no sides, but it did have a roof and the owner spoke some pidgin English. He brought out a pipe—not an opium pipe as that would be illegal—but nevertheless, a most unusual one.

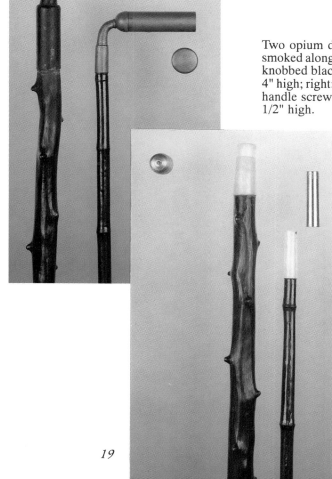

This pipe was made from a thick heavy branch about 5 feet long. How would one reach out to light its antique brass bowl while puffing on the mouthpiece, I thought? Stranger still, how could one drill a hole 4 1/2 feet long through the center of this shaft that had knots, from cut off branches, all along its side. I had for years been trying to have a hole drilled in malacca and rosewood shafts as replacements for broken sword cane sheaths and gun barrels and I, and all the machinists and gunsmiths I consulted, came out the side of the cane in the drilling process, before reaching more than 1 foot deep into the wood. I asked how did they drill such a straight hole? The English speaking shopkeeper said that was a big secret. I wheedled and wheedled and finally he told me a worm eats its way from end to end, eating only the 1/8 inch pith in the center, but I never found out where you get the worm, or whether it was naturally in the wood. But the pipe did work fine if someone lit it for me and in addition to being a pipe, it was a staff that could be used in walking—a real oriental gadget and so well concealed it must at one time have been an oriental opium pipe.

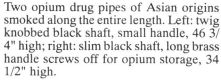

Two opium drug pipes of Asian origins smoked along the entire length. Left: twig knobbed black shaft, small handle, 46 3/4" high; right: slim black shaft, long brass handle screws off for opium storage, 34 1/2" high.

A similar method was used by the American Indians in the southwest desert area. There they would make beautiful canes from 2 inch thick cacti—that had holes down the center and through the sides every 1/4 inch apart, up and down the stick. The wood is very hard and holes are not circular so they were not drilled. It seems that the stick is the skeleton of that particular cactus and is so strong that the cactus can't be bent or broken while growing straight up. All the holes are originally there—in the center of the live cactus and in the sides but filled with an organic substance softer than the skeleton, much as our flesh is over the bones of our own bodies. A skin covers the whole cactus. The Indians found that, by removing the skin and soaking the cactus in honey or sugar water and then laying it alongside an anthill for a few weeks, all the organic material would be eaten out of the entire cactus, leaving a beautifully and randomly perforated stick, tough enough to be used as a walking stick or cane.

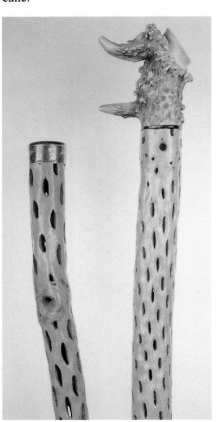

Two cactus shaft canes, left: with silver handle, right: with horn handle. Left: 37 1/2" high; right: 35 3/4" high. Shafts were de-barked and then soaked in honey or sugar water and placed on ant hills. Ants ate out the centers and "windows."

I'll never forget the surprise of receiving a long distance call from Switzerland about 20 years ago when the operator asked for Dr. Monek. I replied they must be asking for my son who owns an international medical and pharmaceutical manufacturing and supply company. Another voice interjected and said, "No, I want the cane man." He then got on and said he had heard of my collection all over Europe and could he please come and see it. Thinking really that he was kidding, I said, "When do you want to come?" He said how about Tuesday of next week and I agreed and remained home that day. He arrived early in the morning, examining each cane all day long and in the evening he drove back to the airport and took a plane home! All that distance - over 3,000 miles just to see my canes! He was a chemist in animal foods and so successful in his business that his doctor told him he was heading for a heart attack and he better take up a hobby so he started collecting canes. He must have liked what he saw for not only did he come again, but he brought his wife and child along a few months later.

The word gets around, for shortly thereafter I received a call from Frankfurt, Germany. This man was a banker who knew the above mentioned Swiss Industrialist and could he too come and view my collection? He did, with his wife, sister-in-law and another, and he too was a most avid collector for his health's sake.

Shortly thereafter, I received a call from California by a Japanese representative of a Tokyo television company. Would I consent to appear on Japanese TV about my canes. Arrangements were suggested that I bring all my canes to the Japanese station in Tokyo to appear "live" on their TV. I said, "You must not understand. How could I bring all my canes? I've got over 2,000" (that was then). He said, "Never you mind, we pay for it all, just come and bring the canes." I finally refused as I was too busy with my law practice and couldn't take off the time and dreaded the jet lag and customs hassle with such a load of canes. He then said, "All right, then I'll have them come to your house from Tokyo." They surely must be kidding I thought, but sure enough, about 10 days later seven Japanese, including one Japanese movie actress and a translator, arrived. They spent the whole day shooting movies of me and

my sticks and then left. They were most gracious and generous and, true to their offer, paid cash in advance for the interview and sent me a full cassette of the show which appeared nationally in Japan - with all 10 minutes of me! I have found the Japanese much more reliable on keeping their promises than our American radio and TV stations, who after getting everything they can - including meals too, forget entirely about the conditions previously agreed upon to supply copies of all film and records made.

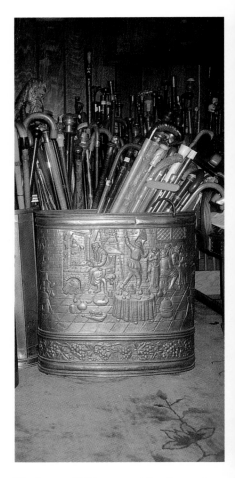

I had over 2000 canes at the time a Japanese television station offered to transport me — and all my canes — to Japan to appear on live TV.

Chapter 2
The Evolution of the Cane

When primitive man reared off all fours and first stood erect, it was probably with the aid of a stick, which successively became his walking stick, his cudgel, and then his flint-tipped spear. As man became more civilized, this stick-weapon in the hands of the chief evolved into a badge of office as a staff. Subsequently, as the world divided into secular and religious society, all leaders, be they kings or bishops, carried scepters or crosiers and their minions such as judges, magistrates, officers and abbots, even the lowly municipal watchmen, carried staffs as symbols of their authority.

It is not however, with these staffs, scepters, crosiers, or batons that we are here concerned, except in studying the evolution of the walking stick as an item of fashion or utility and as a collectable object.

Monkey playing wind instrument on black cane and a simple cat with brads for eyes on an unpainted stick. Both canes are made of a single piece of wood. Monkey: 39" high; cat: 38 1/2" high.

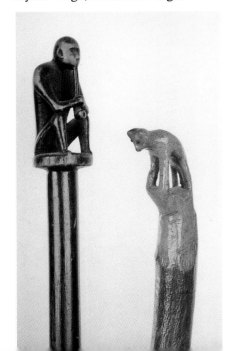

Origin of the Name "Cane"

Some antiquarians claimed that the name cane arose from the fact that Cain, the son of Adam and Eve slew his brother Able with his staff thus CAINING him to death. Many modern writers have, however, asserted that the name CANE was adapted from the use of rattans by such a name in the Far East. I, however,

Canes sizes over the centuries. The earliest staffs were the largest and the size of canes has diminished over time down to the small swagger stick.

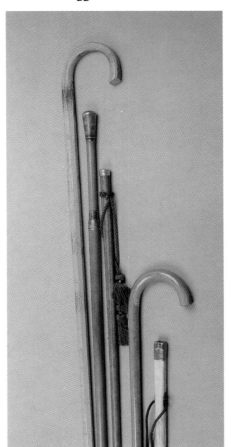

am convinced that the name CANE was first used by the Romans long before the birth of Christ.

On this subject, J.H. Ingram in 1838 wrote in his essay on canes that:

"It is well known to classical readers that from the time of Romulus and Remus, dogs in great numbers have infested the streets of Roman or Ital-

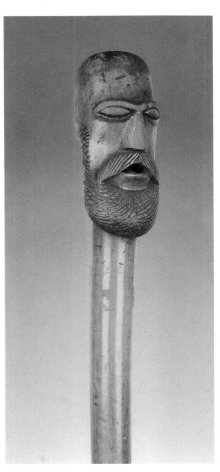

Some claim the name cane arose from the fact that Cain slew his brother with his staff. Folk art cane featuring a bald-headed, bearded man with his mouth open, 35" high.

ian cities Vide, in attestation of this, T. Pomp, Atticus, the epistle of Demmocritus, the Greek: the letters of Cadmus; the Annibal's commentaries on the battle of Apulia, wherein he asserts, that from the adjacent village of Cannae, so called from the multitude of its dogs (canes) there did issue after the battle from the gates of the town, thirty thousand of these animals, which being attracted hither by the dead, did cover with their vast numbers all the plain, and appall the very gods with their howls."

"This being the condition of things in an obscure Roman town, how great must have been the multitude of these brutes in Rome itself! That their number was so large as to defy census, and remain altogether unknown, may be gathered from Ceasar in his letter to Tullus Brutus; informing him of the death of his sister Appicia by hydrophobia and also, by inference, from the third oration of Cicero against Cateline; further Junius Brutus is recorded by C. Laelius to have been pursued on horseback by a pack of hungry dogs ***and barely escaped with his life*** Such being the danger of the streets of Rome, it became customary for pedestrians to go provided with stout birchen cudgels, armed at one extremity with a short, sharp pike, for the purpose of defending themselves against these demi-savage animals. This cudgel, by a natural substitution of cause for effect, was called CANI, the dative singular for CANIS, which meant literally "for a dog." A more significant and befitting term than which could not have been chosen. The plural of CANIS is CANES and this is the precise appellation by which they are now known.***"

"The introduction of the CANI into Rome, we learn from Nevius Metellus was in the year 67 B.C. Within the two weeks immediately preceding the ides of August the same year, we are told by the same author, no less than eighty thousand dogs were killed with this instrument alone besides nine thousand supposed to have been torn to pieces by their species in fighting over the carcasses of the slain. But a sweeping pestilence succeeding this exposure of so vast a quantity of animal matter to the sun of the dog days, and, on account of the alarming increase of murders among the common people with this weapon, with which all men went armed and readily used

in the slightest quarrel, the emperor was forced to promulgate an edict prohibiting anyone beneath the patrician rank from carrying the CANI. This imperial edict at once made it a privileged thing, and forthwith it was taken into high favor by the aristocracy of Rome."

And the author went on at great length telling how the fashion took hold, sizes and decorations, and shapes changed and "that half of Rome thought and dreamt of nothing besides the shape and fashion of the CANI." He tells further that in the 5th Century, the cane was introduced into England but limited to the patrician rank.

The later non-historical use of the word "cane" arises from the fact that many of the sticks are canes in the botanical sense as rattan and bamboo which grows like sugar cane, tall and wavy. Malacca in the botanical sense is a "cane". It is very strong, light, smooth and has no stub marks of branches.

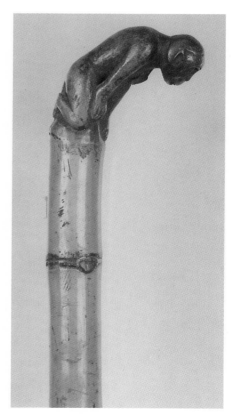

Bowing monkey on one knee, bamboo shaft, 41 1/2" high.

People today try to make a distinction between canes and walking sticks. I personally think it an unnecessary sophistication. The finest differentiation was made by the essayist Odell Shepherd in "The Harvest of a Quiet Eye" in 1927:

"— Generally speaking, the cane is recognizable by its glossy smoothness and by its handle of gold or silver, whereas the stick goes in rather for serviceability than for any gauds of outward appearance. There is a look of honesty about all genuine sticks seldom to be observed in canes. It should be remembered that the two things have come down to us along utterly different lines of descent and that they have always kept very different company. The cane is a lineal descendant of the scepter, the baton, the sword, the rapier, and it bears even today the sinister marks of that ancestry. But the forebears of the walking stick are the countryman's cudgel, the single stick, the leaping pole, the pilgrim's staff, and the shepherd's crook. Its aristocracy that is to say, is intrinsic and real - not based like the canes, upon mere public opinion. Instead of having deteriorated from a long line of slaughterous side-arms and futile badges of office, it is today what it has always been: a third leg, a longer arm, a weapon fit for an honest man's use, and a friend. Let the cane vaunt itself as it may, the walking sticks ancestry is far more ancient. Scipio Africanus was named after it, Socrates always carried it, Abraham the Patrioch never stirred abroad without one. No, the cane, by comparison, is mere upstart."

A simpler differentiation might be that the cane has an upright handle whereas the walking stick has a handle that juts out at an angle or curve.

Webster's Universities Dictionary gives this definition for a stick:

"Walking Stick: A cane, staff, or stick carried in the hand as part of a man's costume, or for support or diversion in walking."

A more precise and accurate definition or description cannot be made.

The Cane in Ancient History

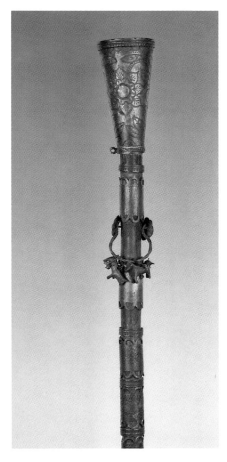

Ancient Peruvian cane, said to be an Alcalde or mayor's cane from shortly after the Spanish conquest, c. 1533. Taken from an old tomb. Silver and wood with Catholic medals and various symbology. I have seen an identical cane in the museum in Lima, Peru. 43" high.

The cane obviously became an implement of support early in the history of man when he traveled solely on foot and, being his constant companion, it became an article of dress whereupon artistry and craft were devoted to making it a desirable object.

As a walking stick, it probably first became known in antiquity in the riddle of Greek mythology when that terrible half man, half beast monster, the sphinx, propounded a riddle (Diodorus I,Iv c VI): "What animal walks on four legs in the morning, two at noon, and three in the evening." Only Oedipus was able to solve it and cause the suicide of the sphinx when he answered that it was man that creeps on all fours as a child, walks erect in adult-hood, and supports his infirmities in the sunset of his life on a staff or cane.

Greek amphorae depict many uses of the cane and staff, and in Egyptian hieroglyphics we always recognize the king with this token of sovereignty. Upon the opening of the tomb of the youthful King Tutankhamen at Luxor in 1923, two gold sticks were found carefully wrapped in linen and one of these was an elaborate cane with a gold statuette of the young king on top. This was in the year 1358 B.C., more than 3300 years ago.

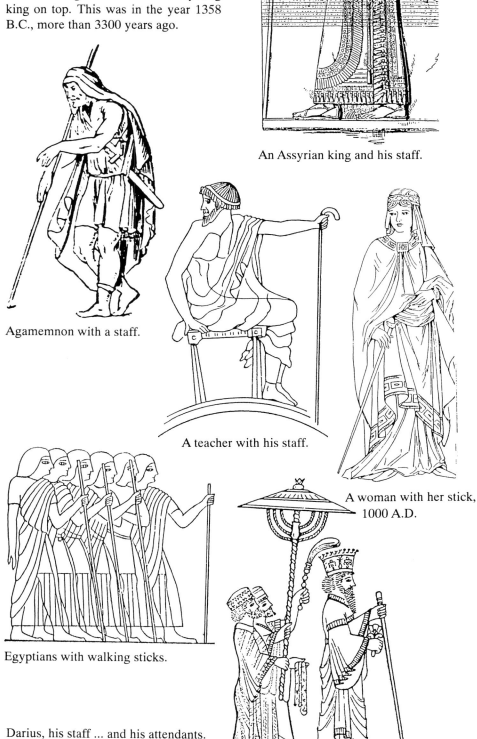

An Assyrian king and his staff.

Agamemnon with a staff.

A teacher with his staff.

A woman with her stick, 1000 A.D.

Egyptians with walking sticks.

Darius, his staff ... and his attendants.

23

Many references are made to the cane in the Old Testament: Jacob said, "With this staff I passed over Jordan," Genesis XXX, 10; and in Hebrew XI, 21, there is another allusion, "...worshipped leaning upon the top of his staff." In Exodus VII, 10-12, it is stated, "And Aaron (the brother of Moses) cast down his rod before Pharaoh and before his servants, and it became a serpent...and they (the Pharaoh's sorcerers) cast down every man his rod, and they became serpents, but Aaron's rod swallowed up their rods." In the beautiful hymn of the 23 Psalm, it is said, "Thy rod and thy staff, they comfort me," and in Exodus XIV, Moses on the flight from Egypt lifted his rod over the sea and divided it so his followers could pass through, and in Exodus XVII 6, he quenched the thirst of his followers, when he, obedient to the Lord's command, struck the rock with his staff and water gushed forth.

In the New Testament (Mark VI, 8), mindful of its extreme usefulness, Jesus commended his twelve apostles to start their ministry of preaching, and to go out in pairs, forbidding them to take any bread, haversack, or money, not even a spare tunic, nothing but a staff only.

Rameses I, had a collection of fine walking sticks, and 12 of them are portrayed on the walls of the Temple of Karnak outside Luxor and are depicted likewise in the Temple of Karma, where the Egyptian Pharaohs are buried.

The Cane in The Middle Ages

The cane marched on in history up to and through the Middle Ages with hundreds of thousands of pilgrims and Crusaders who traveled to the Holy Land. At this time, it was a stout, strong stick about five feet high with a pointed metal spike at the bottom to dig into the earth on steep inclines and to fend off ferocious animals and dangerous brigands. About ten inches from the top there was a protuberance upon which to rest the hand so it would not slip downwards in traveling. This pilgrim's cane was called a *bourdon* and it soon evolved to where the top portion was designed to be hollow and could be unscrewed from the lower portion to conceal therein religious relics and valuables. Already it was becoming a dual purpose cane.

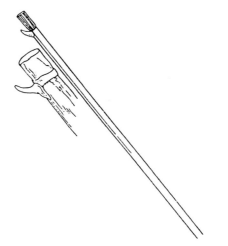

Figure 8. A walking stick found in Thebes, Egypt. A bag or bottle was suspended from the upper peg.

In 1853 in the book called "The Leisure Hour" we can read a fine history of the cane at that time and learn that in even earlier centuries the streets of Dover and the highways of the Continent were thronged with pedestrian pilgrims enroute to the Holy Land,

Figure 9. A 14th century pilgrim's staff.

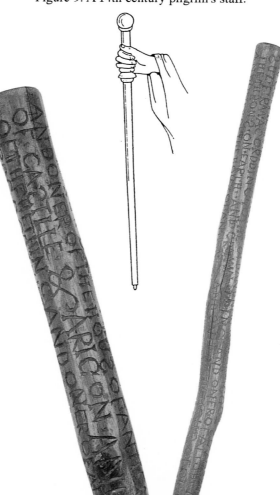

"each equipped with his bourdon - a strong stout stick about 5' high with a spiked foot to aid its possessor in the ascent of steep and perilous places. About a foot from the top was a handle to facilitate a powerful grasp, or bring down from the trees adjacent to the road refreshing fruit. Glad to avoid all encumbrances on his —- journey —- the pilgrim skillfully entrived to make this staff almost the sole receptacle of his chattels —- Half way down the Bourdon was a joint, which unscrewed and revealed the upper half hollowed for the reception of treasures. Here were the relics the wayfarer had purchased from the imposing guardians of foreign shrines; in this snug receptacle was the silent lute, which, as occasion served, would be drawn forth to earn a scanty meal in the towns through which he passed or to charm the denizens of a wayside hostelerie. In this curious crevice, too, many a boon was smuggled which became a source of private wealth and even national advantage —- in a pilgrims staff was brought over from Greece the first head of saffron, at a

Artist with a great deal to say, carved an inscription down the entire length of the shaft and completely around it. "Know all men women and children of thes presents that Lord John Joseph Augustinus Adolphus Ferdinand Cood Suz firm acordding to the old and new Wricht Cood sowz Will Whitch civs. to Lord Cood Suz Imppol. Prince Cood sowz. Regent of all The 'Throns' on earth and Crown Prince and over of all the crowns on earth and over and prince of the Royal Hous of Apsburg/ And over of the hous of antients and over of the hous of orang and over of the . of orlenes Hous and over of the antchent Hous/ of . Castile. & Arigon. and over of the hous . of. Tiber and over of all other Houses on the faze of all the earth and over of all the lands/ Of the hethin C and over of all the Crown. Titles and over of the Whol Twelv plates and over of all the Gold Silver Brass iron steel and E.C.S./ Lord Cood suez New Empire and over of the Clob His Vane Estate Ferm of Sir John J.A.F.R. Cood suz Zwas & Ion o Cood suz E.S. Lord/F.C.S. Title. 43" high.

time when it was death to take a plant out of that country —- In the same manner, a solitary silkworm found its way into the south of Europe and made the wealth of the Italian valleys —- Upon a hook near the top of his staff hung the travelers water bottle and the whole was surrounded by a hollow globe. A bunch of palm tied around the head of the bourdon, denoted the travelers return."

From very old illuminated missals of the middle ages we see illustrations of the bishop's pastoral stick, adapted from the shepherd's crook as a symbol of his being shepherd of his flock, having a hanging piece of cloth dependent from its top. As at the time, the bishop would travel around diocese on foot, this was meant to wipe his heated brow, another practical dual purpose cane.

Many of the portraits of eminent personages of that period and throughout the sixteenth century show the richness of the walking sticks being used. Canes were now becoming such an essential part of one's dress that different canes were used for separate costumes and were collected for their own beauty.

Many of the portraits of eminent personages from the Middle Ages show the richness of the walking sticks being used.

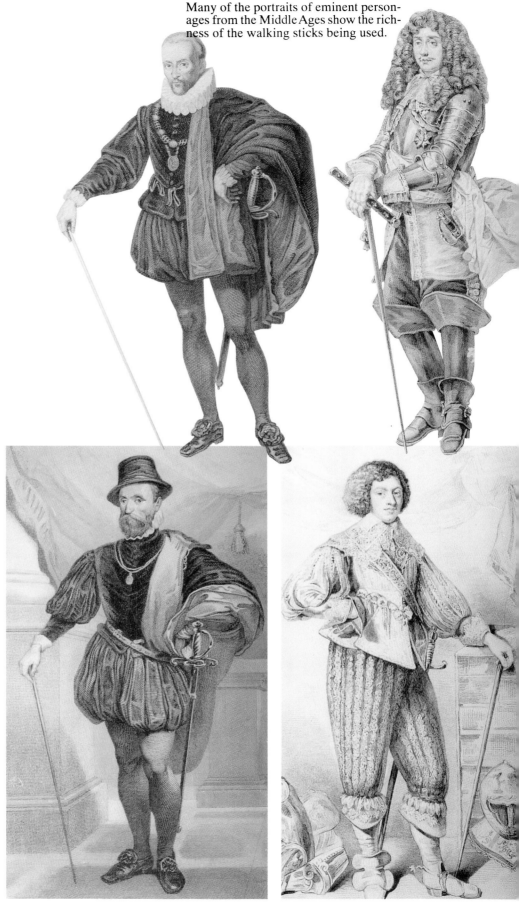

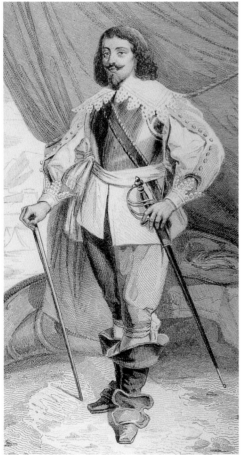

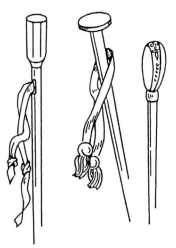

Canes from the 1600s.

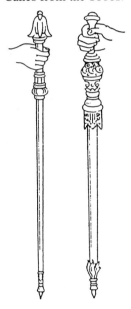

Staffs of office, c. 1578. Metal work and guilt from brass in Canterbury Cathedral, 1578, with a portrait of C. G. Hart, 1587.

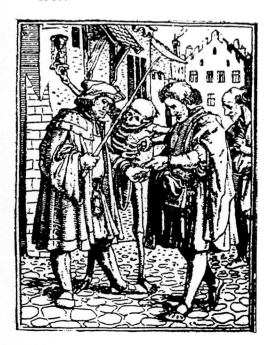

Charles V of France, in the fifteenth century, had a large collection of canes and two of them are itemized in the inventory of his belongings. In the seventeenth century paintings of Henry VIII's time, England's king and his nobles are shown with richly embellished canes. Canes and staffs are so often part of the portraits of the period that they are named "cane-staff pictures."

The Cane in Europe

The aristocracy, who lead a life of leisure, had shorter canes than the travelers, for we see from old English prints of the seventeenth and eighteenth century that the simple pedestrian had a stick more like a staff and as high as his head to enable him to leap over the ditches, gullies and ruts that scarred the roads. There, the cane was used as a fighting staff, a vaulting pole, and a sounding stick in fording unbridged streams.

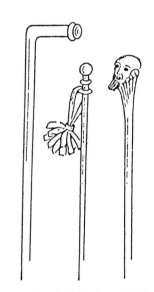

Examples of sticks from 1500-1730.

Image of a magistrate with his walking stick from the "Dance of Death" by Hans Holbein.

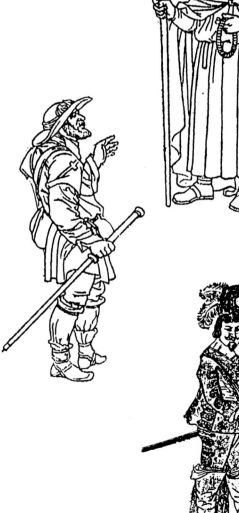

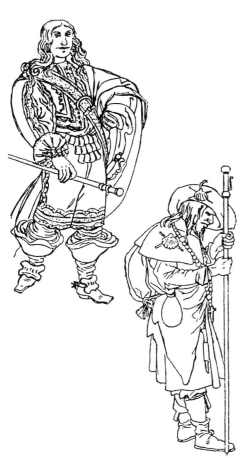

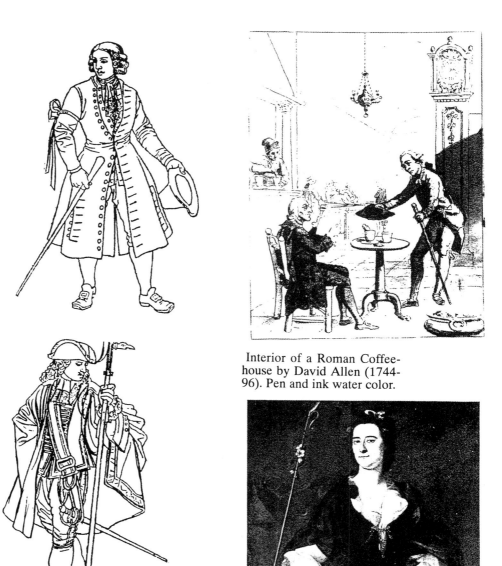

Interior of a Roman Coffee-house by David Allen (1744-96). Pen and ink water color.

In the seventeenth and eighteenth centuries, the stick became a sartorial extravagance in England and on the Continent. One English writer in 1897, in speaking of that period, was no less extravagant when he rhapsodized:

"such sparkings there were from precious stones embroidering in lavish loveliness the ivory, gold or silver of the stick, such flutterings of gay bunched ribbons lightly hung round beruffled wrists, so that dependent cane might not be lost.

Chelsea, Battersea, and all the china works deluxe provided heads for canes, jewelers designed exquisitely modeled snuff boxes; there were silver framed looking glasses, grotesque Punchinello heads, rare enamels, etc."

Mary Sylvester (American) in a French shepherdess' outfit complete with a shepherds crook, by Joseph Blackburn (c. 1754).

An Englishman with his stick, c. 1650.

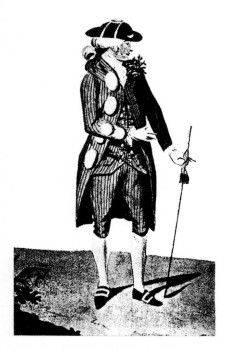

"Foreign Fashionable" c. 1773.

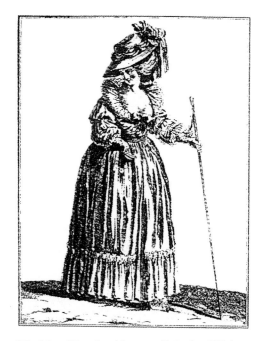

"Fashion Plate" with a staff, Paris, 1784.

Madame de Maintenon. King Frederick I of Prussia had dozens of canes and his successor, Frederick William I, had equally as many in the 1700s, all embellished with precious stones.

It is reported that a person of wealth would spend up to 40,000 francs a year on walking sticks. A sartorial gentleman had as many canes as a modern gentleman has neckties.

Napoleon was a cane fancier and collector with a large and elaborate collection; Voltaire had over 75 canes; and Rousseau, who was considered a poor man, felt it necessary to have 40 walking sticks.

In Germany, a Prime Minister was reported to have 300 canes, one to match each of his elaborate suits, and even more extravagant snuff boxes. King Frederick the Great of Prussia, notoriously penurious with his court, spent immense sums on his collection of canes.

As with the aristocracy, the carrying of a cane, even if not elaborate, was slavishly aped by the public. This discovery of the New World, with its exotic new woods had added impetus to the craze and one could now have a beautiful stick even without the addition of gold and precious stones.

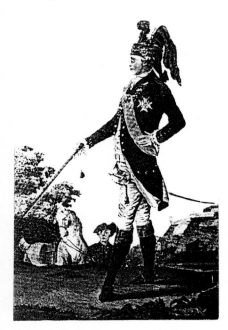

Colonel of the French Artois Dragoons, 1778.

The cane was now a collectible item, a requisite for fashionable dress. Louis XIII of France had elaborate canes in abundance. Richeleu, his Prime Minister, was almost as extravagant. Canes were splendid examples of the jeweler's art, and sticks were decorated with precious stones and chased gold, often with miniature enameled portraits of one's favorite lady concealed in the handle. Louis XIV on May 31, 1680, according to one cane's inscription, gave such a gift to

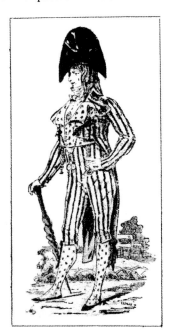

A French " Incroyable" of the 1790s.

The reign of Louis XIV (1695) of France was noted for its extravagances. As he wore very high heels, the king carried a long cane to keep his balance in walking, a practice soon imitated by his court.

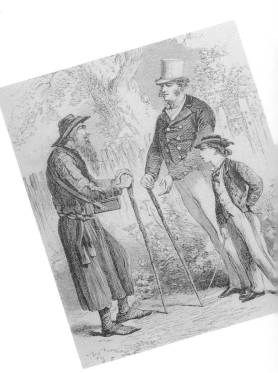

As with the aristocracy, the carrying of a cane, even if not elaborate, was slavishly aped by the public.

They said a man with a cane was truly a gentleman, "who toils not, neither does he spin."

By the way, one never carries a cane, one wears one. This is a universally used phrase by cane collectors, but very few know that in the middle ages, men had two buttons sewn on their clothing from which to hang the wrist cord of their canes to actually wear their stick as it hung from the buttons.

So much were canes in demand, that canes were sold on the very streets of London and Paris, much as newspapers are hawked today. A vendor's sales song from 1790 has been recorded:

"I've sticks and canes for young and old
To either are they handy
In driving off a barking cur
Or chastising a dandy."

One old English cane was reported to contain the following inscription:

"John Alcock is my name, England is my nation, Markham is my dwelling place, and Christ is my salvation.
When I be dead and in my grave And all my bones be rotten, Here's this to see upon this stick, That I am not forgotten 1644."

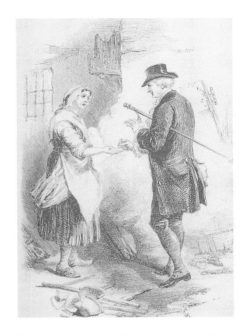

They said a man with a cane was truly a gentleman, "who toils not, neither does he spin."

The demand for walking sticks was so great that the ingenuity of it's craftsmen, jewelers and manufacturers were stretched to the utmost. From 1851 and on, Hamburg, Berlin and Vienna were the center of cane manufacturing, employing thousands of people. In the 1870s the English were strong competitors. To list just the exotic and varied woods used would unduly lengthen this book, but the world was combed for different woods. Animal substances such as ivory, tortoise shell, rhinoceros hide, ram's horn, shark's spine, narwhal bone, serpent skins all were used.

A tortoise shell shaft topped with a gold handle marked "AC," gold eyelets, 34 1/2" high.

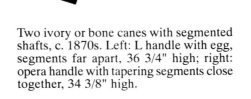

Two ivory or bone canes with segmented shafts, c. 1870s. Left: L handle with egg, segments far apart, 36 3/4" high; right: opera handle with tapering segments close together, 34 3/8" high.

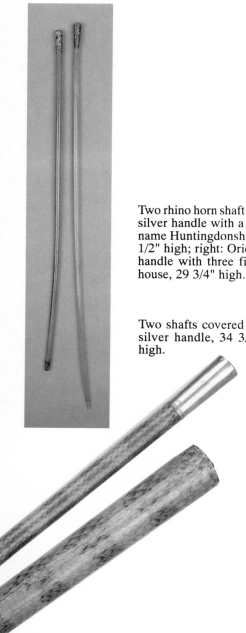

Two rhino horn shaft swagger sticks. Left: silver handle with a rearing stag and the name Huntingdonshire on the handle, 26 1/2" high; right: Oriental scene on silver handle with three figures, a tree, and a house, 29 3/4" high.

Two shafts covered in snake skin. Left: silver handle, 34 3/4" high; right: 35" high.

Again quoting from "Leisure Hour" (supra), the 1853 author states:

"The commonest and cheapest stick previous to sale passes through at least twenty pairs of hands. The forest and hedgerows of the entire world and every shrub and tree have been placed under contribution for woods of various qualities —- The common curved handle is formed by softening the wood in hot <u>damp</u> sand after which it retains the required curvature. —- The wood is straightened in a similar manner, after being steeped in <u>hot</u> dry sand. When the bark is not retained, the stick is boiled for an hour or two and then it is easily peeled with the fingers. In order to polish the article,

it is brought to a very smooth surface by means of emery paper and fish skin, then it is dyed according to the taste of the maker and the demand of the market"

Sticks were sold in London in the street. It was estimated over 200 hawkers of walking sticks were on the main avenues on Sunday, like balloon vendors 30 years ago on American streets and as now

in Mexico City. In 1898, it was reported that 2 to 3,000,000 rough and unfinished chestnut sticks alone were imported into the United States from Austria to be made into Congo sticks. In London, new samples of new woods were always being prepared for several seasons ahead, such was the demand for canes. One wholesaler in London sold 509,000 walking stick in just one year. In 1893 in England, there were over 4,000 people employed in the walking stick trade. Wood was imported to England for canes from all over the world: olive from America, Queensland (Australia) and South Africa; Pimento from Jamaica in quantities of 3 to 4,000 bundles annually, each bundle containing 500 to 800 sticks.

Whole farms and plantations were devoted to growing sticks. Most walking sticks were grown upside down, the roots becoming the handle and the tops becoming the bottoms. They were trained as they grew to conform with the fashion demand of the day. As they grew, many small trees were lanced with an instrument that cut the skin of the young tree. This caused the skin to bleed sap and puff up like keloid scars on a human being. A few years more of growth and one had a very interesting staff or cane. In the Orient, other trees of hardwood, after being cut for canes, were allowed to dry for several years and then were acid etched into beautiful designs.

Also we read in "Hand Me Down My Walking Stick" by Frank Farrington (March 1945) in *Hobbies,*

"in the 18th Century they (canes) were 4 feet long and had a bunch of ribbons near the top —- Merely to list the novelties in canes, ancient or modern, would require pages. It is this endless variety varying from the ugliest bludgeon-like weapon to the slenderest rattan wand that prevents the collection from ever reaching the saturation point in varieties secured —- The first tulip bulb introduced into Holland came in (a hollowed cane). Asparagus was introduced into England in the space in a Templar's staff. Seeds of melon, quince, tomato, cauliflower, onion, apricot came to European gardens in the same manner"

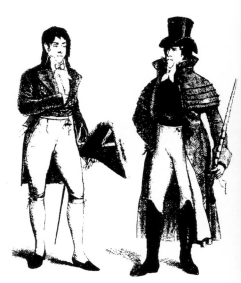

19th century gentlemen, (c.1805), complete with a cane.

A 19th century gentleman with his cane.

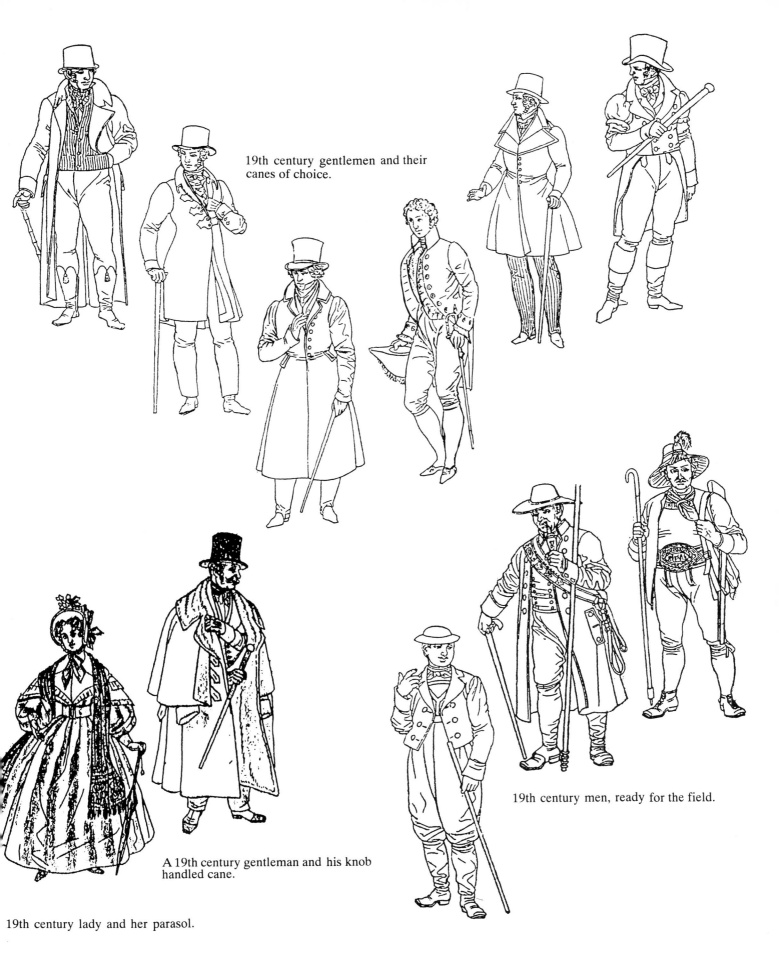

19th century gentlemen and their canes of choice.

A 19th century gentleman and his knob handled cane.

19th century lady and her parasol.

19th century men, ready for the field.

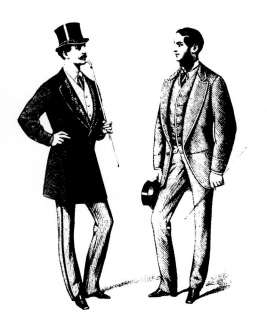

19th century gentlemen with swagger sticks.

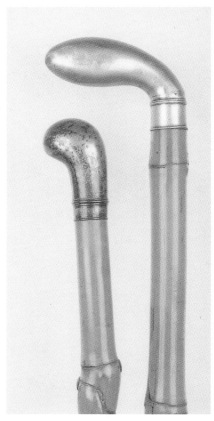

Two silver handled pistol grips, both on rare bamboo. Lower with smaller handle, 34 3/4" high; upper, 33 3/4" high.

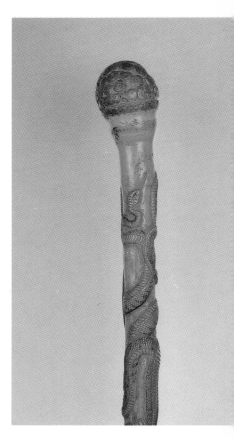

Bamboo intricately carved with many twining snakes. The handle is the root of the bamboo, 35" high.

"In the latter half of the 19th Century canes reached their most widespread popularity and in Hamburg, Berlin, Vienna, thousands of artisans were employed in their manufacture. One family —- the Meyers —— absorbed all competition and then proceeded to undersell the Chinese, Arabians and Egyptians in their own countries — Canes became fashionable in Paris, London, Naples, Madrid, Algers. The Meyers crowded local canes out of South America where the Belgians had formerly monopolized that trade. In the United States —- Californians were the first to adopt canes generally and from there they came to Chicago and New York —- The Germans reached out and swallowed American production and by 1870, Meyers canes had displaced English crab-sticks, carved Brussels thorns and all others —-"

Two Chinese carved canes, the left shaft is made of bamboo, the right is made of bone. Left: 35" high; right: 35 1/2" high.

Four silver handled Thai Royalty canes, left to right: 1870, 37" high; 1890, 38 3/8" high; 1890, rare wood (light color), 38" high; 1890, bamboo shaft, 37" high.

Thai Royal swagger stick with silver handle, bulbous with a pointed tip, full stick shown, 28" high.

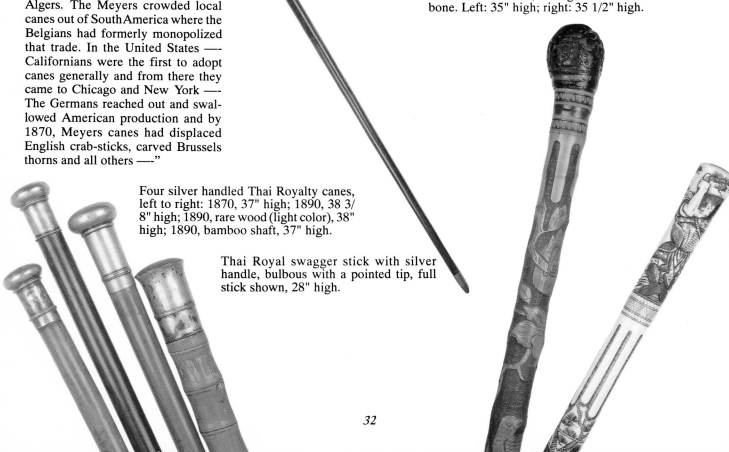

Stick making was a very important industry in England in 1871 and the process of making sticks is best explained in *Chamber's Journal* (a British publication) of February 11, 1871 in describing a "Stick Factory":

"At Mr. Dangerfield's mill, sticks are manufactured both from large timber of from two to six feet width, and from small underwood of about the thickness of a man's thumb. The timber, which is chiefly beech, is first sawn into battens of about three feet in length and as many inches in width; and from each of these battens are afterwards cut two square sticks with square heads in opposite directions, so that the middle portion is waste wood. The corners of each stick are afterwards rounded off by a planing process called 'trapping' and the square head is reduced by a small saw to a curve or rectangular bend, so as to form a convenient handle. When a number of sticks are brought in this way to the exact size and pattern, they are polished with great care, are finely varnished, and packed in boxes or bundles for the market. Many sawn sticks, however, are supplied with bone and horn handles, which are fastened on with glue; and then of course there is less wood-waste, as a larger number of them may be cut from one batten."

* * * * * * * * *

"A very different process takes place in the manufacture of sticks from small underwood, in which there is no sawing required. The rough unfashioned sticks, which are generally of hazel, ash, oak and thorn, are cut with a bill in the same way as kidney-bean sticks, and are brought to the factory in large bavins or bundles, piled on a timber tug. There must, of course, be some little care in their selection, yet it is evident that the woodmen are not very particular on this score, for they have in general an ungainly appearance, and many are so crooked and rough, that no drover or country boy would think it worth while to polish the like of them with his knife. Having arrived at this place, however, their numerous imperfections are soon pruned away, and their ugliness converted into elegance. When sufficiently seasoned and fit for working, they are first laid to soak in wet sand, and rendered more tough and pliable; a workman then takes them one by one, and, securing them with an iron stock bends them skillfully this way and that, so as to bring out their natural crooks, and render them at last all straight even rods. If they are now required to be knotted, they next go to the 'trapper', who puts them through a kind of circular plane, which takes off their knots, and renders them uniformly smooth and round. The most important process of all is that of giving them their elegantly curved handles, for which purpose they are passed over to the 'crooker'. Every child knows that if we bend a tough stick moderately, when the pressure is discontinued it will soon fly back, more or less to its former position; and if we bend it very much, it will break. Now the crooker professes to accomplish the miracle of bending a stick as it might be an iron wire, so that it shall neither break nor 'backen'. To prevent the breaking, the wood is rendered pliant by further soaking in wet sand; and a flexible band of metal is clamped down firmly to that portion of the stick that will form the outside of the curve; the top end then being fitted into a grooved iron shoulder which determines the size of the crook, the other end is brought round so as to point in the opposite direction, the metal band during this process binding with increasing tightness against the stretching fibers of the wood, so that they cannot snap or give way under the strain. The crook having been made, the next thing is to fix it, or remove from the fibers the reaction of elasticity, which would otherwise, on the cessation of the bending force, cause it to 'backen' more or less, and undo the work. With the old process of crooking by steam, as timber-bending is effected, the stick was merely left till it was cold to acquire a permanent set; but in the new process, for which Mr. Dangerfield has a patent, a more permanent set is given by turning the handle about briskly over a jet of gas. The sticks being now fashioned, it only remains to polish and stain or varnish them; and they are sometimes scorched or burned brown, and carved with foliage, animal heads, and other devices; but this kind of ornamentation is more generally employed on the sawn sticks, and especially on those which are used for umbrellas and parasols."

In *Chamber's Journal* for May 1893, it is interesting to note the vast manufacturing technique used in England in gathering, making, and selling canes and walking sticks:

"The raw material from which are produced the almost countless varieties of sticks in the market is brought from nearly every part of the earth. There is a large quantity grown in England, but the bulk is foreign. To get an idea of the vast quantity of foreign sticks imported into England, one should visit the London Docks, East Smithfield Entrance Warehouse, No. 1, which is one of the largest storehouses of the kind in England. Here, piled from floor to ceiling, are all sorts of sticks imaginable: pimento, olive, myrtle, hazel, oak, ash, orange, bamboo, Tonquin canes, and a host of others in such profusion as to be bewildering. It must be seen to be realized, by any person outside the trade. It would be impossible to name all the different kinds of raw material; but the following are the names of the most important: Olives from America, Queensland, and South Africa. Pimento from the West Indies, chiefly Jamaica, from each island from three to four thousand bundles, each containing from five to eight hundred sticks, are imported annually. Many of these sticks are sawn up into half-a-dozen smaller ones. Myrtle from South Europe, and most of the countries situated round the Mediterranean Sea. Ash from America, South Europe, and South Africa. Cornel or cornelian cherry from Mid and South Europe and some parts of Asia. This wood is very tough, and was used extensively when the 'acacia' became popular. Also several varieties of each of the following: Oak, orange, cherry, hazel, thorn, Ceylon vines, supplejacks, palm, orange, crab, birch, beech, sycamore, lancewood, ebony, Amboyna, tulip-tree, snakewood, rosewood, Whangee, Jambeze, Penang, Rajah, Partridge, bamboo, Tonquin, betel, Malacca, Nana, Madagascar, Whampoa canes, bird's-eye maple, greenheart, etc. The chief produce of Great Britain are: Oak, ash, furze, birch, hazel, thorn, beech, crab, sycamore, cherry, and many other minor varieties. This list will show the great amount of skill required to become a judge of the raw material only."

"Many pieces of very rare wood are made into walking sticks - pieces of old ships, etc., beside scarce specimens of wood almost unknown, such as Myall wood, Australian black wood, muskwood, Cypress pine, Zebra wood, kauri pine, deodar wood, calamander, sabicu, and occasional pieces of lignum vitae. The 'modus operandi' whereby sticks which grow crooked are made straight is not generally known, and has been the subject of some curious speculation. We do not remember to have met with a satisfactory account anywhere in print, although at different times sage advice has been given on the subject through the press, in answer to correspondents. All such advice, so far as we know, has been more or less erroneous and absurd. The main object is to render the wood or cane soft and pliable; to do this, it is plunged into heated sand. Woods such as oak, ash, orange, etc., require wet sand; while olives, pimento, and all varieties of cane, require dry sand. In addition to this, a contrivance called 'a horse' is used, which consists of a plank of beech two inches thick set up on one end at an angle of forty-five to sixty degrees. Out of the two edges of this plank, pieces are cut, to allow the insertion of the stick. When sufficiently heated, the stick is taken from the sand, and, using it as a lever, it is bent here and bent there until it is perfectly straight. This process is repeated at a later stage, which is called 'baking.' For this second process, dry sand is used; and the stick is not only made quite straight, but as stiff as it is possible to make it. The success of this process depends entirely upon the judgment of the workman, who is known as a 'kilnman.' He must determine how much heat is required, and whether wet or dry sand. If he gives too much heat, the stick becomes stunned, and in most cases is useless, as it will rarely come straight after. If, on the other hand, he does not make it hot enough, it is liable to break in halves."

"Wet sand is also used for bending purposes; but a more improved method for sticks requiring moist heat is to boil them in water. For bending canes and wood requiring dry heat, a powerful gas jet is used. All such work requires an extensive knowledge of the nature and growth of the material to be operated upon, and a large amount of skill in the process."

The Cane in America

In the eighteenth century, contrary to the magnificence of the continent, the early colonists followed more conservative patterns in clothes and accessories. But, even our Pilgrim fathers, despising frills, are never depicted without a walking stick, though it may be just a sturdy and practical oaken stave.

As we see, the English and Continental fashion dictated that canes were for gentlemen; a man carrying a cane could not, and need not, perform manual labor. So much was the cane a symbol of gentlemen, that all portraits of aristocrats, European or American, depict them with their favorite walking stick.

The walking stick indicated rank and was adopted by the learned professions. Doctors particularly were known for their gold-headed canes.

Canes in Wills

So fond were some men of their personal walking sticks that they made sure these sticks were well taken care of after their deaths. If these men were not interred with their canes, as very many were, they provided by their wills who should be the post-death custodians of their most prized possessions.

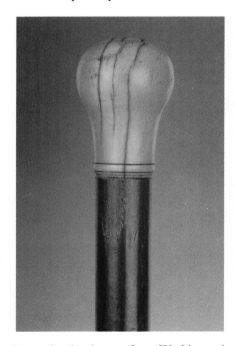

Ivory doorknob cane from Washington's carriage.

Herbert R. Collins and David B. Weaver in a book called *Wills of U.S. Presidents,* (Communication Channel, Inc. 1976) noted that the cane is the most frequently bequeathed object of our presidents. Thus:

"George Washington left to his brother Charles the goldheaded cane that Benjamin Franklin had left to him in 1790. James Madison left two canes, one of them a "walking staff made from the timber of the frigate U.S.S. Constitution and presented me by Commodore Elliot, her present commander." Madison's other cane had been left to him by Thomas Jefferson.

Thomas Jefferson...[bequeathed] "to my friend James Madison of Montpellier my gold-mounted walking staff of animal horn, as a token of cordial and affectionate friendship." John Adam's—-son. John Quincy, bequeathed 4. — (canes)

Andrew Jackson crisply says, "Lastly, I leave to my beloved son all my walking canes."

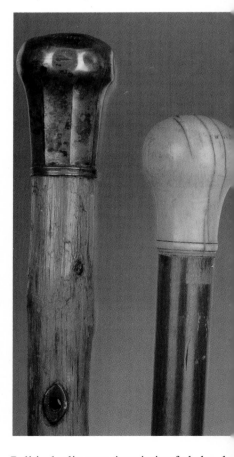

Political relic cane, inscription faded and largely illegible, but it is engraved "George Washington" and is the ivory doorknob from Washington's carriage.

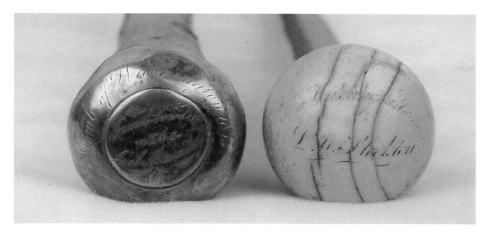

Ivory knob - very faint inscription due to wear reads "George Washington, L.W. Stockhill," said to be the knob from Washington's carriage.

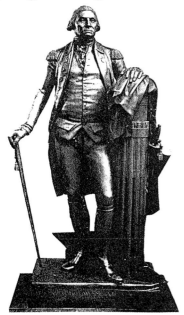

George Washington in bronze complete with his cane. Note the wrist cord visible below the handle.

It is not generally known that President George Washington died as a result of medically induced bleeding to cure an illness, the symptoms of which were sore throat and general malaise. It is, however, known that there is a rivalry and sometimes outright antagonism (caused by our representation of their injured patients) between doctors and lawyers about the respective merits of our professions.

On more than one occasion, I have had to remind some doctors that while the leading exponents of their medical profession were causing the death of our beloved first president with their primitive and barbaric bleeding treatment, members of the legal profession were creating and drafting the Constitution of the United States, the greatest document ever devised for the protection of the freedom and welfare of humanity and which has been a model for, and is emulated by, all democracies in the world since then.

Paul J. Reale writes that John Quincy Adams bequeathed to his grandson a gold-headed cane cut from the timbers of the frigate Constitution and to another grandson another such cane from the Constitution given him by its commodore Isaac Hull in 1836, to another grandson he left a cane made from olive from Mount Olivet in Jerusalem.

Presidents Franklin Pierce and James Madison each had canes cut from the frigate Constitution. President Pierce also had one from "Ironside" and a bone cane which once belonged to General Lafayette. All of these canes were bequeathed to favorite heirs.

"Benjamin Harrison was fond of "my Grand Army Cane" and Andrew Jackson willed "to my beloved son, all my walking sticks."

The former owner of Uncle Sam's Umbrella Shop, Norman Simon told me canes were owned by all modern presidents, Roosevelt, Truman, Eisenhower and Kennedy. All of these canes were made by Uncle Sam's Umbrella Shop at 110 W 45th Street, New York City. He also regularly made sword canes for Sammy Davis Jr. and Charlie Chaplin. Chaplin's more well known stick was made of wangee wood, and is the most expensive and beautiful bamboo-type available, particularly known for its suppleness.

Although men have been buried with their favorite stick or sticks like the pharaohs of old, this did not stop the cupidity of some collectors. The story is told by William J. Burtscher in his book *The Romance Behind Walking Sticks* that a certain Negro ex-slave owned a stick cut from the Hermitage estate of the deceased President Jackson where the latter was buried. This ex-slave known as Uncle Deb wore the stick for fifty years until he died in Dickson County, Tennessee about 1907. An avid collector had tried to buy it frequently but was unsuccessful. While still trying, he learned the Negro had died and had been interred with his stick. The author says, "There is a 'Hermitage' cane in a certain private collection which will illustrate the length to which some collectors will go in order to get what they want — (after the Negro's death) the collector still yearned for the cane. So one night, when the moon was down, he stole quietly into the graveyard, dug into Uncles Deb's grave and filched out the cane — thus, at last adding the much coveted prize to his collection." Disgusting, but then others may say "haven't we done the same to King Tut? And aren't we doing the same to the Mayas in Central America today in stealing their skulls and other parts from their graves? At least the cane collector left Uncle Deb his skull!" To which we reply "Here we must distinguish between the avaricious collector and the true scientist who by his digging advances the historical and scientific knowledge of the world."

The Henry Clay Cane

Henry Clay (1777-1852), Kentucky, Whig, was one of the five Immortals of the United States Senate. The others were John C. Calhoun (1782-1850), South Carolina, Democrat; Daniel Webster (1782-1852), Massachusetts, Whig; Robert LaFollette (1855-1925), Wisconsin, Progressive Republican; and Robert A. Taft (1889-1953), Ohio, Republican.

Clay was called the resourceful expert of the art of the impossible.

In April 1957, a special committee of the Senate selected these five outstanding U.S. Senators from over 2,000 men who had served in the Senate up to that time. The committee's choices were confirmed by the Senate as a whole and portraits of the five were to be painted and placed in the Senate reception room where five oval spaces designed for the portraits of outstanding Americans had been empty ever since the Capital was finished in 1859.

Physicians' Canes

Clay was a great orator, and he, with Webster and Calhoun, dominated the American political scene at that early time.

The cane I have has a thick, heavy satin-wood shaft with a long ferrule. The silver tulip handle has engraved on the top:

To
J. F. Cook
New Brunswick, N. J.
By
H. Clay
June 10, 1849

Below the handle a wide silver band has been added. It is engraved:

To
H. R. Kent
By
Mrs. J. F. Cook
Aug. 24, 1910

Henry Clay gave the cane to Mr. Cook and on his death, his widow gave it to Henry R. Kent who was her nephew. From Kent's widow it sold to Bennett W. Cooke in 1949 and thence through the latter's son to me.

Presentation cane from Senator H. Clay.

In England, where the custom of gold-headed canes for the medical profession was initiated, an interesting biography of such a stick has been written, tracing its history for 150 years from 1689 as it was carried professionally by a series of prominent London physicians. "The Gold-Headed Cane", published by Dr. William Macmichael in 1827, is the story of a celebrated walking stick that now occupies a conspicuous position in a glass case in the Royal College of Physicians in Pall Mall, and was carried by five distinguished physicians.

It is the story of the most famous cane connected with the medical profession and should be read by every cane collector and every physician. The canes adventures are told as it is successively owned and carried by:

Dr. John Radcliff, who lived from 1650 to 1714
Dr. Richard Mead, who lived from 1673 to 1745
Dr. Anthony Askew, who lived from 1722 to 1774
Dr. David Pitcurn, who lived from 1749 to 1809
Dr. Matthew Baille, who lived from 1761 to 1823

Presentation cane with a silver knob handle inscribed on top "To J.F. Cook New Brunswick, NJ by H. Clay, June 10th, 1849." Underneath the handle on a silver band is inscribed "To H.R. Kent by Mrs. J. F. Cook, Aug 24, 1910." Exceedingly fine stick shaft of heavy, light colored wood, 35" high.

When the latter died, his widow presented the cane to the College of Physicians in London where it should still be on display. The cane, which contrary to the straight gold handles of the canes carried by American doctors, had a T-shaped handle (called a cross bar by some) and is decorated with the coat of arms of the various doctors who used it.

In the third edition of "The Gold-Headed Cane", edited by Dr. William Munk and published in 1884, is mentioned the custom of every physician carrying a cane and the historical origin of this practice is explored.

A presently viable doctors' cane is famous in the Chicago area. This is called "The Silver Cane" and was made to order for Dr. Joseph C. Beck, 1870-1942. He was an outstanding eye, ear, nose, and throat doctor in Chicago and had the cane so constructed that its handle held three ear, nose, and throat instruments, plus a reflecting mirror. He used it in his daily work in the class room, clinics, and in his examining room. As a member of the Chicago Larynological Society and the Otological Society he decreed that on his death it should pass on to the oldest active member of that medical group and upon that person's death it should be bestowed upon the next oldest. Each mans name is engraved upon the cane when he receives it. To date, it has been possessed by eight outstanding professionals in that field:

Dr. T. Melville Hardie
Dr. J. Gordon Wilson
Dr. George Shambaugh
Dr. Alfred Lewy
Dr. Tom Galloway
Dr. John Lindsey
Dr. Stenton Friedberg
Dr. Robert Lewy, the present holder.

I first learned of this cane in 1980. I was able to photograph it at Dr. Lindsey's home. Over the years I lost the pictures; however, I have the poem that is read upon its presentation to the new custodian. It was composed by Dr. Waller H. Theobald who never became the keeper of the cane, but was Secretary of the Society for many years.

The cane was possessed at different times by the distinguished heads of the departments of Otolaryngology of all the four leading medical Schools of Chicago. The poem reads as follows:

This is not the Cain that slew brother Abel.
In that time so long ago,
It's a noble cane --- an illustrious cane
That belonged to good old brother Joe.

It has its secret pocket -- And instruments
It does hold,
It's made of sturdy hickory --- with a top
That shines like gold.

It's been to many a clinic, and to meetings
of the "Clan".
It holds a lot of memories of a kind
And gifted man.

But its story isn't ended with its placement
On the shelf.
The wish of its last owner, was told
To my very self.

He said, "Please pass this on to my senior
In succession
I know he'll guard it tenderly as a dearly
Prized possession."

Now in compliance with that request and
With my eyes a little dewy.
I hand it to the next in line,
And that is Alfred Lewy.

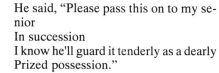

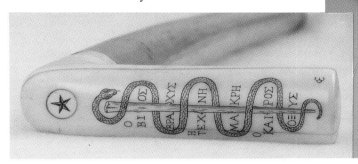

Top view, L handle medical cane of the Caduceus with a snake, stick, star, and Greek text.

Physician's sword cane, ivory handle with snake, ebony shaft, c. 1840, 34 3/4" high.

L handle medical cane with a Greek Caduceus on top and the date 1899 on the silver ferrule, 35" high.

Three physicians canes: left: bone handle with a snake entwined on the shaft, 34 1/2" high; center: hollow brass handle opens to reveal instruments, the shaft holds medical instruments and medicines, 36 1/2" high; right: American patented gutta-percha cane, part of this cane reassembles to form a stethoscope and the rest holds medicines, 35 1/2" high.

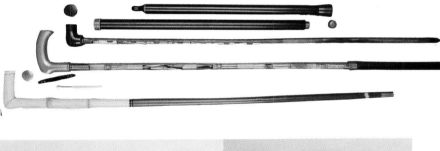

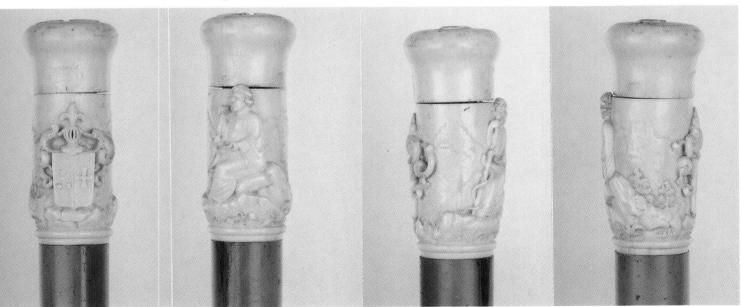

Ivory handled doctor's cane with a crest, an image of Hypocities, and inscribed "Dr. D" on top, malacca shaft, 38" high.

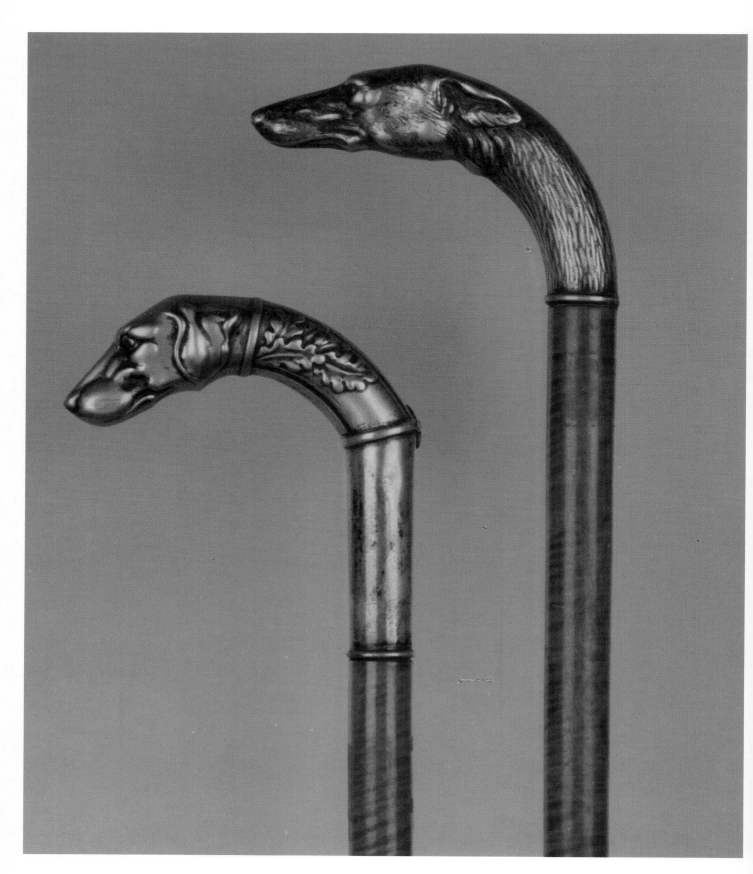

38

Chapter 3
Nomenclature for Parts of a Cane and a Walking Stick

Handles

Early canes, even to the present time, had handles made from deer or elk horn and there is nothing finer than a well-balanced, tapered shaft of wood crowned by such a horn. Costlier canes had handles made of silver and gold and woods rarer than those used for the shaft. Ivory and bone and eastern water buffalo horn have always been much in demand. I have some canes with rhinoceros horn handles (and shafts too) and this was always considered the most desirable. Tortoise shell, another rarity, is almost as desirable.

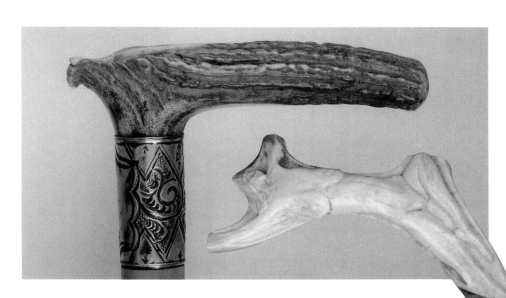

Antler handle, silver collar with an open space for inscription, malacca shaft, c. 1870, 36" high.

Folk art reclining nude carved in an antler horn handle, 37 1/2" high.

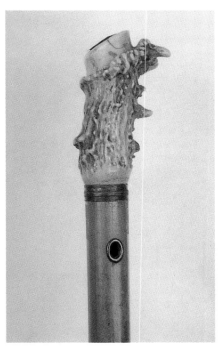

Many canes had handles made from deer or elk horn. Antler handle (somewhat figural in profile) fitted with a crest, silver collar, and eyelets, on a malacca shaft, c. 1700, 35 1/4" high.

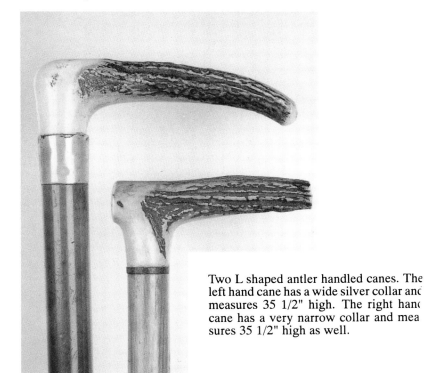

Two L shaped antler handled canes. The left hand cane has a wide silver collar and measures 35 1/2" high. The right hand cane has a very narrow collar and measures 35 1/2" high as well.

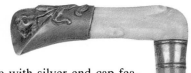

Bone L handle with silver end cap featuring Art Nouveau style flowers, silver collar, step partridge wood shaft, 35 3/4" high.

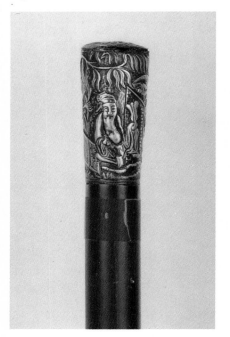

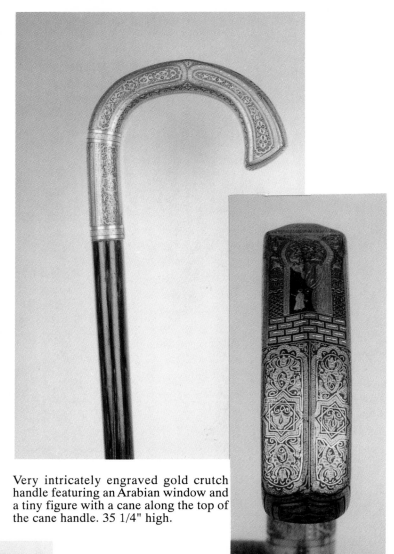

Costlier canes had handles made of silver and gold. Chinese cane with silver handle with figure and ebony shaft, 36" high.

Very intricately engraved gold crutch handle featuring an Arabian window and a tiny figure with a cane along the top of the cane handle. 35 1/4" high.

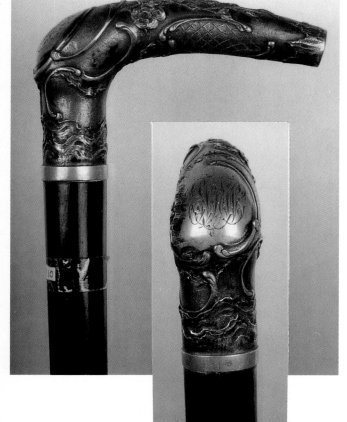

Ornate foliated silver handle, monogrammed. Ebony shaft, German silver ferrule on this French cane dating from c. 1890. 36 1/2" high.

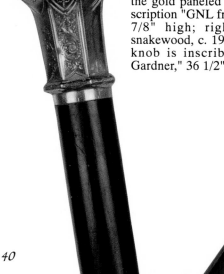

Two formal canes with gold handles. Left gold quartz stone mounted at the top of the gold paneled handle bearing the inscription "GNL from MEB," c. 1888, 36 7/8" high; right: gold handle on snakewood, c. 1900, the top of the gold knob is inscribed "H.C.F. to Peter Gardner," 36 1/2" high.

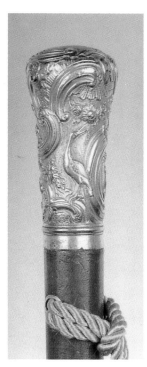
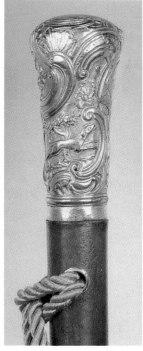
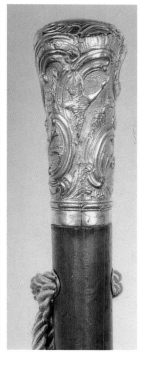
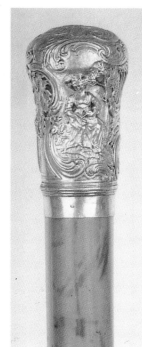
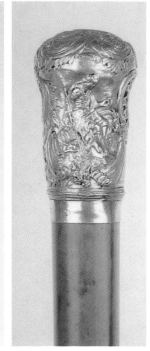

Gold elongated foliated straight cap handle decorated with a hunting dog and two birds among scrolls and flowers. Gold eyelets. Malacca shaft. The top of the handle has an open area suitable for inscription. French, c. 1870. 37" high.

Ornate Victorian gold handle with seated man and woman on malacca shaft, 36 3/4" high.

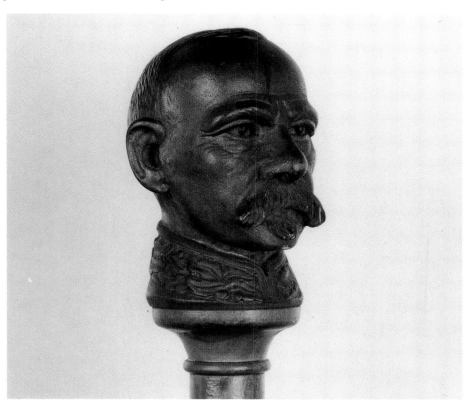

Costlier canes also had handles made of woods more rare than those used in their shafts. Eastern European figural handle of a foreign dignitary with thinning hair, a mustache and a goatee, 35" high.

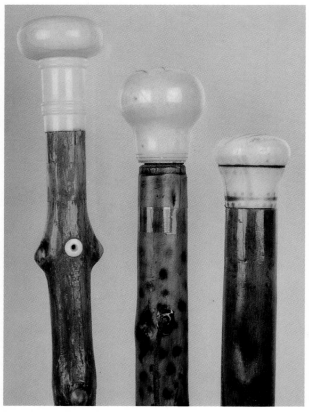

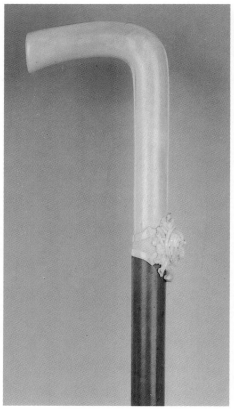

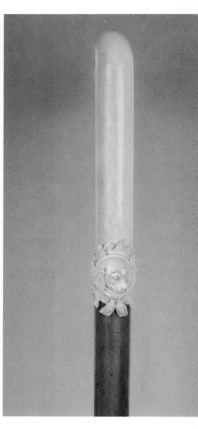

Ivory and bone handles have always been much in demand. Three ivory knob handled canes. The left has eyelets finished with ivory, 36 1/4" high. The center has eyelets finished in silver, 35 1/2" high. Right has no eyelets and a worn dot and band pattern on the side of the knob, 39" high. All three date from c. 1850-1880.

Fine ivory L handled with hunting hound and horn, on fine malacca, 33" high.

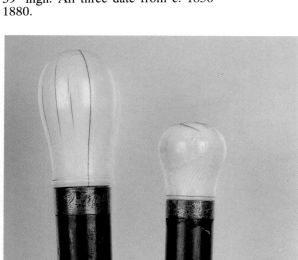

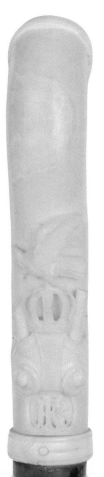

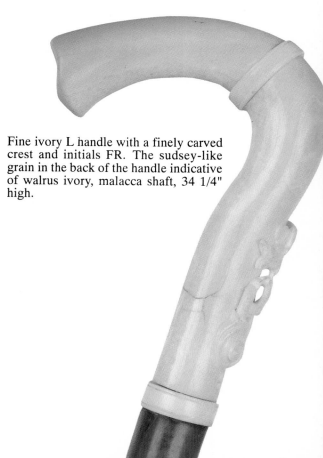

Fine ivory L handle with a finely carved crest and initials FR. The sudsey-like grain in the back of the handle indicative of walrus ivory, malacca shaft, 34 1/4" high.

Two ivory knob handled canes with simple silver collars. The left hand handle has the larger straight knob and a three band pattern just above the collar. Left: 33 1/2" high; right: has a pear shaped knob: 34 1/4" high. Both date from c. 1870.

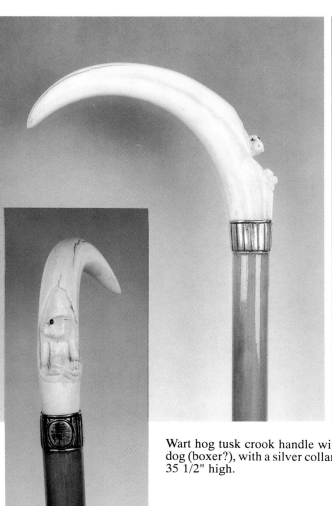

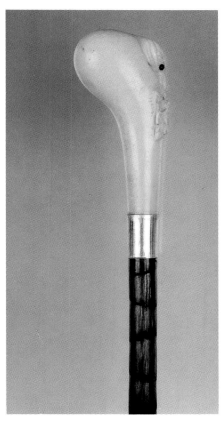

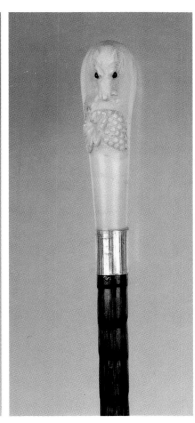

Wart hog tusk crook handle with carved dog (boxer?), with a silver collar, c. 1905, 35 1/2" high.

Pistol grip walrus ivory Aesop's fable fox and grapes with black eyes, Towle Sterling collar, partridge wood shaft, gold ferrule, c. 1900, 36 1/4" high.

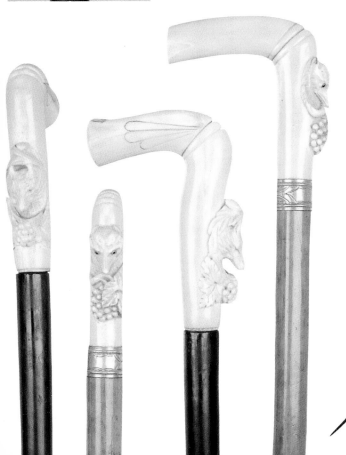

Two ivory Aesop's fable fox and grapes on L handles, left walrus ivory on ebony, right: gold collar on malacca. Left: 35 3/4" high; right: 34 3/8" high.

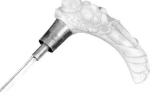

Reclining Chinese woman fashioned on this ivory handled sword cane, 36 5/8" high.

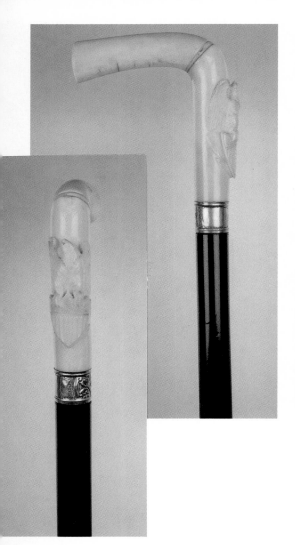

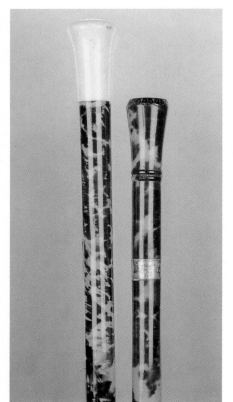

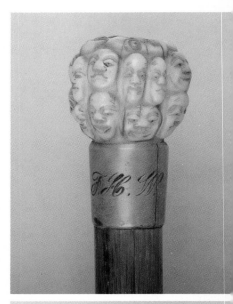

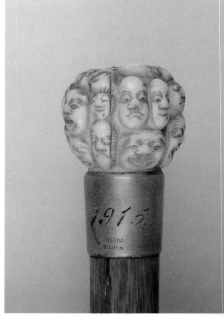

Tortoise shell, another rarity, is also desirable. Two beautiful tortoise shell shaft canes. Left: with ivory handle, 35" high; right: tortoise shell, including handle, top of handle marked CP in gold, silver collar, 34" high.

Ivory American Eagle on shield handle, gold collar with open space for inscription, ebony shaft, 35" high.

The handle is almost the most important part of the cane because it gives a carver an opportunity to show his talent, especially if that handle is ivory or bone. Many intricate ivory carvings in the form of dogs, horses and birds are to be found on fine malacca sticks. Some made with silver trimmings and glass or jeweled eyes are much in demand. In the seventeenth century, even ivory tops were further embellished by being inlaid with silver pique.

Lunatic face in ivory on a wood handle with an ivory collar, malacca shaft, and bone ferrule. 36" high.

The handle gives the carver an opportunity ot show his talent, especially if the handle is ivory or bone. Japanese N Masks or Thousand Faces cane, carv ivory above a silver collar on a reed sha The collar is engraved "F.H.W. 191 Horn ferrule. 33" high.

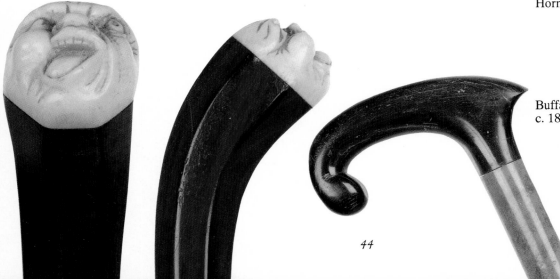

Buffalo horn handle with a malacca sha c. 1890, with a horn ferrule, 35" high.

44

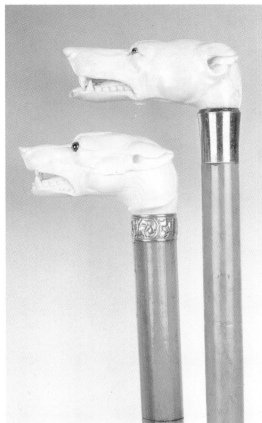

Two snarling hounds in ivory with silver and gold collars. The lower hound, with a twist of the wrist releases a fine Toledo sword blade. Malacca shafts. Produced in Europe and dating form c. 1870-1890. 35 3/4" high sword cane; 34 3/4" high for the silver collared cane.

Many intricate ivory carvings in the form of dogs, horses and birds are to be found on fine malacca sticks. Snarling mastiff in ivory with inset glass eyes above a thin silver collar, c. 1880. 33" high.

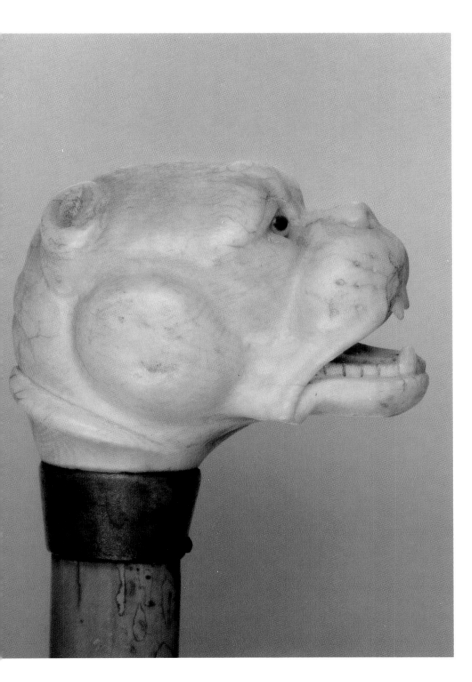

Ivory L handle carved as a bald eagle above a simple silver collar. 35 1/4" high.

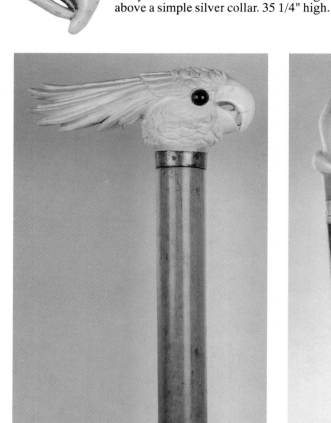

Ivory parrot or cockateel with inset glass eyes above a plain narrow silver collar. Malacca shaft, c. 1900. 35" high.

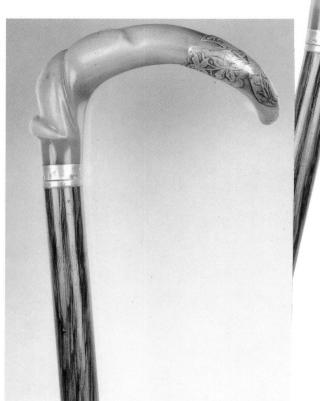

Horn crook handle with silver end cap and collar. The end cap is decorated with a grapevine motif. Horn ferrule. c. 1700. 35" high.

Handles were made of bone, horn, shell, ivory, porcelain, enamel, crystal, glass, onyx, agate, jasper, lapis lazuli, coral, cameos and metal, precious and nonprecious, etched with all the beauty and ingenuity of which the jewelers and craftsmen were capable. Then we have handles intricately carved of eagles, parrots, and other birds, horses, cows, elephants, lions, tigers - whole zoos and dogs and cats and owls.

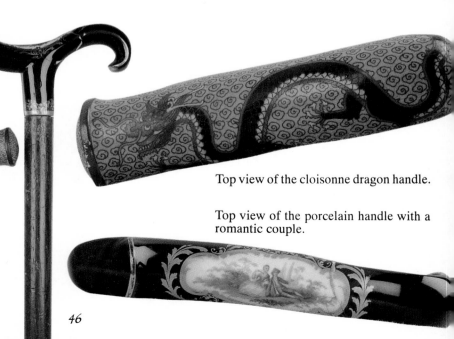

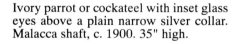

Top view of the cloisonne dragon handle.

Top view of the porcelain handle with a romantic couple.

Left: Cloisonne handle on snakewood shaft, dragon on top of handle, 37" high. Right: porcelain handle with a romantic couple on top, 37" high.

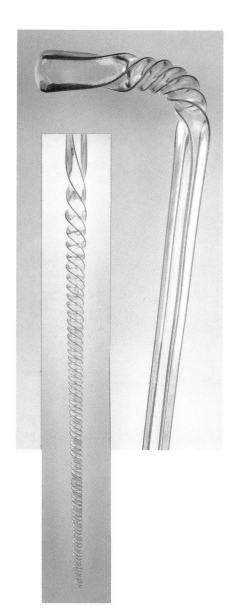

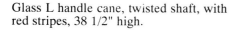

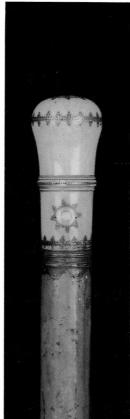

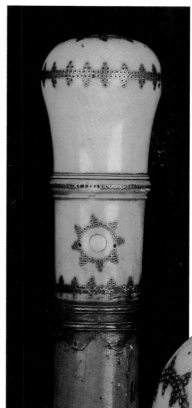

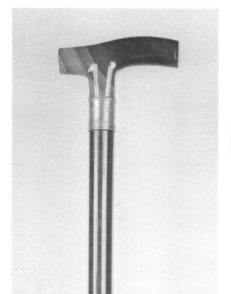

In the seventeenth century, ivory handles were embellished with inlaid silver pique. Old ivory Pique cane with original eyelets in the handle filled, malacca shaft, silver collar. This is an old English cane. The entire shaft is hollow. The top of the handle unscrews. This was originally a container cane but for what? The ferrule states "J. Gillett, Maker, 40 Fetter Lane, London." 36 3/4" high.

Glass L handle cane, twisted shaft, with red stripes, 38 1/2" high.

Straight handle made of a "Boule" of ruby sapphire, man made, 32 3/4" high.

Rare stone handle, brass collar and snakewood shaft, 33 3/4" high.

Rare decorated silver and gold handle and ferrule from Bancock, c. 1880, 35 3/4" high.

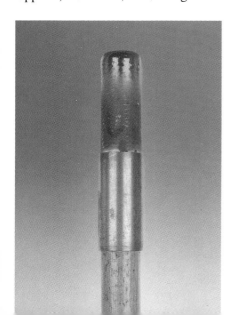

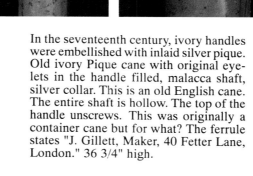

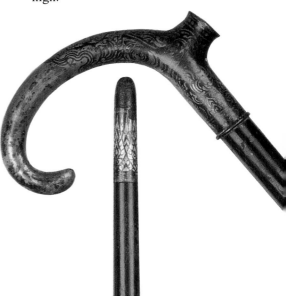

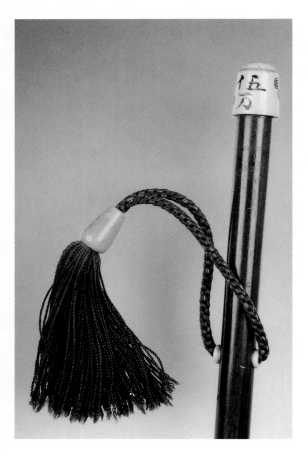

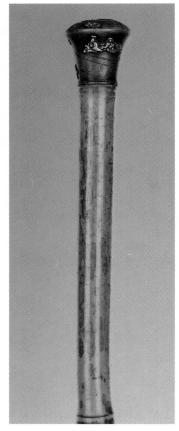

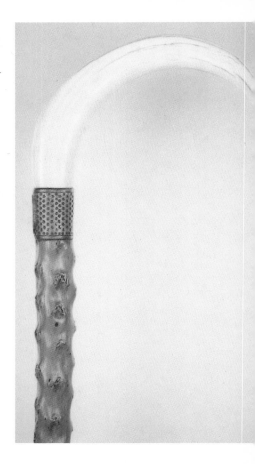

Handles have been made from many materials. Ivorine knob handle carved with Oriental symbols and designs then colored. Features ivory inset eyelets and wrist cord. Ivory ferrule as well. 37 3/8" high.

Japanese brass handled cane with silver figures on the side, bamboo shaft, 35 1/4" high.

Boar's tooth handle, cane of Kaiser Wilhelm, 37 1/2" high.

Two ram's horn handled canes, left: black rams horn on malacca c. 1800, 36 1/2" high; right: Scottish blonde rams horn on hazel wood, c. 1988, 37 1/2" high.

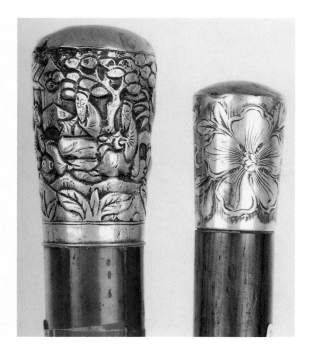

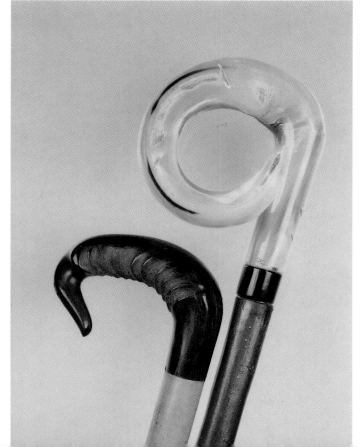

Two Sterling Silver Chinese straight cap handled canes. Left on a malacca shaft. Both have German silver ferrules. Left: 35 1/2" high; right: 36 1/4" high.

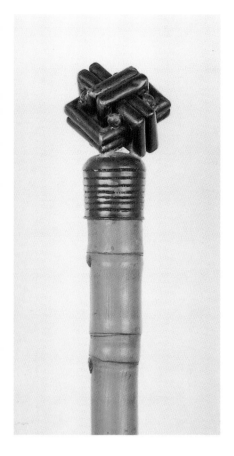

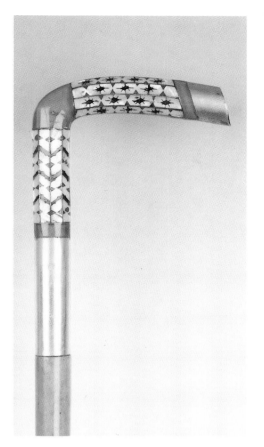

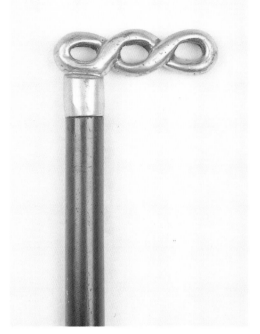

Silver and pewter puzzle cane with rare bamboo shaft, 35 1/2" high.

Inlaid L handle with green, white, red, and black inlay, and a very long brass ferrule. Ferrule: 9" high, cane: 36 1/2" high. Believed to be Latin American.

Simple silver "Odd Fellows" fraternity L handle with three loops. This is a container cane as the handle unscrews and a small secret opening is uncovered. 36 1/2" high.

Then we have handles intricately carved with birds and animals (not to mention reptiles and amphibians). Four birds, polychrome detail, some with glass eyes, ranging from 33 3/4" to 35" high. Left to right: The first and fourth were made by Willard M. Chandler of the Old Soldiers Home in Togus, Maine. They were made prior to 1918. The third is a horn handle on a shaft of paper disks.

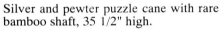

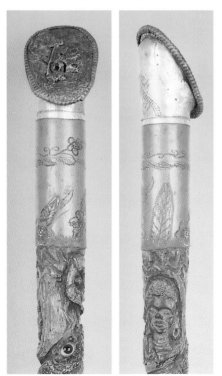

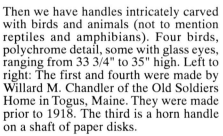

Metal handle, sloping with figure on front, brass collar, and the upper third is carved with a snake and a woman, the snake has a glass eye, 35 1/2" high.

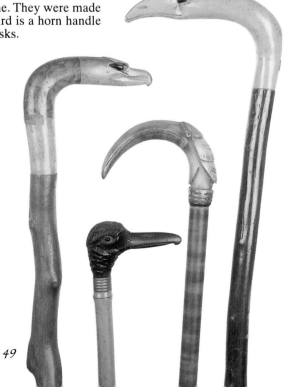

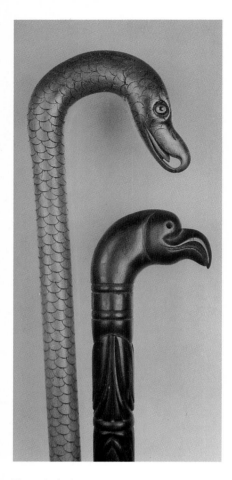

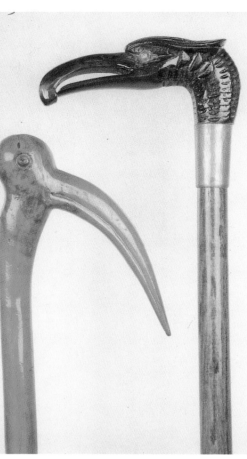

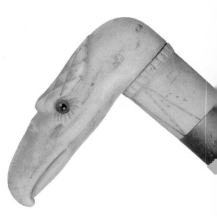

Ivory eagle with inset glass eyes above silver collar inscribed "Dr. S. G. Stevens 33 3/8" high.

Two Asiatic canes of birds: left: with painted feathers, glass inlaid eyes, all from one piece of wood, 35" high; right: painted black with red painted eyes, 35 1/2" high.

Two birds, right hand bird has a "gem" eye and a collar, left hand has a brass ferrule. Left: 34 1/4" high; right: 37 1/4" high.

Ram's horn eagle's head with silver collar and hallmarks on a malacca shaft, by Theo Fossel, c. 1975. 36 1/4" high.

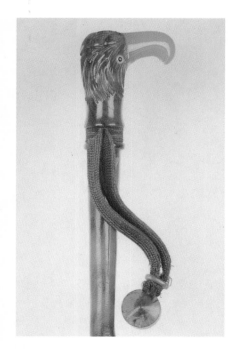

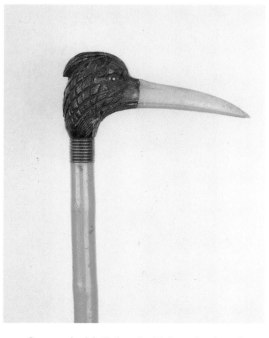

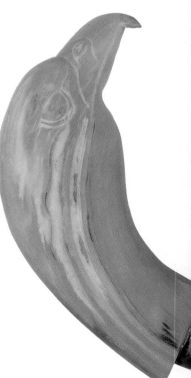

Composite bird with glass eyes, yellow beak, wrist cord, 37 1/2" high.

Composite bird's head with horn beak and inset glass eyes on a bamboo shaft, c. 1885. 32 1/2" high.

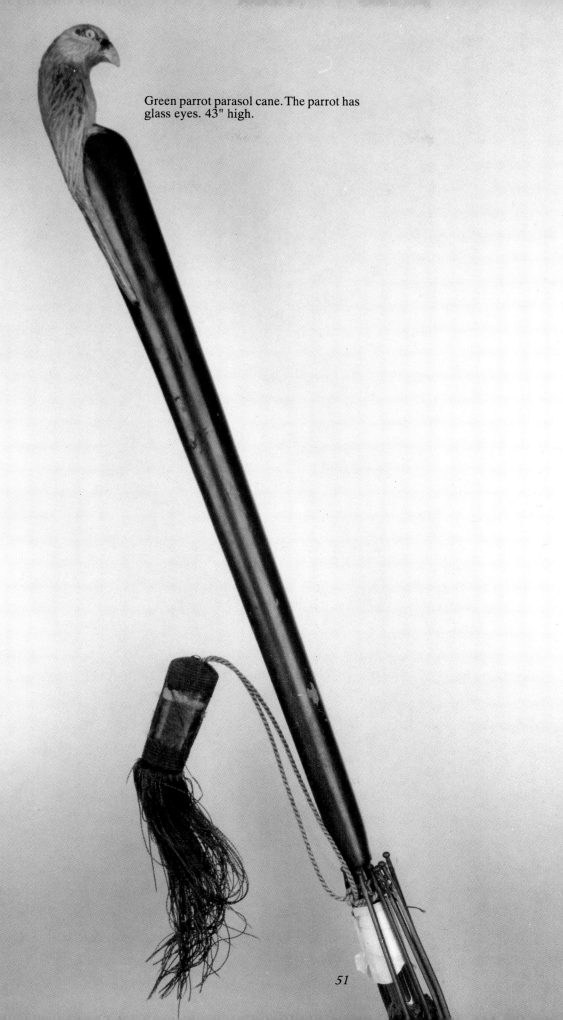

Green parrot parasol cane. The parrot has glass eyes. 43" high.

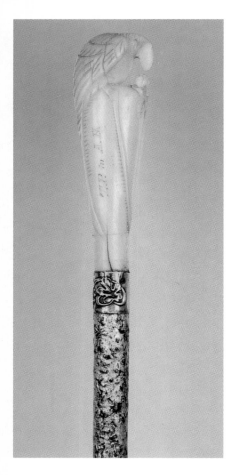

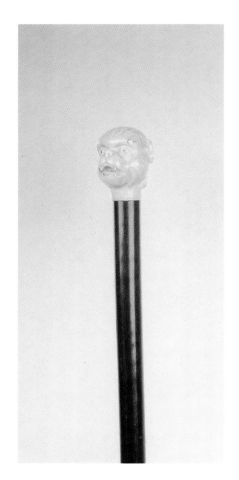

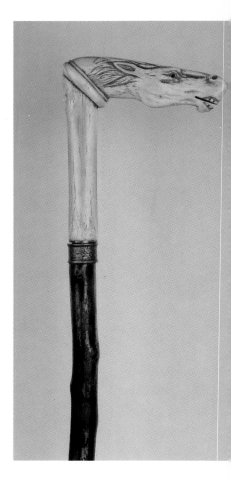

Eagle over lotus blossom ivory handle, a silver collar with grape leaves and a silver sheet covered shaft. The handle is inscribed "T.R. to A.H." This cane is dated to c. 1900. 35" high.

Ivory knob handle, monkey's head with opened mouth on an ebonized black shaft, c. 1870. 34 1/2" high.

Ivory L handle racing horse's head with small glass inset eyes above a narrow decorative collar. 34" high.

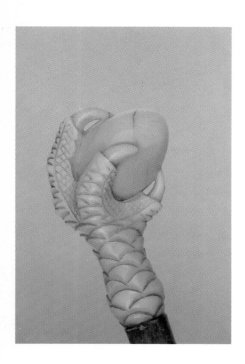

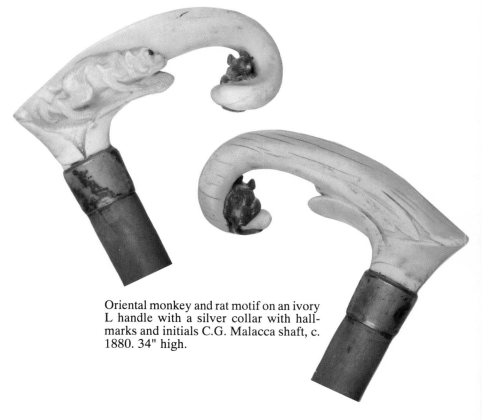

Ivory claw holding egg, straight handle, c. 1880. 39" high.

Oriental monkey and rat motif on an ivory L handle with a silver collar with hallmarks and initials C.G. Malacca shaft, c. 1880. 34" high.

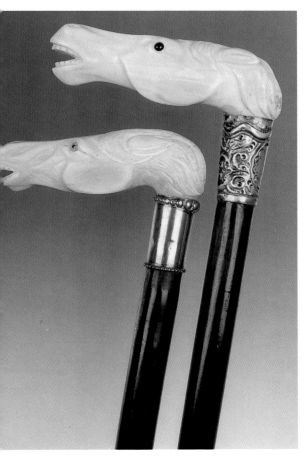

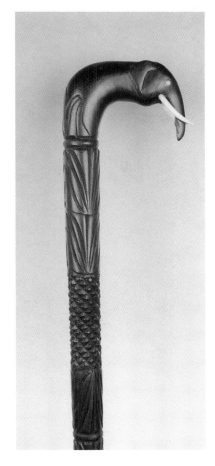

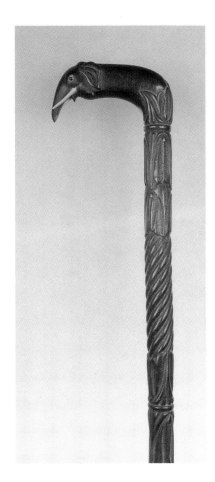

Ivory racing horse canes with glass inset eyes, silver collars and rare snakewood shafts, c. 1870. The right hand collar has an open space for inscriptions. Left: 34 1/4" high; right: 33 1/2" high.

Ebony elephant with ivory tusks and white eyes, 36 1/8" high.

Ebony elephant with white tusks and glass eyes, 35 1/8" high.

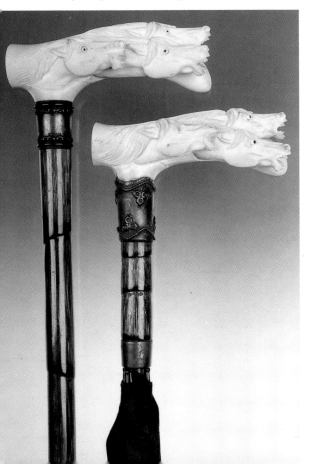

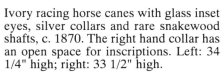

Ivory handled matching set, cane and umbrella, featuring three racing horses with glass eyes, called "dead heat", on a step partridge shaft with silver bands and ferrules, c. 1900. Both 36" high.

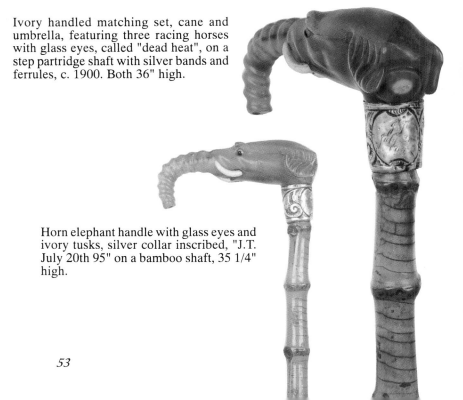

Horn elephant handle with glass eyes and ivory tusks, silver collar inscribed, "J.T. July 20th 95" on a bamboo shaft, 35 1/4" high.

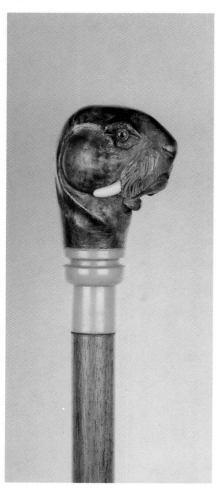

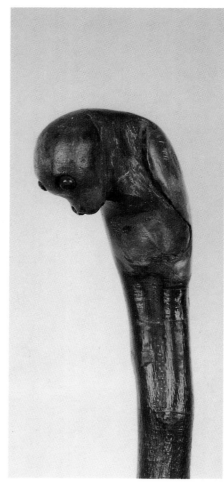

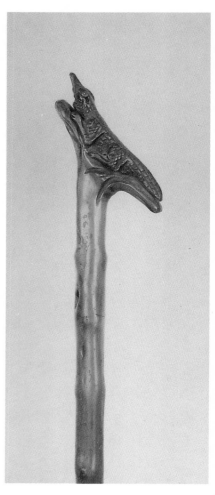

Walrus with glass eyes, ivory tusks, and moving mouth, 40" high.

Crude folk art seal or otter with glass eyes, 36 1/4" high.

Angled alligator on the handle, the cane was produced from a single piece of wood, 35 1/2" high to the tip of his nose.

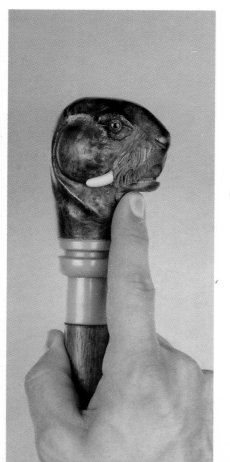

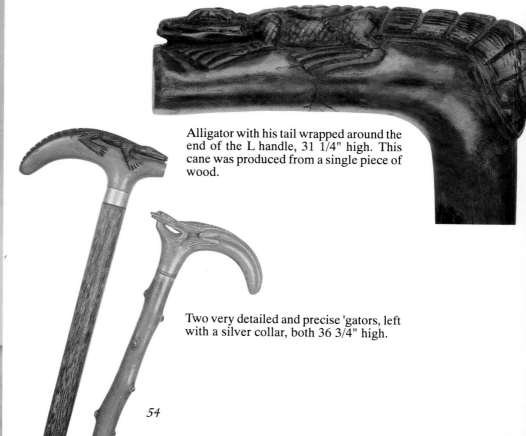

Alligator with his tail wrapped around the end of the L handle, 31 1/4" high. This cane was produced from a single piece of wood.

Two very detailed and precise 'gators, left with a silver collar, both 36 3/4" high.

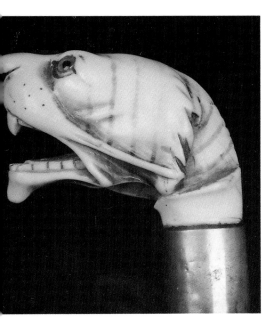

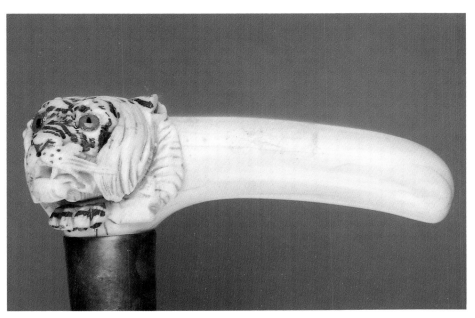

Ivory snarling tiger's head with glass eyes and a sterling silver collar, c. 1860, 36 3/4" high.

Ivory rare Asian white tiger handle with glass inset eyes and a silver collar on an ebony shaft. Made in India, c. 1850. 34 3/4" high.

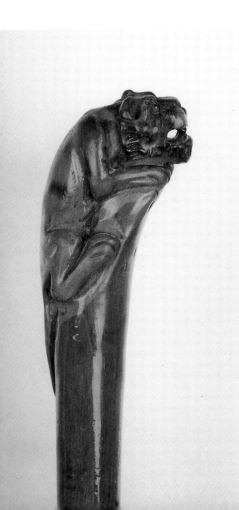

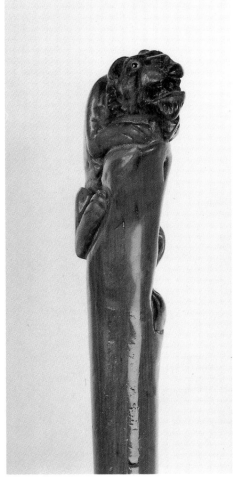

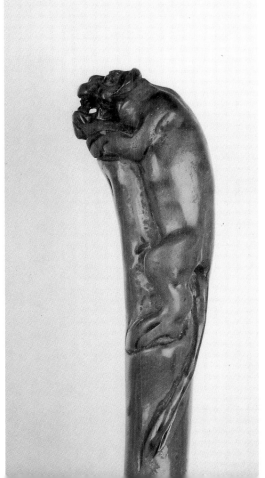

Lion with teeth bared and glass eyes. This cane is made from a single piece of wood. 34 3/4" high.

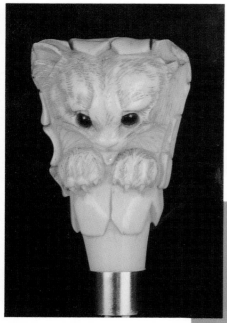

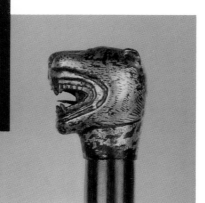

Ivory kitten with glass inset eyes bursts forth, silver collar, c. 1910. 35 3/8" high.

Elegant thin L head in silver shaped as an open-mouthed snake complete with tongue, 37" high.

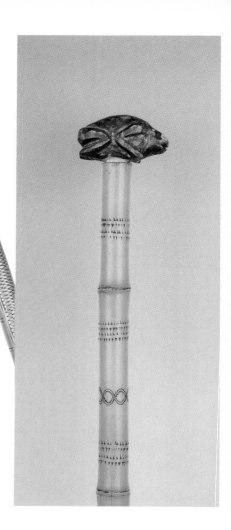

Siamese-Malay lion, rare etching, c. 1890, 34 1/2" high.

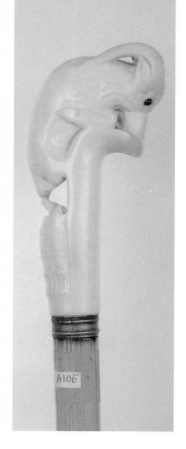

Bamboo shaft with crouching wooden frog as handle. Inked scrimshaw decoration on shaft, 38 3/4" high.

Early advertisement for Bock Beer, ivory goat with black glass eyes standing on a keg drinking from a beer stein, 32 1/2" high.

Rare ivory llama on ebony shaft, glass eyes, engraved silver collar, late 19th century. 35 3/8" high.

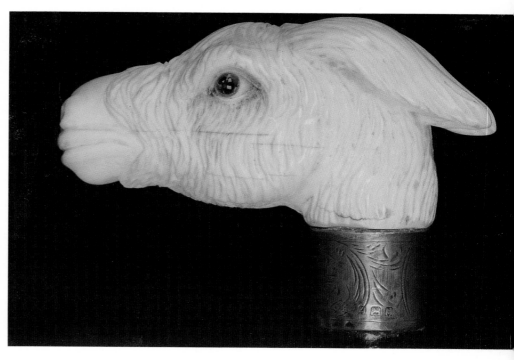

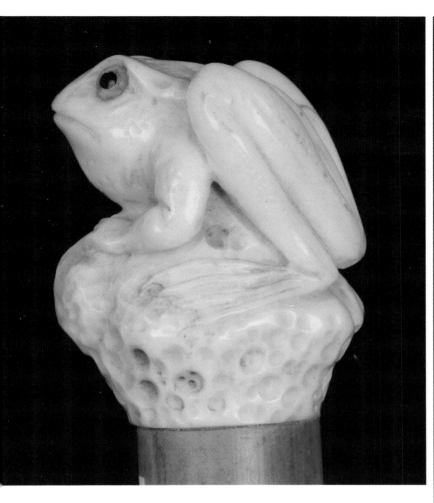

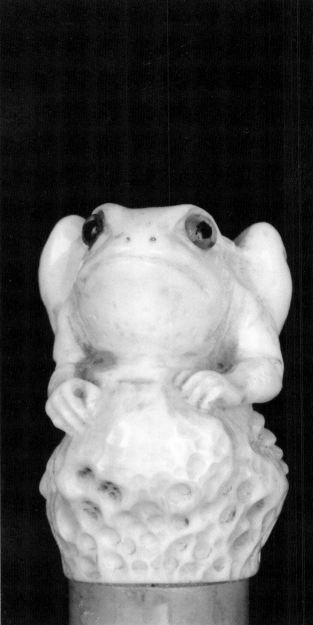

Ivory frog with glass eyes on a blond Malacca shaft, late 19th century. 34 1/2" high.

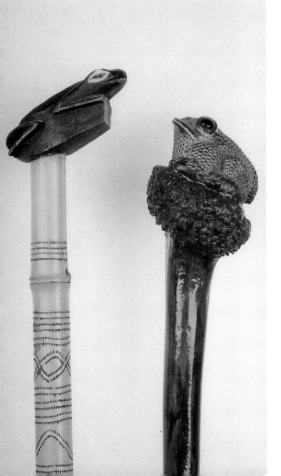

Frog and toad, frog painted on a bamboo shaft, toad carved from a burl and has glass eyes, frog: 36" high, toad: 36 1/2" high.

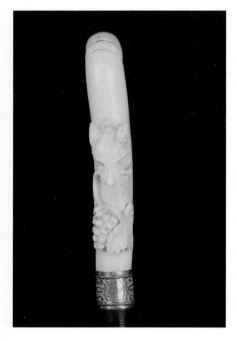

Aesop's fox and grapes in walrus ivory, gold collar and bamboo shaft, late 19th century. 35 1/4" high.

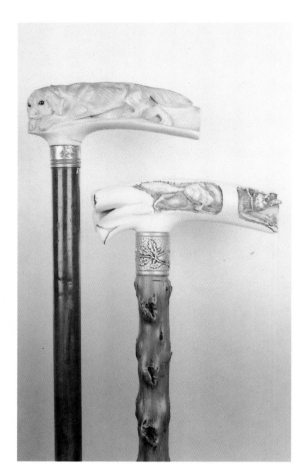

Two ivory L handle canes with collars. Left: a dog with inset glass eyes above a simple gold collar. 32" high. Right: carved fox above a silver collar featuring leaves and a hounds head. 35 1/2" high.

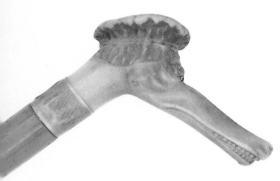

Fanciful horn fox head wearing beret, with inset glass eyes above a silver collar with an oval suitable for inscription. Mottled malacca shaft with a long horn ferrule. 33" high.

Ivory dog's head L-shaped handle with silver collar and a malacca shaft, c. 1880, 34 1/4" high.

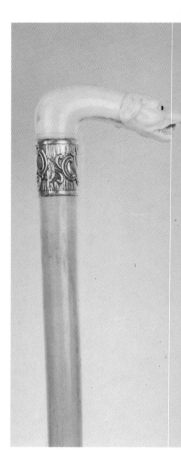

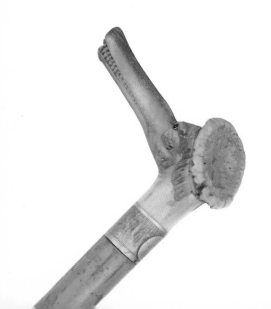

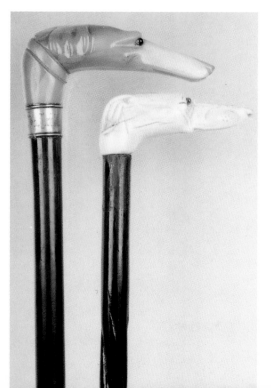

Two greyhound handled canes carve from horn & ivory, both featuring ins glass eyes. Left: horn handle with silv collar inscribed F. O'Neil. Right: has r collar and a twisted ebony shaft. Germa silver ferrule. Left: 35 1/2" high. Righ 37 1/2" high.

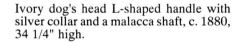

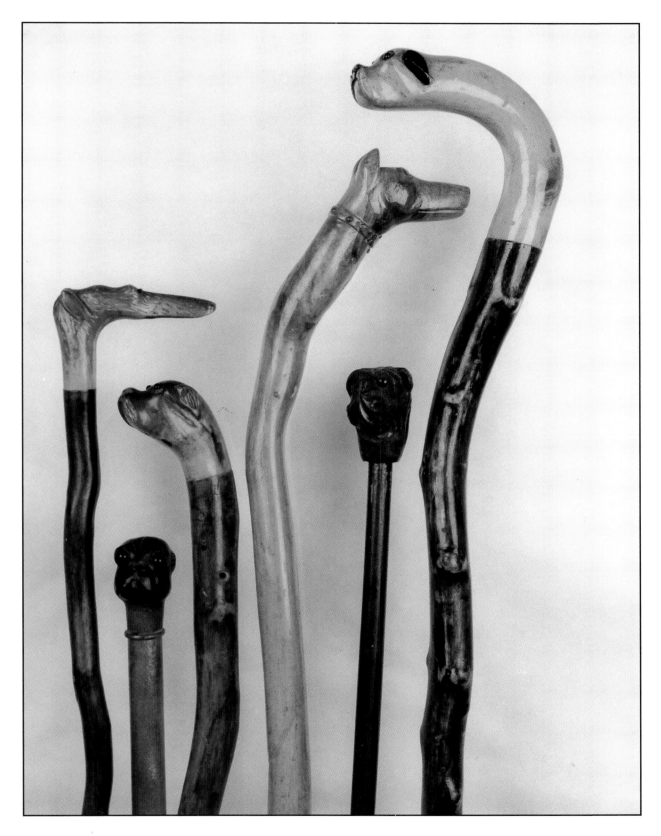

Six dogs, some with polychrome detail,
others with glass eyes, ranging in height
from 34 1/2" to 37". Each are carved from
individual pieces of wood. Left to right:
the first, third and sixth cane were made
prior to 1918 by Willard M. Chandler of
the Old Soldiers Home of Togus, Maine
using only a pocket knife and wood from
the forest surrounding the Home.

Handles contained snuff, tobacco, nutmeg, ginger, disinfectant, perfumed powder, perfumed handkerchiefs, smelling salts and ad infinitum. Some men's canes had compartments with hand warmers that burned charcoal in a little brazier in the handle. Others had a compartment for mustache wax and scent sprays for ladies. Glove holder canes where the glove was taken off one hand and placed in the mouth of a dog handle so that the owner could shake hands.

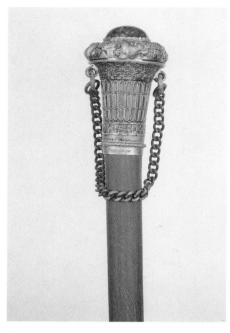

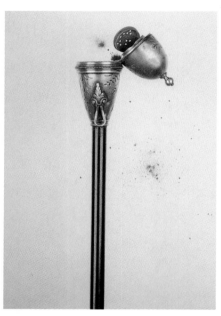

Ladies snuff cane, small silver handle, c. 1900, 36 1/2" high.

Silver handle opens to provide access to a small glass perfume bottle within, purple semi-precious stone on top, small chain attached to handle, 38" high.

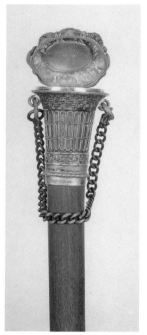

A "glove holder" cane. Dog's head at the end of crook handle, the mouth opens when pressed. 35 3/4" high.

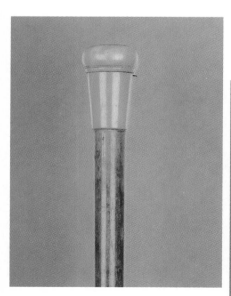

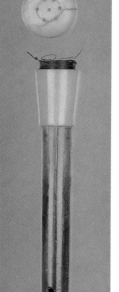

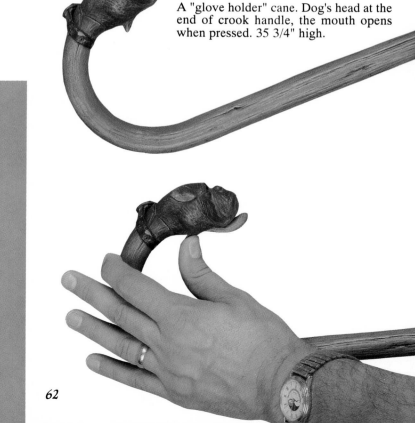

Doctors disinfecting cane — sponge saturated with disinfectant, orange colored ivory handle with holes in top, simple eyelets, 37 1/8" high. The disinfectant is sniffed and also used to disinfect hands.

Shepherd canes - especially the working cane as distinguished from the market cane - had a practical handle that was meant to catch and control their sheep. Almost every trade and profession had its own emblematic handle, and in truth the greatest beauty of a cane is its handle.

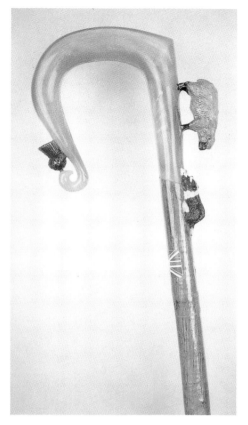

Ram's horn shepherd's market stick (as distinguished from a working stick) with thistle, sheep and sheepdog, 52 3/4" high. Made by a British stickmaker.

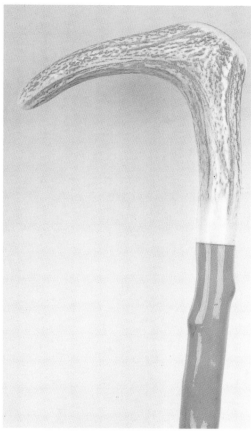

L shaped antler handle English shepherd's market cane with no collar, c. 1960. 47" high.

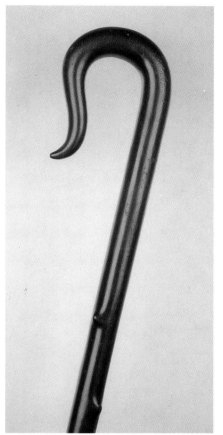

Shepherd canes. Ebony shepherd's leg catching cane, silver ferrule, 37 1/2" high.

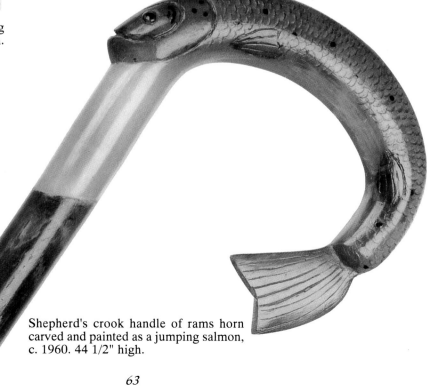

Shepherd's crook handle of rams horn carved and painted as a jumping salmon, c. 1960. 44 1/2" high.

Somewhere I obtained a most interesting cane. The shaft is all white, a color of great dignity among the Japanese, and it has an aluminum handle in the shape of half an anchor, which is called a fluke by mariners. It is 41 1/2" high or long and has Japanese writing under the blade of the fluke and on the forward portion of the rounded shaft of the anchor. Also it has the sacred Japanese flower called a Chrysanthemum on each side of this anchor shaft or handle.

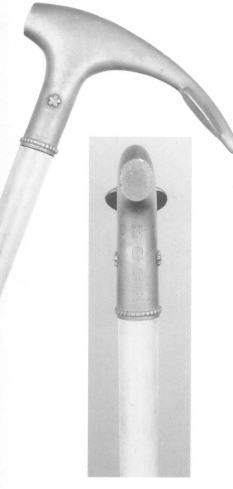

Aluminum whale fluke handle on white shaft, ancient Japanese Admiralty cane of the Secretary of the Navy with Japanese identification on the handle, c. 1820, 41 5/8" high. The Japanese Consul in Washington, D.C. stated in 1968 that the wording down the handle means "Minister for Navy." Characters on the flukes could not be read and may be the artist's signature.

Inasmuch as it is obviously very old, oriental, too high for a cane considering the height of the average Japanese, and because of its color of dignity and it uses the sacred Japanese flower along with its naval motif, this must have been used as a staff of authority by a very high naval authority - possibly a secretary of the navy or the top admiral of the fleet.

The handle, because it is aluminum, in present eyes might cheapen it except for its beautiful construction. If it is from the early 1800's, it certainly is a most valuable item because at that time aluminum was so rare that it was much more costlier than solid gold.

At his coronation as imperial Emperor of France and most of the European continent in 1804, Napoleon Bonoparte snatched the crown out of the hands of Pope Pius VII and placed it on his own head and this crown was alleged to be the most costly in the world at that time because it was made of pure aluminum, then a very rare laboratory specimen. The de-velopment of a commercial process for production of aluminum was first made possible by a French scientist, Henri Sainte Claire Deville, in the early 1800's. (Encyclopedia of America) Vol. I, p. 450 & Vol 19, p. 698.

I had written to the Japanese Embassy in Washington for information on this cane, as I had also inquired of the Japanese TV crew that interviewed me. Both groups said the Japanese writing is ancient and indecipherable by modern Japanese, but it seemingly was the staff of the Secretary of the Japanese Navy from well over a hundred years ago.

Handle Shapes

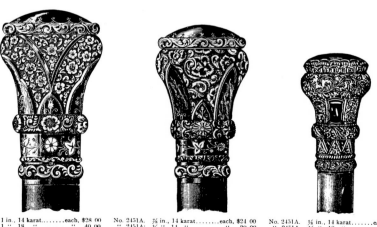

Figure 45. Advertisement for gold handled canes from the 1893-94 Marshall Field & Company's catalogue.

No. 249A. 1 in....each, $20 00   No. 249A. ⅞ in..each,$18 00   No. 249A. ¾ in.each, $16 00   No. 249A. ⅝ in: each...,$14 00   No. 249A. ½ in; each........$12 00

FINELY CHASED 14 & 18 KARAT OCTAGON PEAR SHAPED HEAD.

No. 2451A. 1 in., 14 karat........each, $28 00
" 2451A. 1 " 18 " 40 00

No. 2451A. ⅞ in., 14 karat........each, $24 00
" 2451A. ⅞ " 18 " 20 00
" 2451A. ¾ " 14 " 36 00
" 2451A. ¾ " 18 " 32 00

No. 2451A. ⅝ in., 14 karat........each, $17 00
" 2451A. ⅝ " 18 " 28 00

All Canes less 50 per cent. Discount.

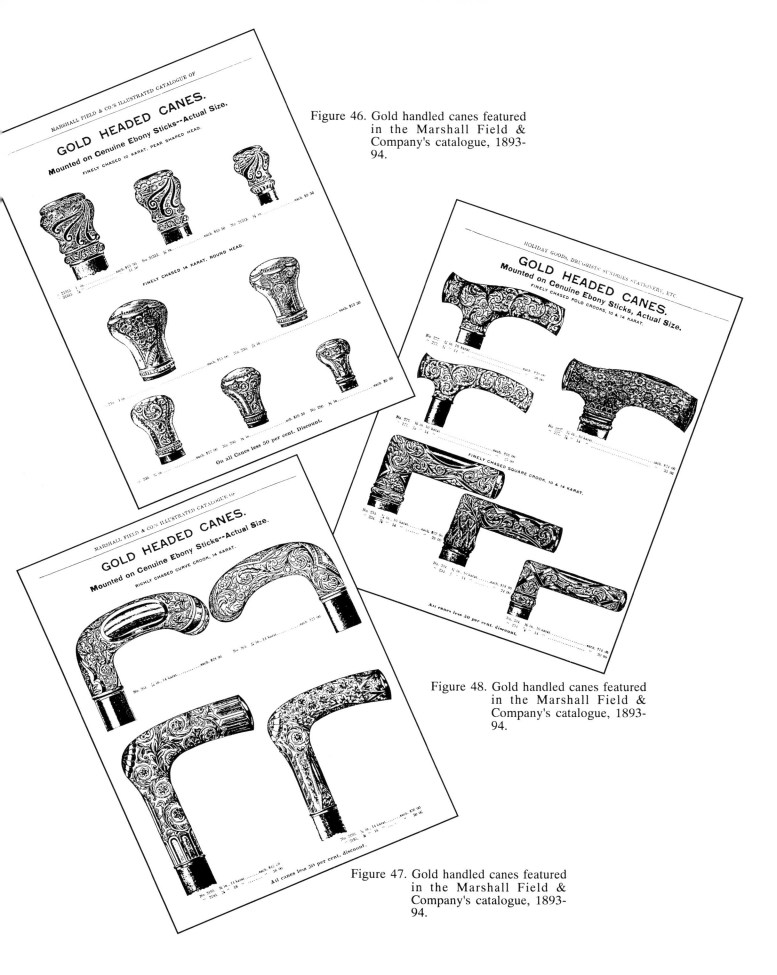

Figure 46. Gold handled canes featured in the Marshall Field & Company's catalogue, 1893-94.

Figure 48. Gold handled canes featured in the Marshall Field & Company's catalogue, 1893-94.

Figure 47. Gold handled canes featured in the Marshall Field & Company's catalogue, 1893-94.

Ivory L handle, jovial bearded man, step partridge wood shaft, c. 1870. 37" high.

Walrus ivory L handled with small patterned band and malacca shaft, c. 1840, bone ferrule. 33 3/4" high.

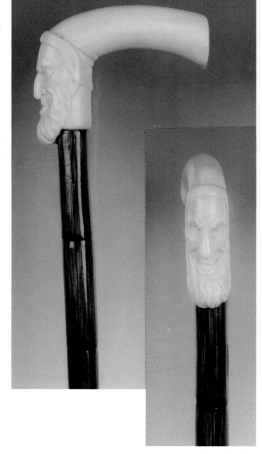

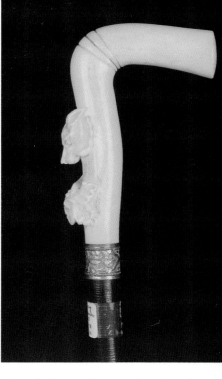

Aesop's fox and grapes in walrus ivory, gold collar and bamboo shaft, late 19th century. 35 1/4" high.

Ivory L handle with a fine ivory double strand collar on a black shaft, 36" high.

Ivory L handle with an ivory collar in the shape of a belt, malacca shaft and a 3" high bone ferrule. 33 1/2" high cane.

L-shaped ivory handle, sterling band signed Stephen J. Young, malacca shaft, and eyelets, c. 1870. 34" high.

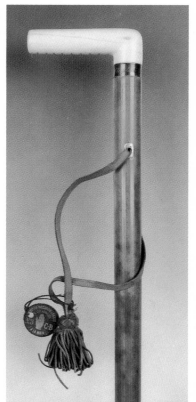

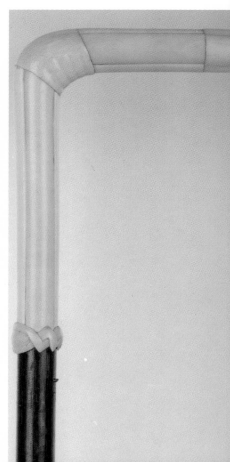

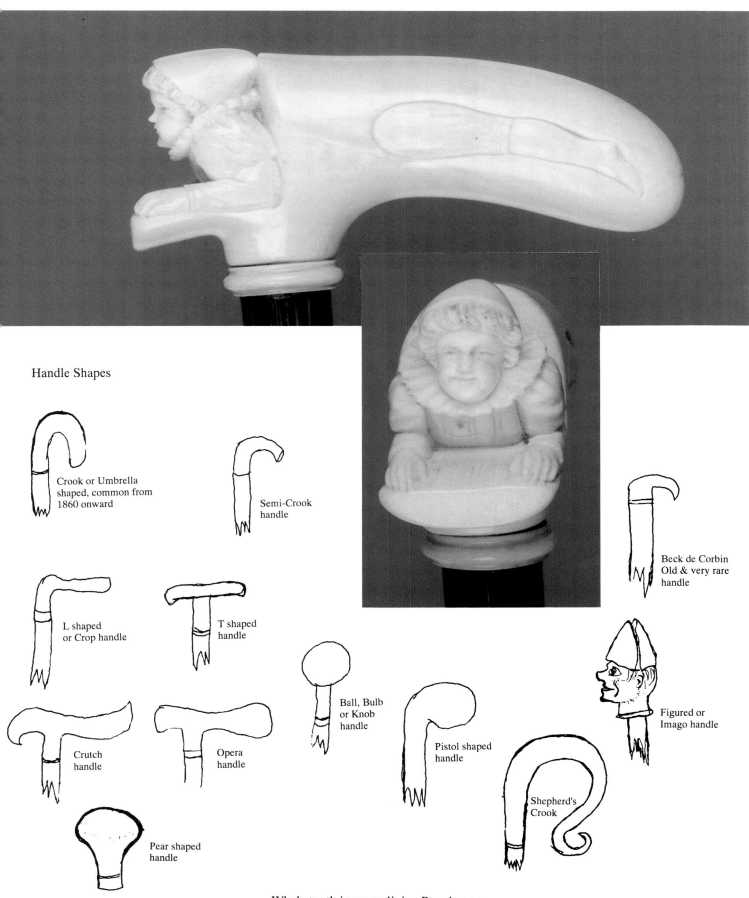

Handle Shapes

Crook or Umbrella shaped, common from 1860 onward

Semi-Crook handle

Beck de Corbin Old & very rare handle

L shaped or Crop handle

T shaped handle

Ball, Bulb or Knob handle

Figured or Imago handle

Crutch handle

Opera handle

Pistol shaped handle

Shepherd's Crook

Pear shaped handle

Whale tooth ivory reclining Renaissance figure on a partridge wood shaft, c. 1860. 35" high.

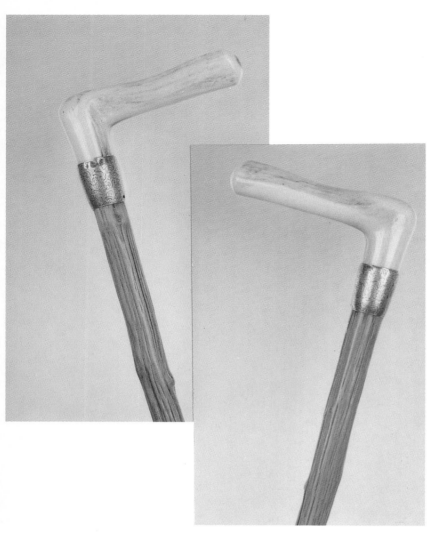

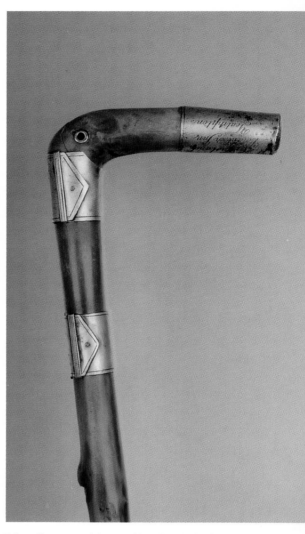

Simple antler L-shaped handle with an engraved silver collar featuring an oval of undecorated silver suitable for inscriptions, 34 1/4" high.

L handle cane with two silver bands fashioned as belts, eyelets of silver, silver end cap with inscription on it "W.H. Husband. Volunteer Inn, Yealmpton." 32 1/2" high.

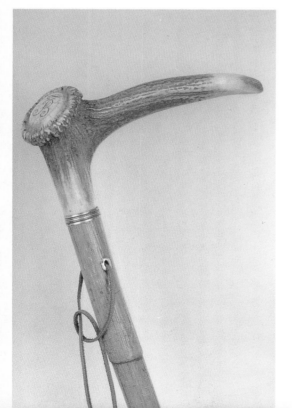

Black L handle with three ring collar, bone ferrule, 35 3/4" high.

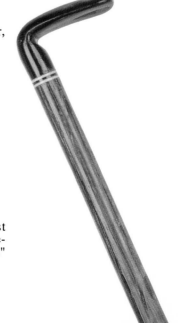

Large L antler handle with crest monogrammed FB, silver collar and eyelets, on step bamboo, c. 1780, 36 1/2" high.

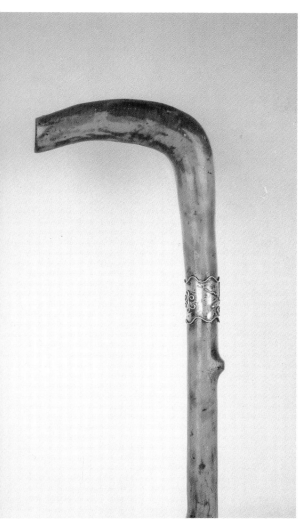

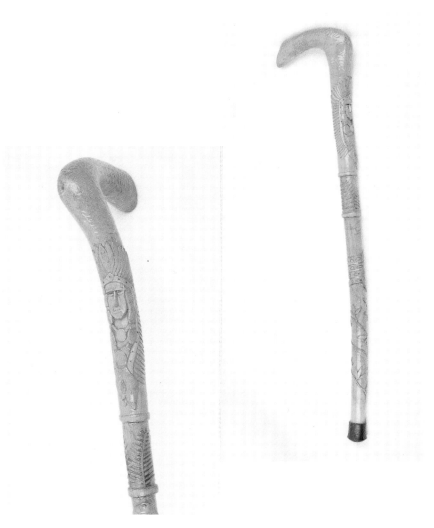

Rustic L handle with a silver collar featuring two designs, made from a single piece of wood, 35 1/2" high.

Indian in full head dress with coiled snake below, folk art, 34 1/4" high.

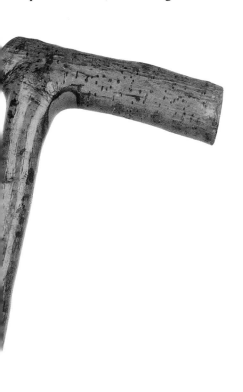

Golden chestnut L handle, c. 1900, 33" high.

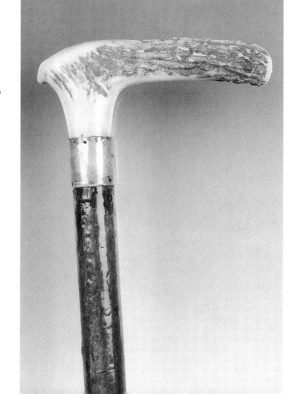

Antler L handle with a silver collar and a hazel wood shaft, c. 1870, 37" high.

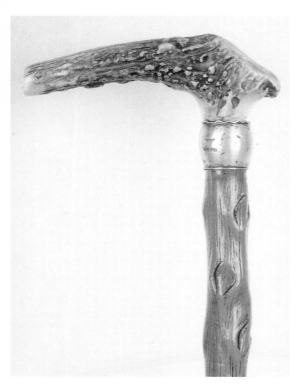

Antler **L handle** with a silver collar stamped STERLING, vine shaft, 33" high.

These are the handle names in general usage in 1890 by Henry Howell & Co. of London established in 1832 and said to be the largest manufacturers, importers and exporters of canes in the world and having over 500 employees:

Straight Butt	Brighton Crook
Root	Tam O'Shanter
Pistol Butt	Crook
Prince of Wales	Shepherd's Crook
Knob	Cross Handle
Grafton Knob	Rustic Cross Handle
Round Hook	Bent Cross Handle
Scarboro Crook	Crutch Handle
	Rustic Crutch Handle

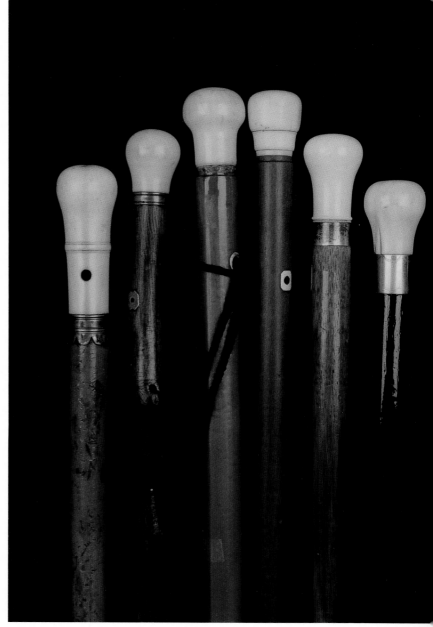

Six ivory knob handled canes changing style over time. Left to right: 1) eyelets in the handle itself, Georgian, silver collar, malacca shaft, 35" high; 2) much smaller knob, silver eyelets in the shaft, silver collar, 3 3/4" long ferrule, 33 3/4" high; 3) elephant ivory knob, silver eyelet and a wrist cord in place, malacca shaft, c. 1790, 33 1/2" high; 4) whale ivory kn silver eyelets, c. 1810, 35 5/8" high; ivory knob, eyelets cease to be used, ver collar with a dedication, lignum tae, c. 1870, 33 3/4" high; 6) ivory kr with silver collar on a mahogany shaft 1890, 33 1/8" high.

Ivory knob handle with stepped malacca shaft, silver eyelets, and a very long ferrule, c. 1850, 34" high.

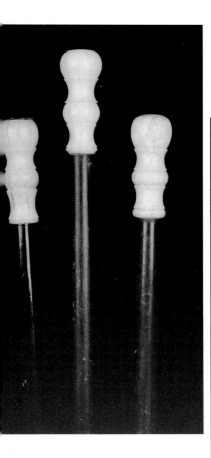

Three elongated straight bone knob handled canes, the left hand cane fixed with a brass American eagle on top. Left to right: 34 3/4" high, 36 1/4" high, 35 1/4" high.

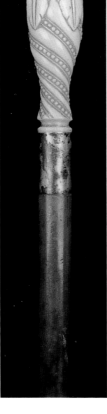

Old English ivory elongated straight knob handled cane with foliate, spiral band, and dot designs, silver collar and a malacca shaft, c. 1850. 34 1/2" high.

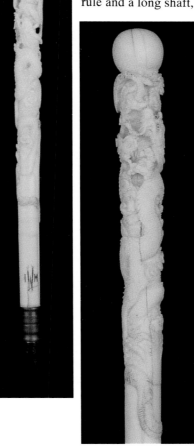

Intricate Oriental ivory carved dragon with monogram "IMW" with a bone ferrule and a long shaft, 46 5/8" high.

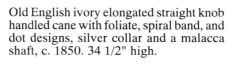

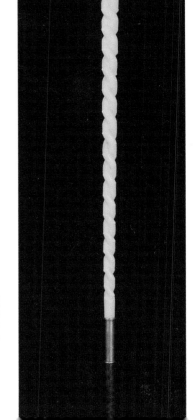

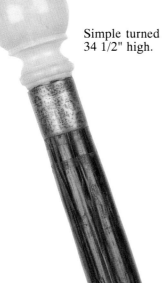

Simple turned ivory knob, silver collar, 34 1/2" high.

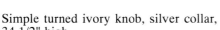

Straight butt. Ivory entwined branches with a long silver collar on a snakewood shaft. Very thin, woman's cane or swagger stick? Ferrule of ivory as well. Dating from the early 1900s. 33" high.

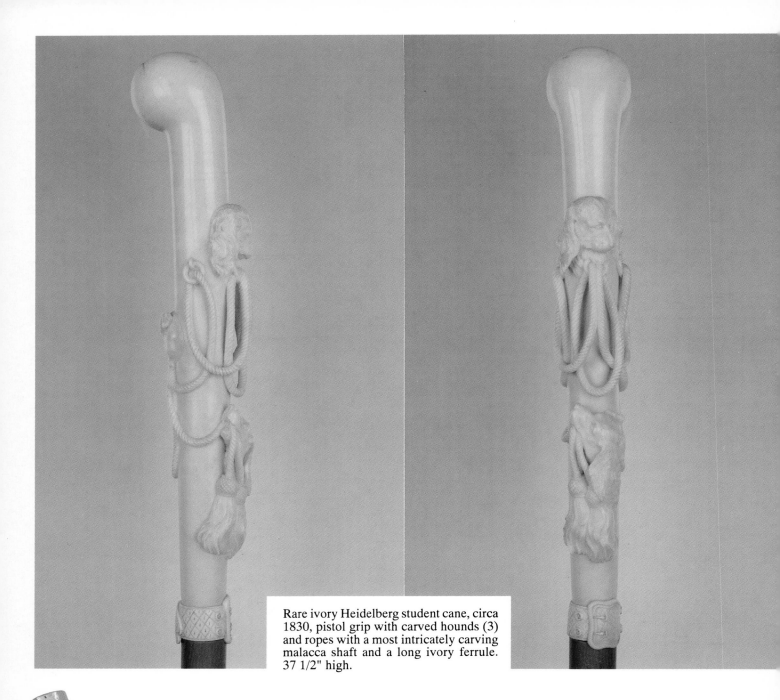

Rare ivory Heidelberg student cane, circa 1830, pistol grip with carved hounds (3) and ropes with a most intricately carving malacca shaft and a long ivory ferrule. 37 1/2" high.

Sterling Silver ladies cane, marked Silver on faceted side, 36 5/8" high.

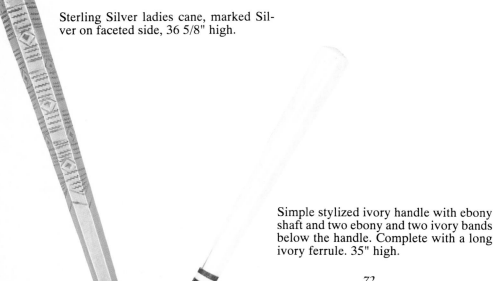

Simple stylized ivory handle with ebony shaft and two ebony and two ivory bands below the handle. Complete with a long ivory ferrule. 35" high.

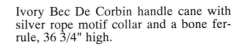
Ivory Bec De Corbin handle cane with silver rope motif collar and a bone ferrule, 36 3/4" high.

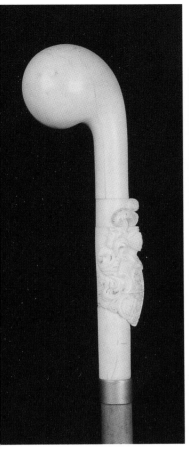

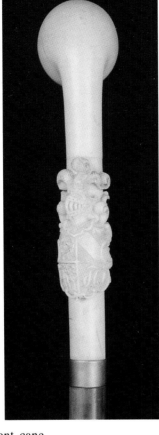

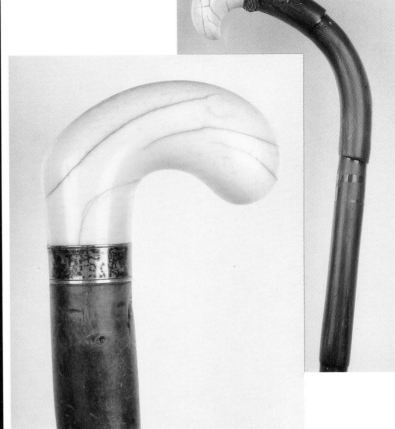

Pistol grip ivory German student cane with a finely engraved crest, a silver collar and a malacca shaft, c. 1870. 35" high.

Small ivory semi-crook handle with a silver collar and a 3" metal ferrule, 36 1/4" high.

Pistol grip shaped L handles, lower with a gold collar, silver handle and rare wood, 34 3/4" high; upper with silver handle and rare wood shaft, 35 3/4" high.

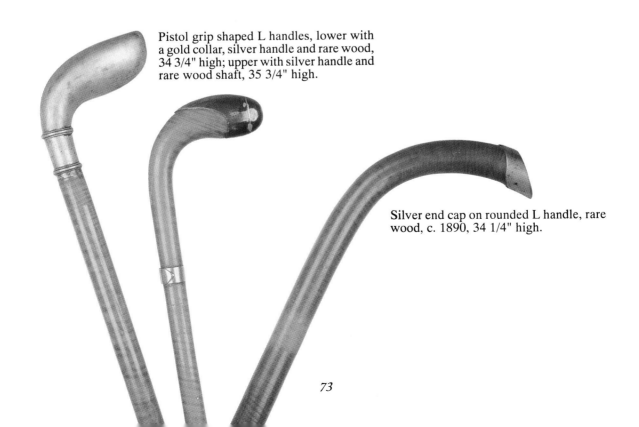

Silver end cap on rounded L handle, rare wood, c. 1890, 34 1/4" high.

73

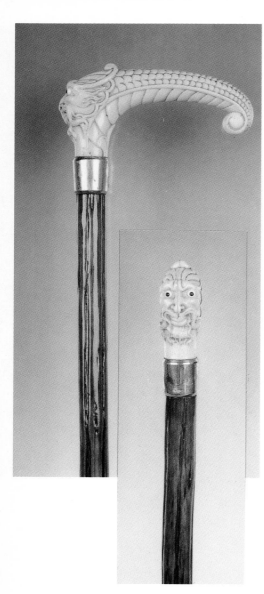

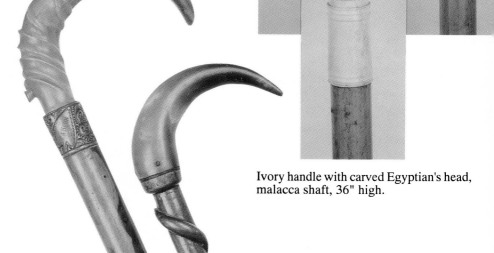

Ivory handle with carved Egyptian's head, malacca shaft, 36" high.

Ivorine grinning bearded gargoyle with glass eyes and with a signed gold collar (signed Dide), vine shaft with a silver ferrule, c. 1880. 32 1/2" high.

Two crook horn handled canes, the left has lignum vitae shaft and a collar with the name R.A. HORN, the right has a snake winding up the shaft.

Whale ivory handle with inset metal disks, rounded silver collar, whale bone shaft, 33" high.

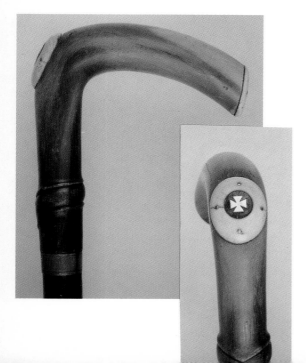

Horn L handle with bone end cap and disc with silver formée cross in its center, 34" high.

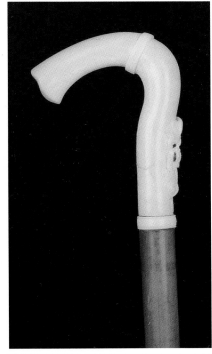

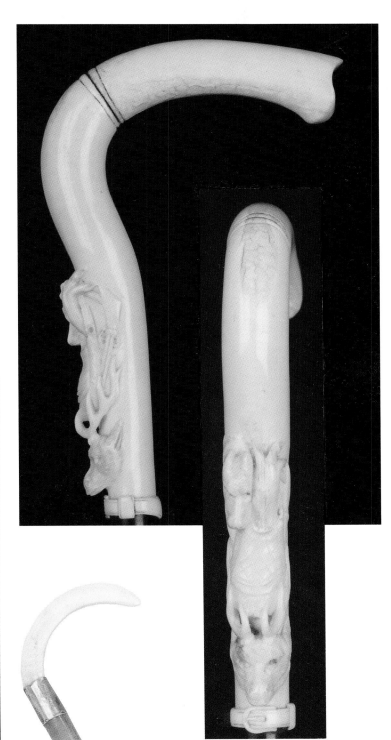

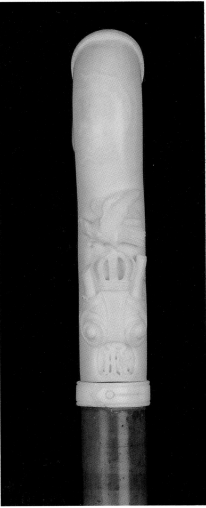

Hunter's cane with dog, backpack, rifle, sword, and elk carved in ivory. Ivory collar in the shape of a belt, ebony shaft, late 19th century. 33 3/4" high.

Walrus ivory crook handled cane engraved with an eagle and crown crest and the monogram "FR" on a malacca shaft, c. 1890. 34 3/8" high.

Tusk handle, the shaft follows the ridges of the tusk, silver collar, 35 3/4" high.

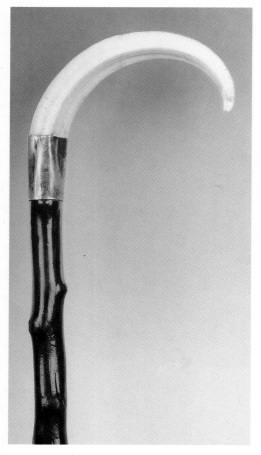

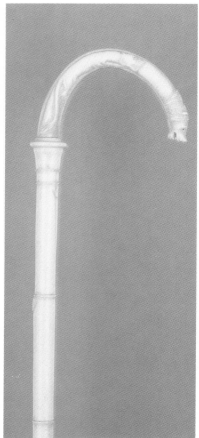

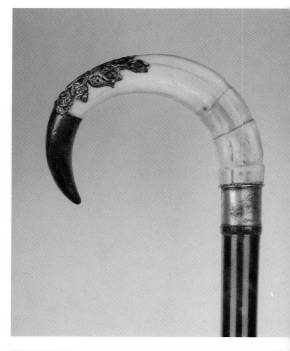

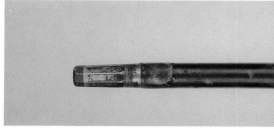

Wart hog tusk, crook handled cane with silver collar and ferrule, knobby shaft, 36 3/4" high.

Segmented ivory crook handle with fox on the side of the handle, 32" high.

Tooth or tusk with silver end cap and silver collar on tortoise shell shaft, with faceted silver end cap, 36" high.

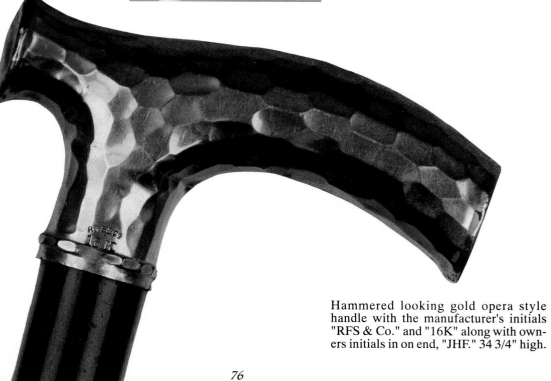

Hammered looking gold opera style handle with the manufacturer's initials "RFS & Co." and "16K" along with owners initials in on end, "JHF." 34 3/4" high.

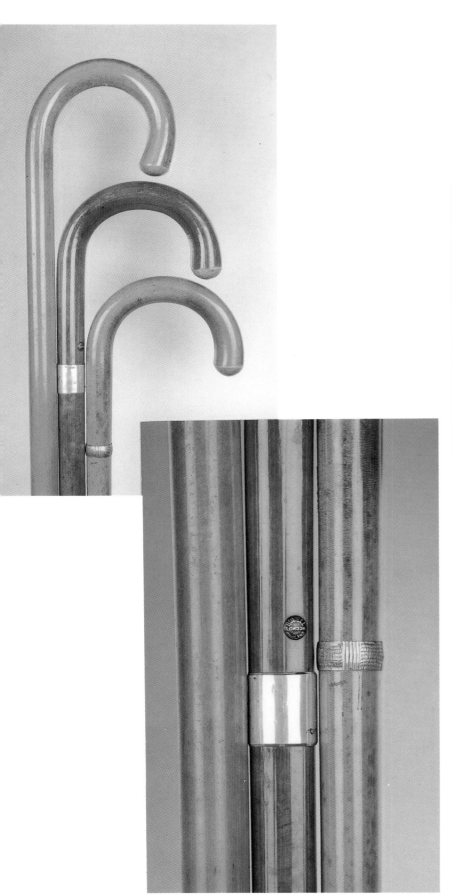

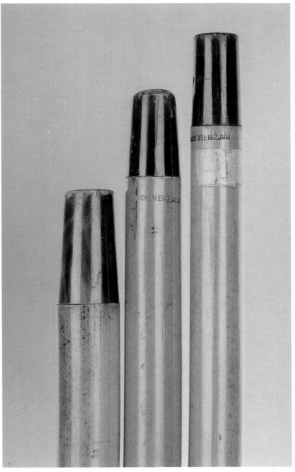

Three malacca crook handled canes from
England with horn ferrules, One with
HOWELL LONDON ENGLAND and
two marked MADE IN ENGLAND.
From 36" to 36 1/2" high.

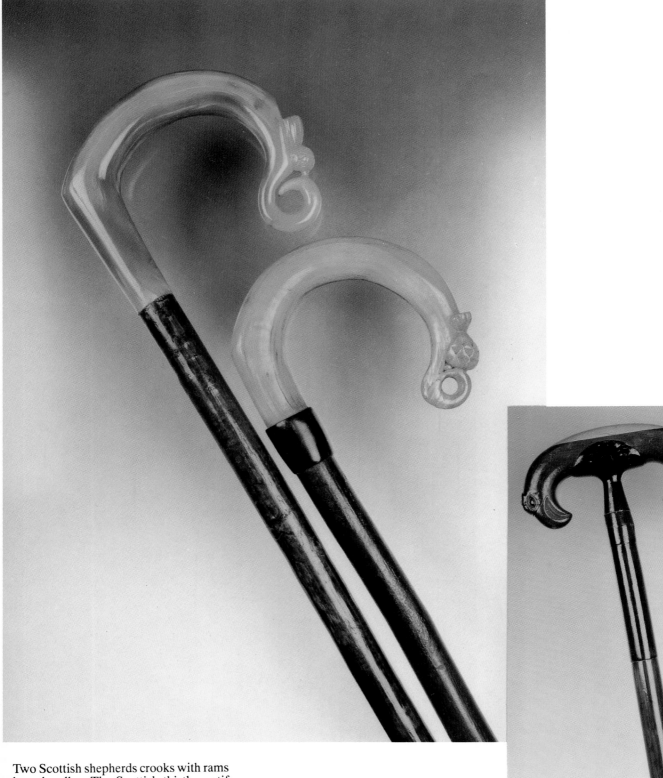

Two Scottish shepherds crooks with rams horn handles. The Scottish thistle motif is carved on the end of the carved handle. These date from c. 1950. Top: 47" high; bottom: 57" high.

Double eagle's head walnut handle cane on a partridge wood shaft, painted details of eyes and beak, 35 1/4" high.

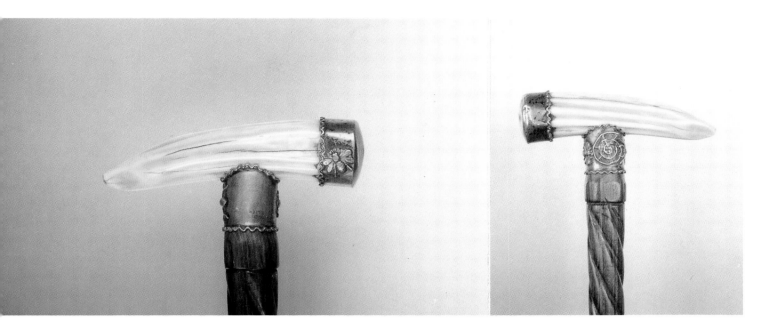

Tusk handle with silver end cap and collar. The collar features the spider and the fly with a central web, the back of the end cap features another fly. The back of the collar is marked silver. The upper third of the shaft is spirally carved. 36 1/4" high.

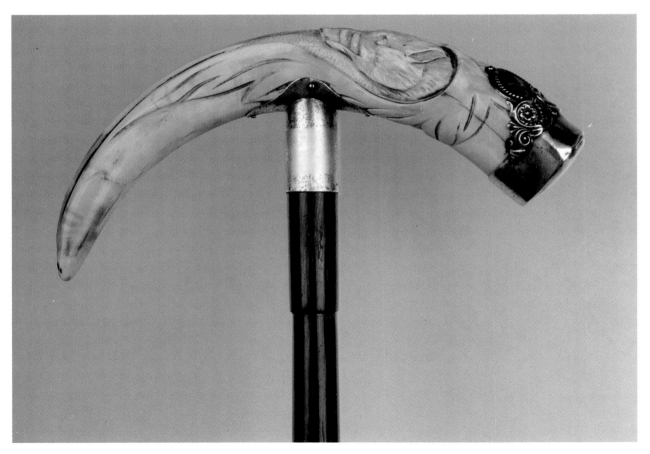

Wart Hog tusk cross bar shaped L handle with silver end cap and collar on stepped partridge wood, c. 1880, 35 1/2" high.

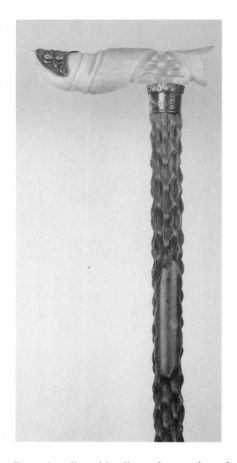

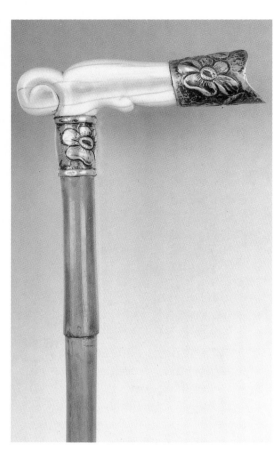

The gold and silver cap mounts were called:

Straight Cap
Pear Shaped Cap
George III Cap

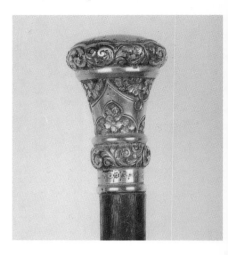

Bone handle with silver shamrock and silver collar with inscribed name John G. Kranzlein. 35" high.

Ivory L handle with silver collar and end cap featuring floral motifs on a stepped rattan shaft. German silver ferrule. 35 1/2" high.

Gold handle presentation cane inscribed: "Presented to Fred E. Gaus DDGC by friends in Stittville Council OUF 279 Aug. 10th 1892." Ebony shaft. German silver ferrule. 34 1/4" high.

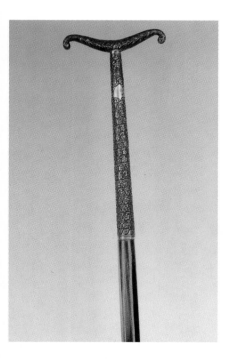

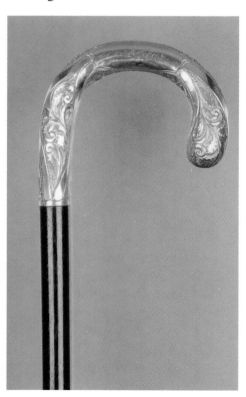

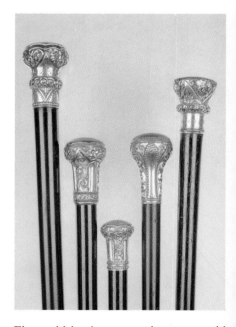

Silver religious staff from India with a crutch handle, wood shaft cut in panels, 45" high.

Gold filled handle on a rustic stick, 38 1/2" high.

Five gold knob presentation canes with ebony shafts, all inscribed: left to right: 1) From R.M. to John Martin; 2) EEP; 3) PSG 1887; 4) To AL from his friends, Thanksgiving 1887; 5) Wm. Corbett, Trinity Church, Christmas, 1897. These canes range in size from 35 1/4" to 36 1/2" high.

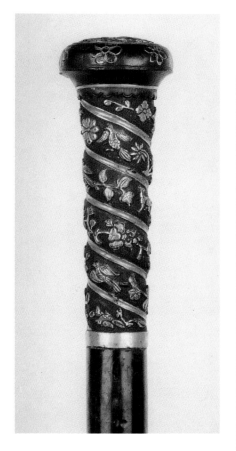

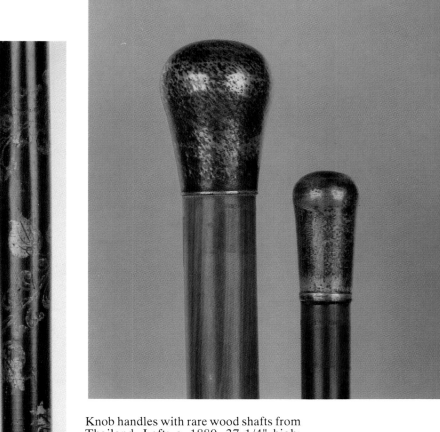

French black cane with raised and gold gilt decoration on handle and shaft, c. 1750, 40 1/4" high.

The handle can be made of most anything-including metal (such as brass or iron), organic or inorganic material, precious stones, bone, or ivory.

Knob handles with rare wood shafts from Thailand. Left: c. 1880, 37 1/4" high; right: c. 1890, 35" high.

Thai Royalty knob handle with panels, silver on rare wood shaft, c. 1890, 34 3/4" high.

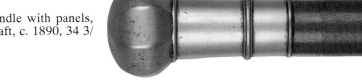

Six silver knob handles in rare woods from Thailand, c. 1890, ranging in height from 33" to 38".

Silver end caps and rare wood shafts: left: c. 1890, 36 3/8" high; right: c. 1900, 34 1/2" high.

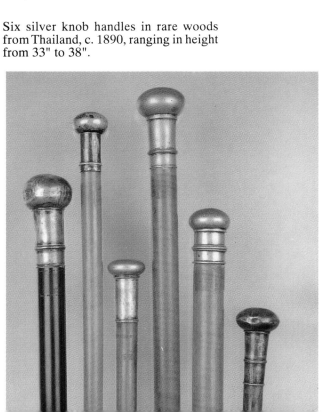

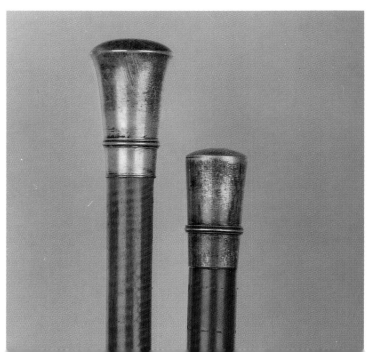

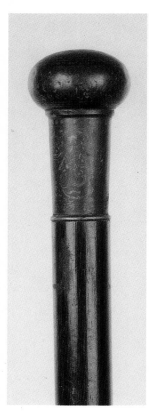

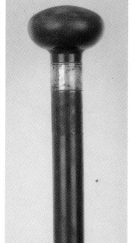

Rare Thai Cane with Niello work handle and ferrule, c. 1870, 35 3/4" high.

Gutta Percha Knob handled cane, c. 1890, hallmarked silver collar, 36 1/4" high.

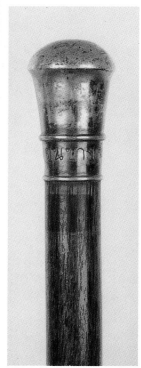

Thai Royal cane, signed, silver & rare wood, c. 1880, 37 1/2" high.

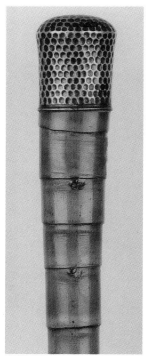

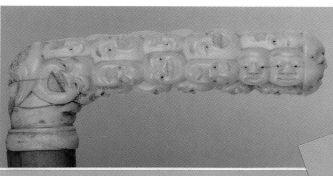

Thai Royal swagger stick with dimpled silver handle on a bamboo shaft, 30 3/4" high.

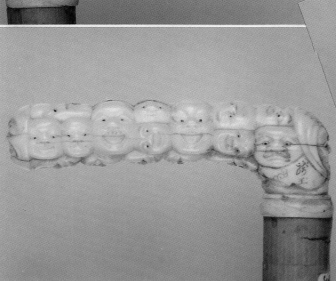

Japanese Noh or Thousand Faces cane in L-shaped ivory handle on a malacca shaft, c. 1870, 33" high.

82

Officious looking gent, possible French gendarme with a small label on the shaft reading: LONDON, L&S STYL, 35 1/4" high.

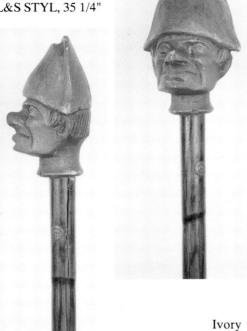

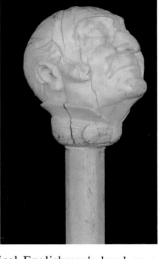

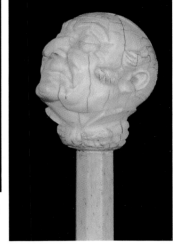

Ivory comical Englishman's head on a whale bone shaft, c. 1800. 35 1/2" high.

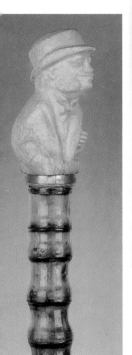

Smug looking Winston Churchill in a bowler and bow tie on a thin silver collar and a reed shaft, 39 3/4" high.

Bearded Oriental man with bone eyelets below, finely carved all from a single piece of vine, 36" high.

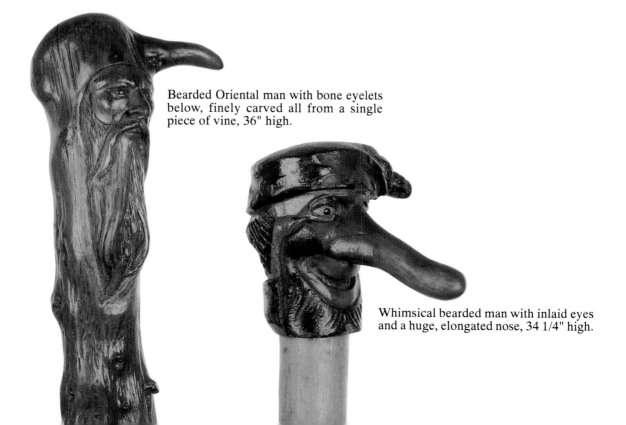

Whimsical bearded man with inlaid eyes and a huge, elongated nose, 34 1/4" high.

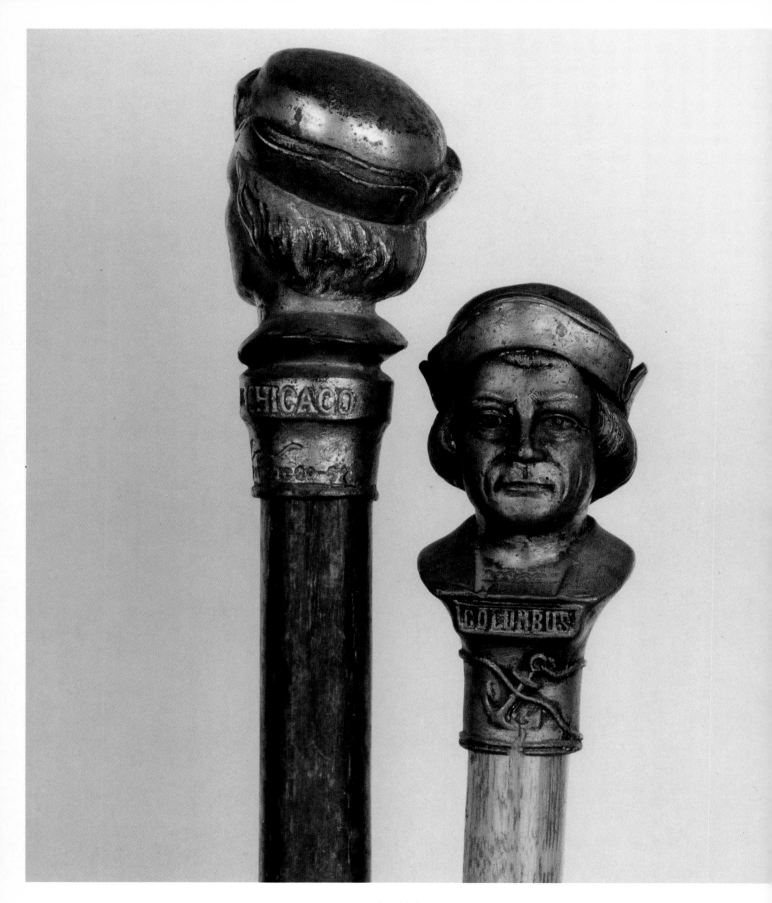

Two commemorative Christopher Columbus handles. The cane on the left is marked Souvenir, Chicago, 1893. Left: 33 3/4" high; right: 37 1/4" high.

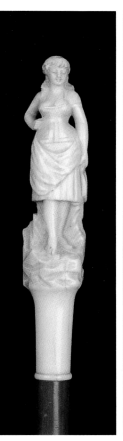
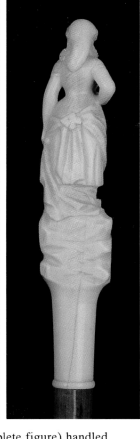

Ivory woman (complete figure) handled cane with a bone ferrule, 34 1/2" high.

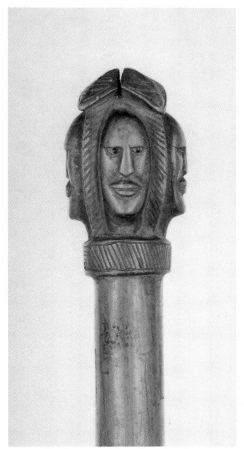

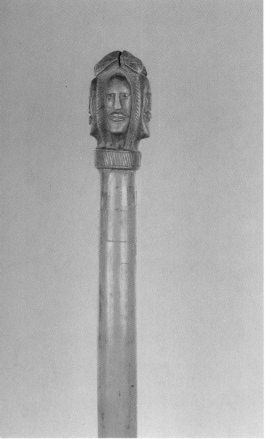

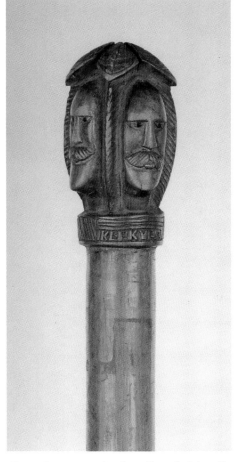

Four faces on the handle of this all wooden cane and the legend KEPKVPA from the Greek Isles, 37" high.

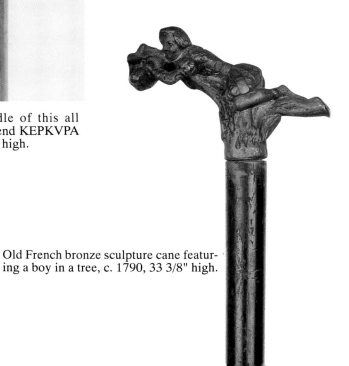

Old French bronze sculpture cane featuring a boy in a tree, c. 1790, 33 3/8" high.

85

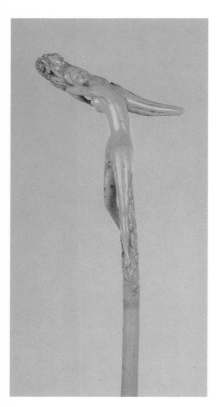

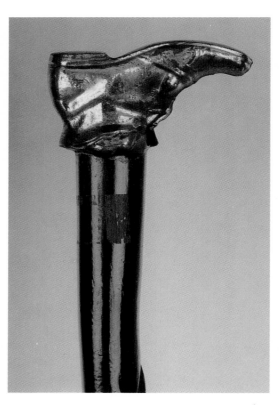

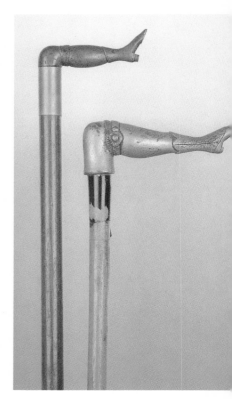

Nude woman, with the exception of a well placed fig leaf, carrying flowers, 38 3/4" high. This folk art cane is carved from a single piece of wood.

Brass shoe handle on a twisted black and brown shaft, c. 1920, 36 1/8" high.

Two canes featuring a woman's leg as the handle, left barefooted with mother-of-pearl and ivory insets into the end of the handle, right with shoe. Left: 35 1/4" high; right: 34 3/4" high.

Two Victorian erotica canes, ladies legs with boots in this case, left: brass L handle with silver collar, 35 1/4" high; right: pewter L handle with flowers on the shin, c. 1880, 33 1/2" high.

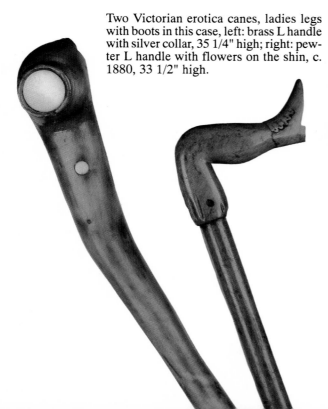

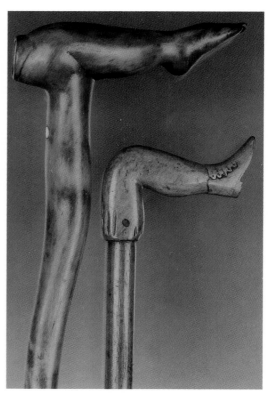

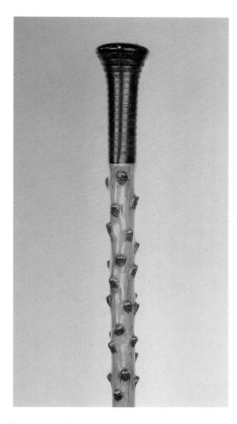

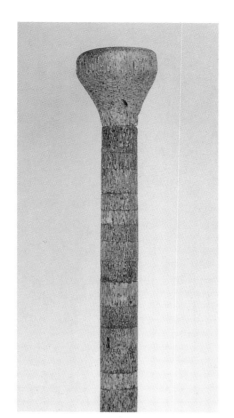

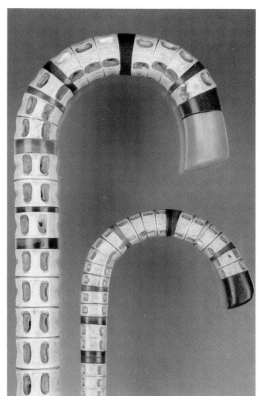

Palmetto shaft cane with leather wrapped wood handle, 33 1/4" high.

Silver serpents head on a large seed pod shaft with a silver ferrule, 39" high. This was a witch doctor's cane.

Knob handled cane of a porous material, fossilized bone-like in quality, the shaft is put together in sections, 32 3/8" high.

Gentle semi-crook shark vertebrae cane with horn handle tip, 35" high.

Two crook handled shark's vertebrae canes. Left: with blonde bone tip; right: with black tip. Left: 36 1/4" high; right: 36 1/2" high.

One horn washer cane (cow, buffalo, etc. horn) with a black handle, 32" high and two knob handled shark vertebrae canes, left with a flaring blonde bone knob, right with black straight sided knob. Left: 32 1/4" high. Right: 34 1/4" high, larger bones.

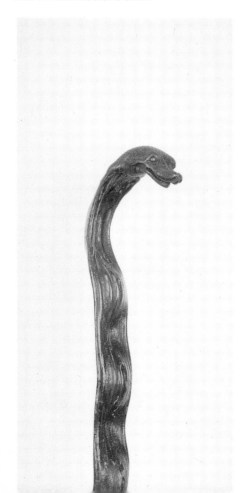

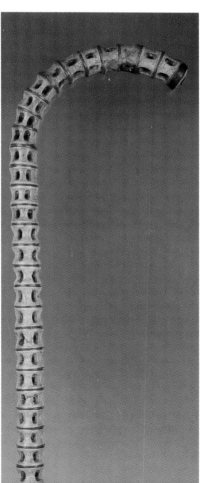

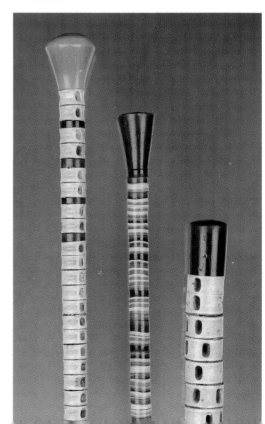

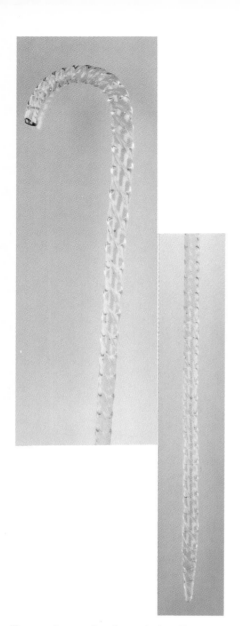

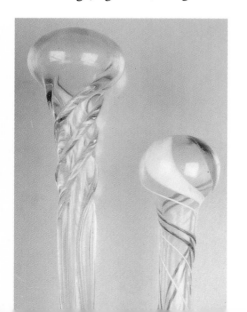

Green glass twisted crook handle cane, c. 1900, 31 1/2" high.

Two glass globe handled canes. Left is clear and right has red & white stripes. Left: 43" high; right: 28 1/2" high.

What is not generally known, and as I have intimated before, is that shafts of wood or vegetable matter are grown upside down - the root end becomes the handle or upper end of the cane and the upper, more tapered portion of the plant is the lower or ferrule end of the walking stick.

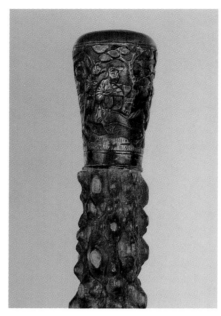

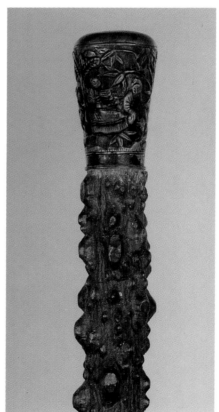

Shaft decorations. Knarled wood with silver handle featuring three Chinese men, 36 3/4" high.

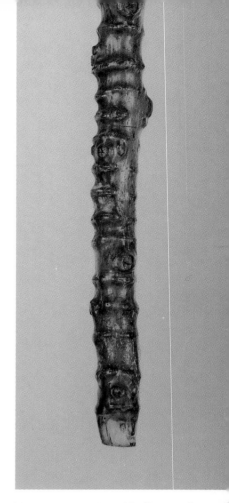

Silver knob handle with silver eyelets and cut branches with horizontal cuts to the shaft, more pronounced in the bottom half of the shaft, 35" high.

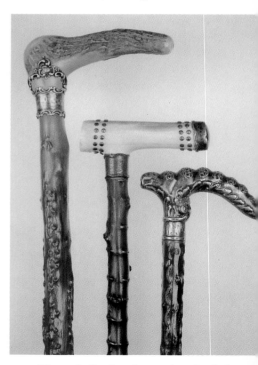

Three shafts showing various healed vertical and horizontal cuts, horn, bone, and silver handles, from 34-37 1/2" high.

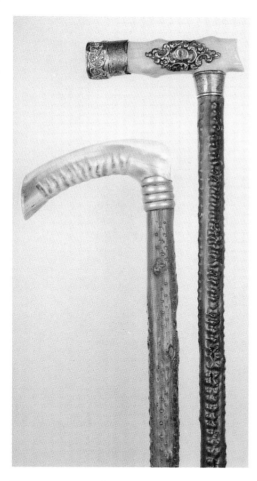

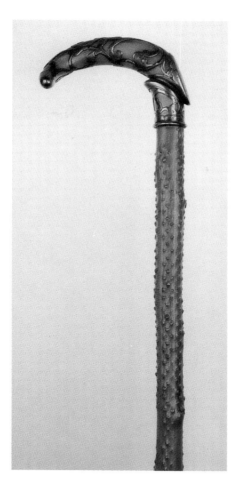

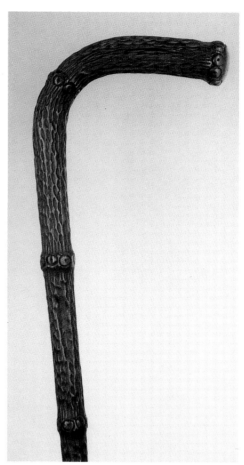

Two more scored and healed shafts with bone & horn handles, top with silver end cap and decoration on bone, 34 3/4" high; bottom 35 1/2" high. Both with silver collars.

Black L handle carved with rings of circles to imitate bamboo, 35 1/4" high.

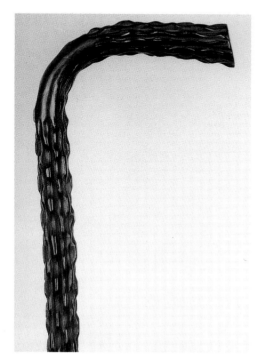

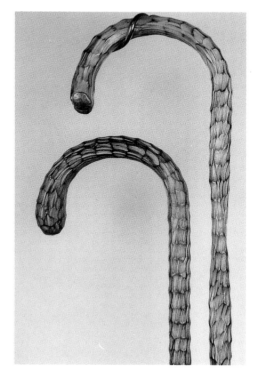

Black ridged shaft with one smooth spot at the curve of the L handle, 35 3/4" high.

Beautiful silver and horn handle on a shaft that has been scored smooth in some spots and allowed to heal while growing, 33 1/4" high.

Two distinctively scalloped shafts with blackened ridges, top crook has a silver snake wrapped around it. Top: 35 1/2"; bottom 36" high.

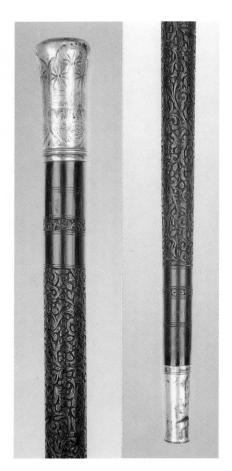

Silver handle with house, palms, and figure with cane, acid etched ebony, 36 1/2" high.

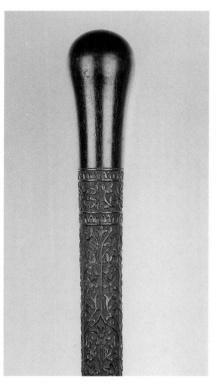

One black ebony cane with acid etched decoration in a foliate pattern, black knob handle, 37 3/4" high.

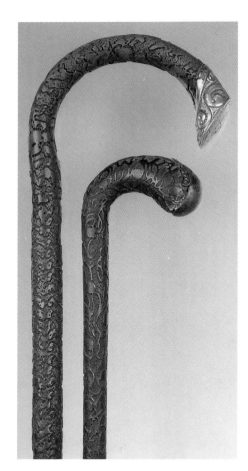

Two acid etched shafts: the top cane is a crook with gold end cap, the bottom is a pistol grip cane with a silver end cap. Top: 36" high; bottom: 35 3/4" high.

In the British Isles and other countries whole farms and plantations were devoted solely to growing shafts for walking sticks and canes. As the young tree grew to about 3-4 feet, the lower branches were cut off close to the stalk and when the young sapling reached 6-8 feet, the constant nipping of its buds left scars that grew over into fine bumps and projections. On some plantations, workmen using special tools that encompassed or encircled the bottom of the sapling, created deep scars in the young bark as the tool was pulled upward. When these had grown over in healing, interesting lines and patterned dots appeared as part of the wood itself in a tattoo-like fashion. All Basque Makilas canes carry these marks on the lower third of their thick shafts. One can see that it really took 1-6 years to grow a proper cane.

Other woods, especially hard woods such as ebony shafts that had been made out of boards and sawed into staves and then tapered into cane shafts, were given an interesting finishing touch. They were covered with a wax and then scratched with an excising needle. The needle scratched through the wax to the wood beneath, where very close and interesting designs were created from top to bottom. These shafts were then placed in vats for an acid bath which ate through the wood for a predetermined time; the canes were then extracted, washed and the wax removed. A very exquisite, lightly carved or engraved cane resulted.

One of the very fine woods for shafts is a very strong, light brown vine called partridge wood. In its natural state, it is smooth and beautiful. It is embellished by a laborious process. Every three to four inches a ridge is carved around the cane and a blackened line is formed, making the stick into what is now called a step-partridge. This wood must be distinguished from the step - malacca which is really grown that way.

Other shafts, instead of being cultivated, were harvested from local woods and forests. In the British Isles, the hedgerows are famous for the quantity and quality of their woods suitable for sticks. When cut, these sticks may have had bends and angles in them which made them so crooked it was unbelievable they would ever become straight and tapered for a cane. However, by application of heat this was accomplished. Most such limbs retain their original bark but many are shaved and colored by exposure to acid fumes into marvelous canes.

Old metallic shafts of aluminum, or cane handles made of aluminum may make the modern collector, who is familiar with the thousands of cheap aluminum pots and pans, reject such a cane outright. He may be missing a most desirable collectable. If it's an old cane from the early 1800s, the aluminum was then actually more costly then gold because of its rarity.

In the 1890s many manufacturers advertised for country boys to grub roots and to cut sticks that could be turned into handles for canes and umbrellas. Ten dollars per thousand was offered. They also paid $12 to $30 a thousand for sticks that could be made into canes. In the United States these canes were birch, dogwood, hickory, maple, oak, red cedar and sheepberry.

Competition among cane dealers for rarities was so keen that every conceivable wood grown any place in the world was sought. The rarer the wood or vine the better thought cane users and collectors.

In the 1940s, the School of Forestry of Yale University was one of the few places in the world where wood from any part of the world - and any time in the worlds recent history — could be sent with reasonable assurance that it could be identified. At that time, they had 5,000 species identified and felt there were about 40,000 woody plants in the world. They also had a fine collection of walking sticks: the *Rudolph Block Collection of Canes* which they received after his death in 1940. He was a wood lover who collected different woods and had them made into canes, ending up with 1400 sticks representing 950 species of trees. Eventually, in about 1960, Yale gave up its collection of woods which went to the U.S. Forest Products Laboratory in Madison, Wisconsin, an equally noted wood laboratory that had 48,000 samples of identified wood. Adding 55,000 samples from Yale made this Wisconsin laboratory the largest wood laboratory in the world. It will identify for industry or interested scientists all wood if a sample of it with its putative origin is sent to them. I assume this would also cover canes - but the cane would have to be cut into and a sample taken for microscopic examination. This service is free of charge for the first five samples. Incidentally, the Rudolph Block cane collection went to the Smithsonian Institute in Washington, D.C.

In checking old English catalogues, I found that the most common woods of 1890 — as listed in *Henry Howell & Co., Manufacturers* established in 1833, London and also in *Briggs & Sons* of London in 1905 — featured the following shafts:

Malacca	Cinnamon	Apse
Ebony	Furze	Ceylon Vine
Snakewood	Orange	Chestnut
Ash	Rattan	Olive
Hazel	Accacia	Pimenta
Oak	Congo	Pamir Vine
Cherry	Dogwood	Bamboo
Whangee	Palmyra	Orange
Thorn	Aucuba	

Mahogany and hickory, in addition to the above, were in great demand in the United States.

Of course, relic canes — such as those from famous structures, ships, flag-

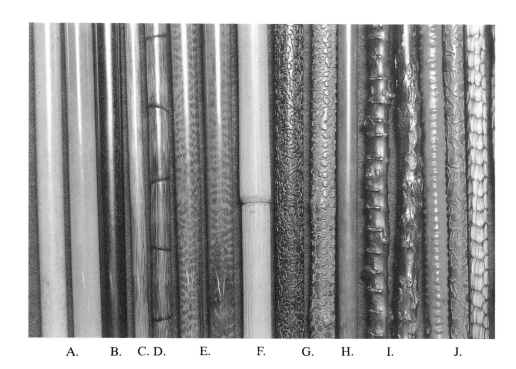

A.   B.   C. D.   E.   F.   G. H.   I.   J.

Examples of different woods and decorations. From left to right: A. two Malacca shafts, B. ebony shaft, C. plain partridge wood, D. step partridge, E. snakewood, F. old step malacca, G. acid etched (the left hand example is etched on an ebony shaft), H. gutta percha, I. lacerated while growing, J. designs carved after the cane has been shaped.

poles, fortifications, old courthouses, homes of famous people, and wood from Philadelphia Independence Hall - all were utilized for the cane mania. If you had to carry a cane, it might as well be an unusual one. And carry a cane you must, because the prevailing opinion was that a person might be a man, but unless he carried or wore a cane, he wasn't a gentleman.

Many a cane that appears to be fine branches or limbs of beautiful trees are in reality boards sawn and shaped into staves, then rounded and tapered into cane shape. They are finally wrapped from top to bottom with thin bark of the tree they are to represent, such as cherry wood.

Some gun canes have 6-10 inches of sectional wooden spindles strung over the barrel and have knot-like formations at the joint to conceal the fact that this is not a single piece of wood bored for its entire length to receive the gun barrel.

Drilling long, deep holes in narrow shafts, without coming out the side, was always difficult so the cane manufacturers drilled short pieces of wood and strung them onto the gun barrel.

This process is particularly noticed in these long, supposedly hollowed, outer sheaths for sword canes in addition to gun canes. Because the cane was too difficult or impossible to drill deeply, the cane was split longitudinally. A channel for the blade or barrel was gouged out and the barrel or blade inserted. Then the two outer pieces were glued together again. To conceal this process, the cane was then wrapped with thin cherry or other bark, resulting in a beautiful sword or gun cane.

Other non-one-piece shafts for canes were made of pieces of wood, horn, leather or combinations of these, in the shape of round washers with a hole in the center. These were then strung on a steel core. Very valuable canes are made in this manner from smaller pieces of rhinoceros horn thimbles strung on a steel core. Some of these canes have alternate pieces of different colored horn strung together, making a most beautiful stick that is much stronger and whippier than all one piece sticks.

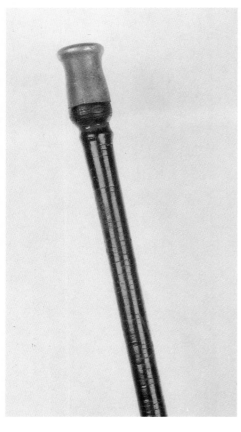

Shafts made of multiple pieces were made with washers of wood, horn, leather, or a combination of these materials. The washers were strung on steel cores. Iron handled leather washer cane, 32 1/2" high.

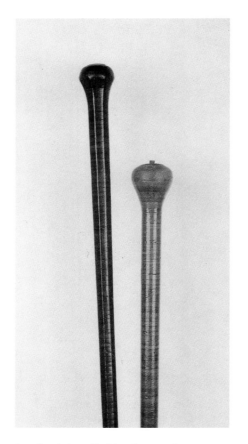

Two knob handled leather washer canes. Left: has enameled plaque on top reading ANCIENT ORDER OF FOREST-ERS, 34" high; right: 34 1/2" high.

Paper cane, 25,000 pieces of paper (said to be stamps) on a steel rod, no glue used, made by men in prison, purchased in Boston in 1922. Brass fittings in the L shaped handle, 32 3/4" high. This is a very effective defensive cane.

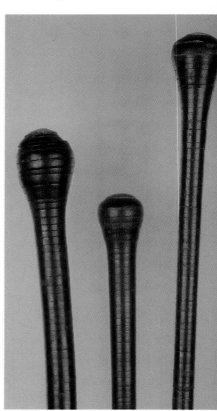

Tight crook handled leather washer cane, 34 1/4" high.

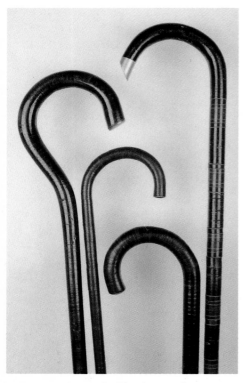

Four crook handled leather washer canes, metal cores, ranging in height from 34 3/4 - 36 1/2".

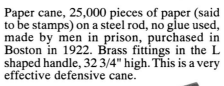

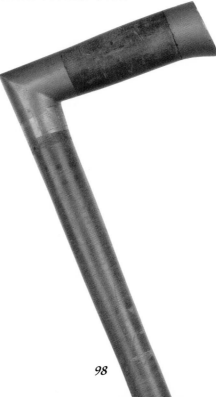

Three knob handled leather washer canes with the metal cores showing through at the top of the handles, ranging from 34-35 1/2" high.

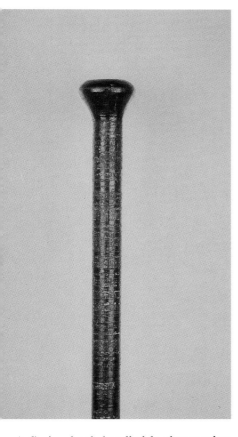

A flaring knob handled leather washer cane, 33 1/2" high.

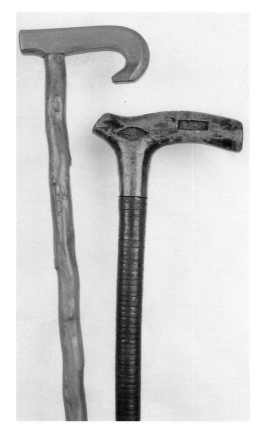

Two simple basically opera handle style canes, right has a metal shaft wrapped in leather washers, and the carvers initials B.R. in the top of the handle. Left: 38" high; right: 35" high.

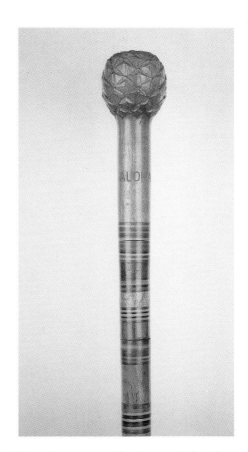

Hawaiian cane with pineapple handle, ALOHA in red on the shaft and the shaft made up of every wood in Hawaii. 35"

Crook handle cow carved in several woods, rudimentary details of eyes and hide painted, 37 1/2" high.

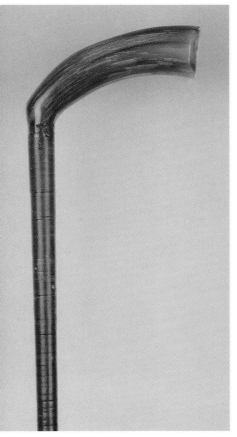

Horn handled leather washer cane, 35 1/2" high.

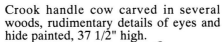

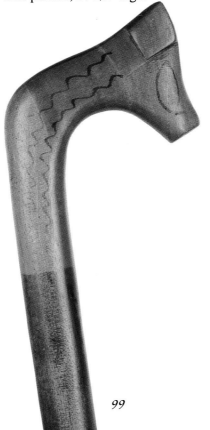

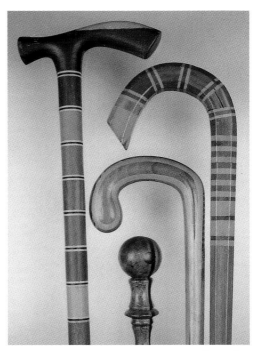

Four canes made from a variety of woods, from 33" to 36 3/4" high. The cane on the left is from Brazil and is composed of all the different native Brazilian woods. The two on the right are examples of "marquetery," inlaid or artistically formed wood out of parts.

99

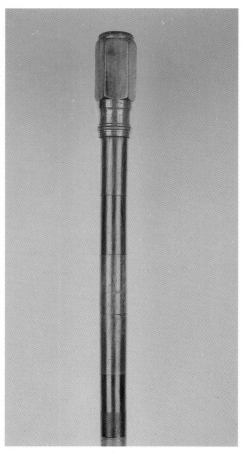

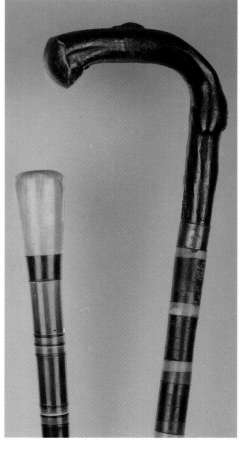

Segmented horn canes, the lower example has a bone knob handle, the upper cane is fitted with a wooden L handle. Lower: 35" high; upper 36 1/2" high.

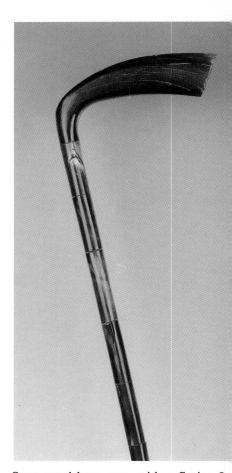

Segmented horn cane with a flaring L handle and zig-zag line etched and painted on top, 35" high.

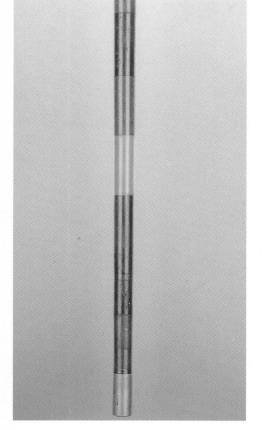

Segmented cane displaying different woods, 35 1/2" high.

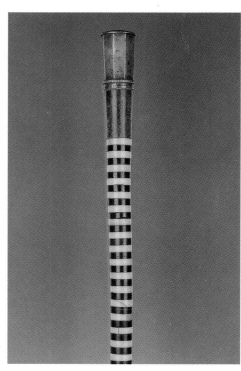

Silver paneled handle with beautiful segmented horn shaft and unusual silver and gun shell ferrule, 33 3/4" high.

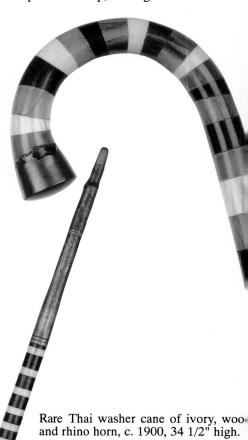

Rare Thai washer cane of ivory, woo and rhino horn, c. 1900, 34 1/2" high.

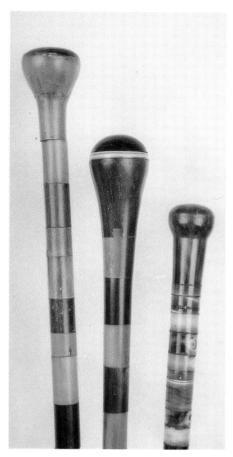

Three knob handled canes made from segmented horn, left & center 34" high, right 35 1/2" high.

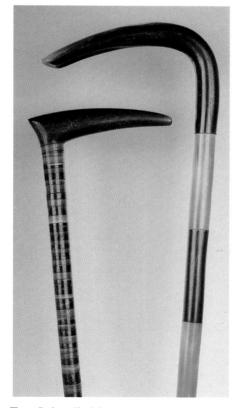

Two L handled horn segmented canes. Left: 35 1/4" high; right: 33 1/4" high.

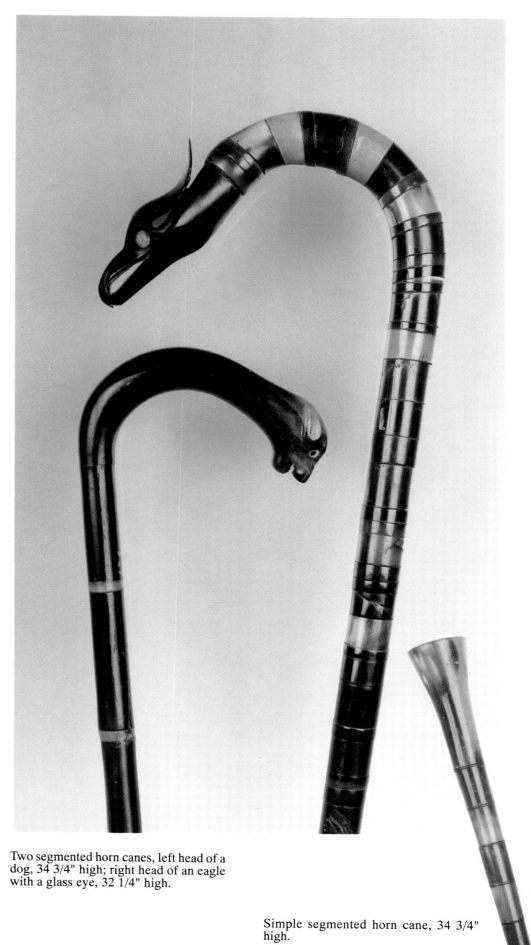

Two segmented horn canes, left head of a dog, 34 3/4" high; right head of an eagle with a glass eye, 32 1/4" high.

Simple segmented horn cane, 34 3/4" high.

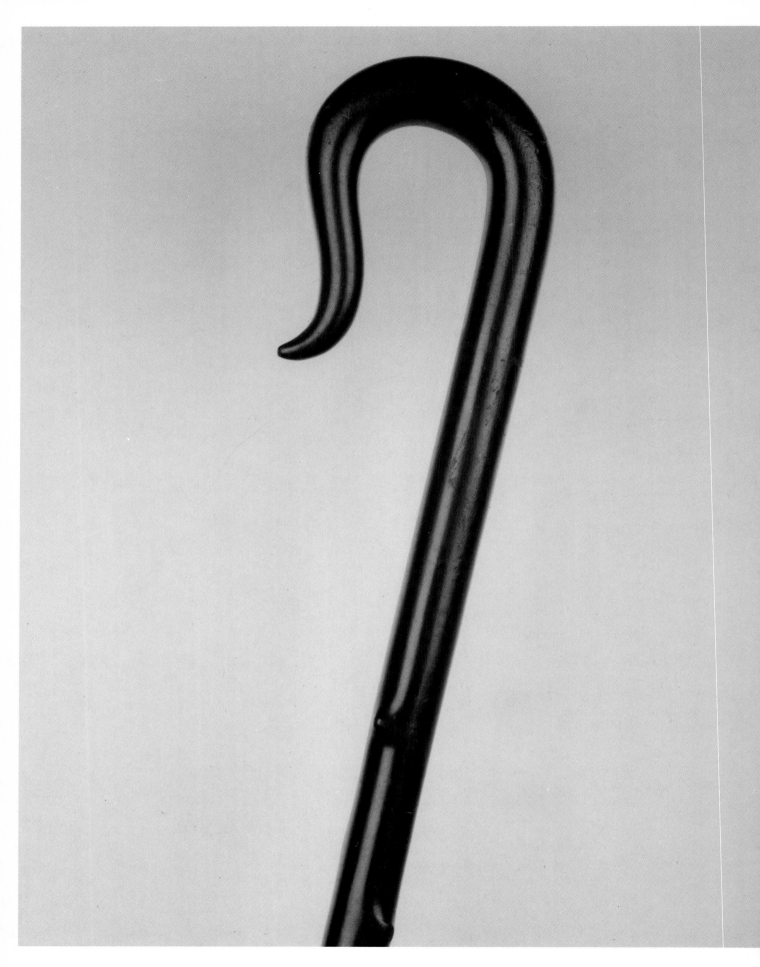

Chapter 4
Shaft Materials

Although most shafts of canes are made of wood, it must be noted that other materials from all the world have been used to make elegant sticks.

Malacca

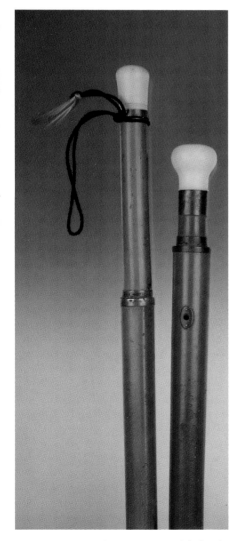

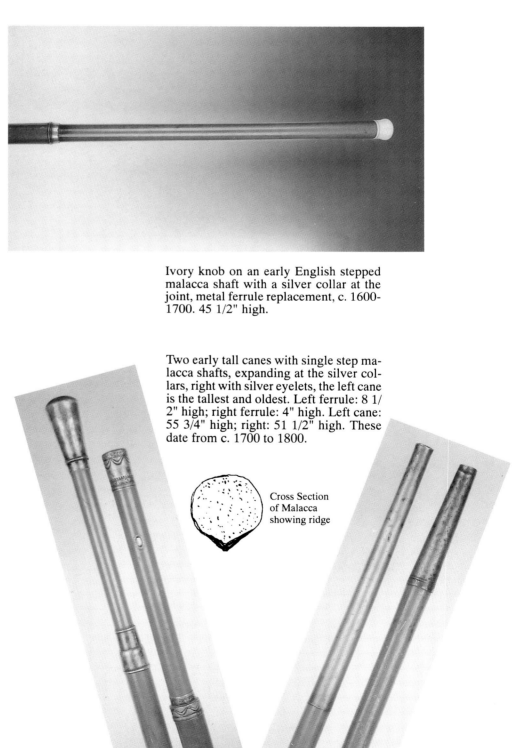

Ivory knob on an early English stepped malacca shaft with a silver collar at the joint, metal ferrule replacement, c. 1600-1700. 45 1/2" high.

Two early tall canes with single step malacca shafts, expanding at the silver collars, right with silver eyelets, the left cane is the tallest and oldest. Left ferrule: 8 1/2" high; right ferrule: 4" high. Left cane: 55 3/4" high; right: 51 1/2" high. These date from c. 1700 to 1800.

Cross Section of Malacca showing ridge

Two stepped malacca canes with knob handles, right with eyelets. Left: 31" high; right: 33 3/4" high.

The famous Spaulding Goldsmiths of Chicago, now extinct, in a booklet published early in this century called "Malacca, the King of Canes". It is actually a cane known as Calamus Asipionum and comes from Siak on the coast of Sumatra. It is extremely light in weight and no two are ever alike in appearance. It is said that out of a shipment of a thousand canes, not over fifty are sufficiently superb to be sought by connoisseurs. This is so because this cane is jointed like bamboo canes and to be a rarity one must have sufficient length between two nodes or joints to make a rare stick. Also it must have throughout its length a proper taper and a perfect bark or skin with a satiny and natural gloss. This perfect stick is commonly called "single bark or all bark Malacca". Upon very close inspection of inferior malaccas, one can find that there is a change in the lower 1/3 of the stick where a knot or node has been shaved down, smoothed over, retapered and then repainted to resemble the top 2/3 of the stick.

Quite distinctive also of a true malacca is that it has a ridge running from top to bottom shaped like an upside down developing tear drop. The more pronounced this spine or ridge is, the more valuable the stick.

If, in addition to the prize malacca, it is a bent malacca, i.e. has a crook handle or umbrella-like handle, then its value is again increased because it takes a much longer single bark malacca to make such a superb stick. Even during the depression, knowledgeable connoisseurs paid as high as $400.00 for such a gem.

The vast majority of malaccas, not being the true single bark bent malacca, are used either to make sticks with attached handles or are shaved and repainted to resemble the honest and valuable gem.

Interestingly, the malacca shaft on American canes always has its spine on the inner or back side of the stick whereas the English and European malacca canes may have this spine on the leading or forward side.

The correct length of a cane was said to be half a person's height plus 2 inches. This made no allowance for the different lengths of the arms of people of the same height and caused orthopedic problems, such as backache, foot pain, and knee discomfort; so now a famous orthopedic sur-

geon says that "as a rough measure a cane should reach above the level of the user's wrist when the arm is hanging at the side. The cane, if for orthopedic use, he continued, should always be held on the side opposite the leg or foot that is injured or weakened.

I have a cane store's "sizing cane" which is used to determine the length of the cane required by the purchaser. The bottom of this cane slides out of the shaft at the bottom. This inner shaft has a calibration in inches. The seller pulls out the ferrule end which is attached to the inner shaft and hands the cane to the purchaser who holds it naturally by the handle and presses down on the handle until the cane length feels most natural to him. The sliding inner shaft stops at this length and designates the exact length of the cane required in inches.

All this concerns only the orthopedic cane, i.e. the stick used to ease or alleviate pain or weakness in the body of the user. It has no merit for the collector or user who wears a cane for fashion. The German word Spatzierstock, meaning strolling stick, best describes the collectible canes as distinguished from the orthopedic sticks.

The proper size of a cane requires that "the elbow must be bent when the stick is held close to the side," according to England's Swaive Odeney Brigg and Sons, Ltd. founded in 1750, "otherwise you cannot reach out as you are walking forward." There would never be any support or ease of swing if the stick were an "arm straight at your side."

From a study of all the canes I have, all I have seen, and all the history I have read about canes, I am of the opinion that the cane or walking stick was originally head high in length. This cane length lasted until the beginning of the middle ages when it shortened to chest high. Thereafter, at the time of George Washington, the cane was about 4' long and in the subsequent years, especially with the crook-type handle, it averaged 32-33 inches and finally, now that canes are no longer worn, they were carried in the past two wars as swagger sticks - about 18-22 inches in length. The Irish Shillelagh was always and is still this size, except it has a very bulbous hammer-like bottom made from the trunk of the tree and the handle is one of the branches. But as they say, what goes around, comes around, and

now the modern cane is either 6' tall as a hiking stick or 32" tall for general use.

Shepherds Canes

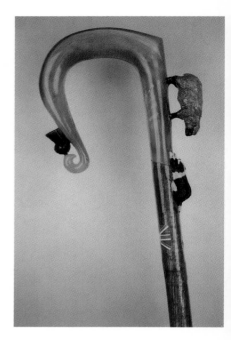

Ram's horn shepherd's market stick (as distinguished from a working stick) with thistle, sheep and sheepdog, 52 3/4" high. Made by a British stickmaker.

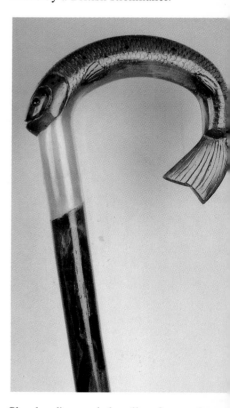

Shepherd's crook handle of rams horn carved and painted as a jumping salmon, c. 1960. 44 1/2" high.

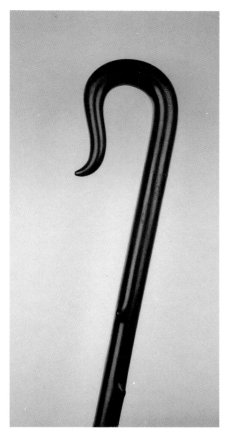

Ebony shepherd's leg catching cane, silver ferrule, 37 1/2" high.

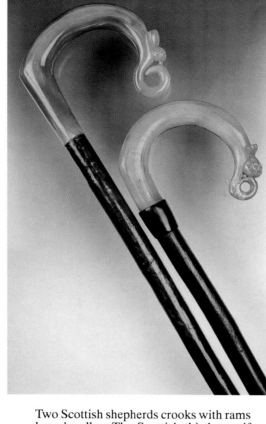

Two Scottish shepherds crooks with rams horn handles. The Scottish thistle motif is carved on the end of the carved handle. These date from c. 1950. Top: 47" high; bottom: 57" high.

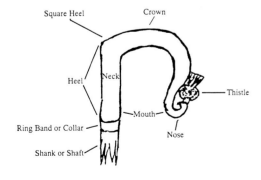

Great Britain is known for its sheep and shepherds. The sheep herders lived lonely lives, accompanied only by their dogs and their staffs. They were separated from their families for long periods of time, living only in tents or one room stone shacks.

They made tall staffs with crook handles used for catching sheep by the neck. Living in isolation, far from villages and stores the shepherd had to use the materials available in his surroundings, thus he used the horn of the ram or the stag for the crook handle, and the wood growing in forests and hedgerows for the staff. All these when seen in the raw would be considered impossible for fashioning a crook or a cane. The rams horn was curved and winding, and the saplings available were bent and crooked.

The herdsmen, however, with simple tools such as a knife and an oil lantern, were able to bend and shape the available material into such beautiful works of art that they were always in great demand at the fair markets.

But the demand exceeded the supply, not all shepherds knew the secrets required and those that did were reluctant to reveal them to outsiders. It was at this time that a woodsman from the continent transplanted to England, a cane carver himself, decided that he would organize all the shepherds and cane carvers into a society where they could exchange their knowledge. In this manner the science of the older craftsmen would not die with them but would be perpetuated for future generations. Theo Fossel traveled all over England, Ireland, Wales and Scotland, visiting every cane maker he heard of. In 1984, he organized the British Stickmakers Guild, like the guilds of old to perpetuate the secrets of the masters. In its first year, the BSG as it is known, had almost 500 members and now it is internationally known amongst stick makers.

The guild publishes a quarterly called "The Stickmaker" which is free to all members. Its stated aim was to provide an information channel between stickmakers and stick collectors. The magazine presently numbered in the 40s (July 1994) contains and publishes articles plus detailed drawings on all problems of stick making from cutting, seasoning and treating shanks, to working horn and wood, tools, methods and renovation and repair of old sticks.

Theo Fossel was president of the guild and became president of the German "Stocksammler", an international Society of Stick Collectors in Munich now headed by Yoseph Kadri. He visited my home before his death and we traded many articles, books and sticks.

So popular had Theo Fossel made his guild that now there are contests and sales by stickmakers at county fairs all over the Isles.

"The Stickmaker" magazine and membership in the guild can be obtained by writing to:

Eileen Dye
Membership Secretary
The British Stickmakers Guild
25 Aldwyck Way
Lowenstoff, Suffolk
NR 33 9J0
England

Anyone interested in the long held secret processes should try to get copies of the first 40 issues of the magazine as they cover the subject most completely.

The shepherd canes of Great Britain are divided into two types: the working stick and the market stick. The working stick is the utilitarian cane with the strength needed to catch a rushing ram; whereas the market stick is a finer, more decorative stick used on market days. The latter are embellished with fine ram's horns in the shape of trout, game birds and other fish or animals striking the owner's fancy. All are at least 5' tall.

Though most working sticks are similar, the shape of the crook is always exactly as indicated previously under handles.

The Stickmaker Magazine advertises all the parts needed for making these various sticks and also lists makers who will sell made-to-order sticks to collectors.

Also in the British Isles is the famous blackthorn. Although known as the Irish Blackthorn, it is not limited only to Ireland as it is also found in Scotland, England and Wales.

Irish Blackthorn

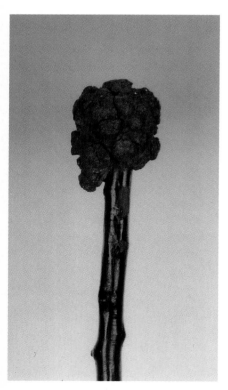

"The Leprechaun." Irish blackthorn with a natural burl in the shape of a face as the handle, 36 3/4" high.

The Blackthorn is a favorite of the Irish. It is used as a regular walking stick but to make it such can be quite a laborious process. The bush or small tree has long thorns on its branches. It is quite hazardous to crawl amongst the thickets and hedgerows to saw or chop a desirable limb and equally as dangerous to exit with eyes, arms and legs unscathed. The perfect blackthorn is said to be only one in a thousand. The thorns must be evenly spaced all around the stick, the stick must be straight, it must be well balanced and have a fine taper. It needs only to have the spurs cut close to the limb and there should be a dimple behind each spur that makes the stick very decorative. The bark is usually left intact and it remains almost forever in its original black or reddish-black color. If the bark is peeled off, an even finer stick will be seen. The spines or thorns grow out from the center of the stick, not like rose thorns that grow out from the bark, and when the peeled blackthorn stick is sanded down, these make a beautiful pattern.

The Irish blackthorn has a romantic history, full of Irish legend. This stick, however, must be distinguished from the shillelagh, which is shorter than a cane or walking stick and is really a weapon.

The shillelagh is also a legend in Irish history as the following poem demonstrates:

The Shillelagh Poem

Oh no its not a walking stick.
It's carried 'neath one's arm
For though it was a weapon
It kept you free from harm.
For long ago invaders came,
To Ireland's pleasant shore.
Those Danes were fearsome fighting men
With sword and shield and more.
To kill or plunder was their aim
And pretty girls to snatch
But when they reached Shillelagh
They found they'd met their match
The peaceful farmers had no swords
Their homesteads to defend
But they knew that on the Black Thorn,
Their lives they could depend.
They cut stout sticks
Then joined the fight
And quickly put the Danes to flight

Most of our knowledge of canes and walking sticks, especially its history, comes from literature in books and articles written over a century ago. So too, all I know I learned by research. Accordingly, I believe more credence and reliance would be granted the facts I'm about to state if I quote verbatim from the author who lived and wrote at the time of the height of the cane craze (1870), rather than if I paraphrase it. Accordingly, we find in Harper New Monthly Magazine, in an article called, "About Walking Sticks and Fans" dated July 1870 - Vol. 41, Pg. 221-224: the situation in 1870:

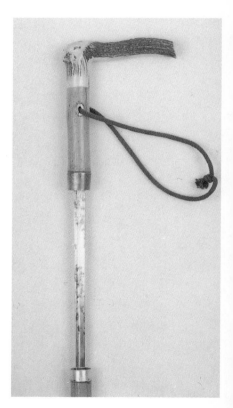

"The English Geographical Society provides its Central African explorers with supplies of ... sword sticks." Antler L-shaped handled sword cane with eyelet and wrist cord, 36 1/2" high.

"The ancient contrivance is not obsolete. Turning from the dead past to the living present, it is found that walking-sticks are still made with hollow centers to answer as repositories. Mustapha Ibrahim, the principal medical man of the Sultan's harem, descends from his carriage, and, accompanied by eunuchs enters the guarded enclosure, supported by a long gold-mounted cane, which contains medicines and surgical instruments. The English Geographical Society provides its Central African explorers with supplies of spring-spear canes and sword-sticks. Alpine travelers now measure altitudes with sextants carried within their alpenstocks; and theodolitea in walking-sticks are one of the present necessary accompaniments of the scientific traveler in Northern Asia."

"Since 1851 commerce in ordinary walking-sticks has more than quadrupled. In Hamburg, Berlin, and Vienna - the present central depots for export - the manufacture employs many thousand of work-people."

* * * * * * * * * * * * *

In the present manufacture of canes great quantities and varieties of materials are consumed. There is scarcely grass or shrub, reed or tree, that has not been employed at one time or another. The blackthorn and crab, cherry-tree and furzebush, sapling oak and Spanish reed (Arundo donar), are the favorites. Then come supple-jacks and pimentos from the West Indies, rattans and palms from Java, white and black bamboo from Singapore, and stems of the bambusa - the gigantic grass of the tropics - from Borneo. All these must be cut at certain seasons, freed from various appendages, scorched to discover defects, assorted into sizes, and thoroughly rid of moisture. A year's seasoning is required for some woods, two for others. Then comes the curious process of manufacture. Twenty different handlings hardly finish the cheapest cane. The bark is to be removed after boiling the stick in water or to be polished after roasting it in ashes; excrescences are to be manipulated into points of beauty; handles straightened and shanks shaped; forms twisted and heads rasped; tops carved or mounted , surfaces charred and scraped, shanks smoothed and varnished, and bottoms shaped and ferruled. Woods, too, have to be studied, lest chemical applications that beautify one might ruin another kind. Some are improved under subjection to intense heat, other destroyed. Malacca canes have frequently to be colored in parts so that stained and natural surfaces are not distinguishable; heads and hoofs for handles are baked to retain their forms; tortoiseshell raspings are conglomerated by pressure into ornamental shapes, and lithographic transfers, done by hand, are extensively used upon walking-sticks for the Parisian market.

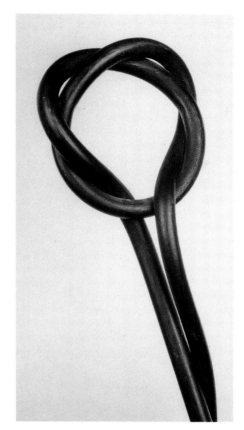

"There is scarcely grass or shrub, reed or tree, that has not been employed at one time or another." Twined vines forming this black painted ebonized cane, 36 1/4" high.

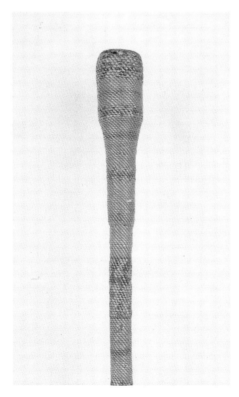

American Indian woven straw covered shaft in a patterned weave from the handle to the ferrule, 35 3/4" high.

Staffs with grotesque heads hold their own in every age. Why, it is difficult to say. Old cynics of Greek memories used them. They were the badge of the tribunes in Rome, whom the better classes despised. Fools and jesters of the Middle Ages carried them as baubles distinctive to their class. The Universal Spectator points them out, in 1730, as "the large oak sticks, with great heads and ugly faces carved thereon, carried at the court end of town by polite young gentleman instead of swords." That draft Highland laird, Robertson of Kincraigie, made himself famous by carving effigies of friends and caricatures of enemies on the upper end of walking-sticks, until the accost, "Wha hae ye up the day, laird?" became a cant phrase for lunacy all over Scotland. The brigands of Italy adopt them. They are favorites with Magyar chiefs in Hungary; and those used by members of Kossuth's train, during his visit to the United States in 1851-52, were objects of particular notice. It would seem that they have been the accompaniments of eccentricity in every age of the world, but for what reason it is difficult to say. Facts, like bon-mots, are not always explicable. Talleyrand, standing in an ante-room through which the Duchesse De Grammont was passing to dinner, looked up and said, "Ah!" In the course of the feast the lady asked him, across the table, why he had uttered the exclamation "Oh!" upon her entrance. The witty statesman replied, "Madame, je n'ai pas dit oh! jai dit ah!

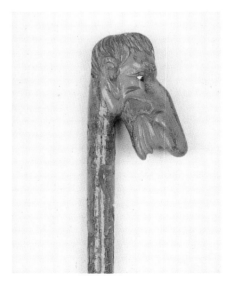

"Staffs with grotesque heads hold their own in every age." Anti-Semitic French grotesque cane, c. 1750 to 1820, 38" high.

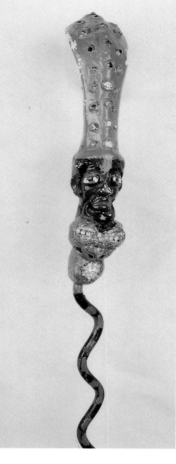
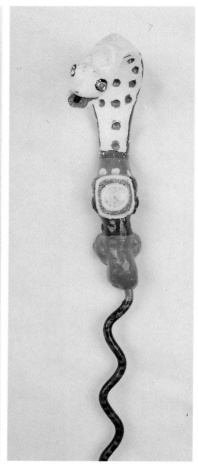
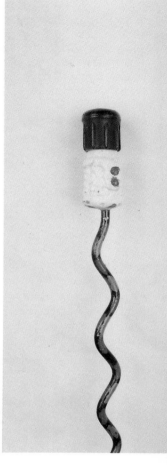

Unusual African-American metal cane with painted decoration featuring a man and a serpent. The man has a clock in the back of his head. 39 3/4" high.

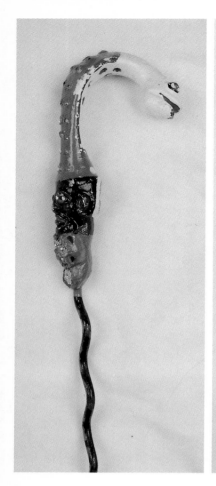

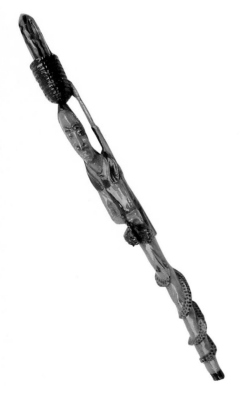

Folk art with polychrome decoration of an Indian carrying a basket on the head with a coiled snake below. 39 1/4" high.

Animal substances have given almost entire place to vegetable in materials used for walking-sticks. Whalebone is exhausted by the umbrella manufacturers; and tortoise-shell, ram's horn, and ivory - once used largely by canemakers - have become too costly a raw material. The horns of animals, which, treated by heat and mechanical appliances, used once to be drawn out into rods, are no longer employed. The hide of the rhinoceros, elastic and tough, submitting readily to chemical agents, and forming a semi-transparent, horn-like substance, is abandoned on account of enhanced cost. Ivory and bone, also, have become too valuable for other manufactures to compete with vegetable products as materials for walking-sticks.

When Goodyear, five-and-twenty years ago, introduced his hard, vulcanized India rubber to the arts, for cutlery handles, harness trimmings, furniture, and boudoir ornaments, it was expected to supersede all other materials in the manufacture of walking-sticks. It vies with ebony in color. No known substance is capable of higher polish. Neither heat nor frost affects it. Closeness of texture, freedom from brittleness, lightness of weight, and imperviousness to abrasion, gave it extraordinary advantages. For several years it became the haut bon of London, Paris, and Berlin. Even now, to elderly gentlemen of mode, who affect gold heads surmounting stout and serviceable staffs, it is distinguished above all others. But its cost killed it. For general use it was never much introduced. Besides, it lacks elasticity - an essential element in walking-sticks - hence is never likely to compete with the various woods.

The highly ornamented and decorated sticks used by the rajahs of the East, exhibited at the Paris Exposition, can hardly be considered as articles of commerce. Bamboo canes richly mounted in gold and silver, sandal-woods enriched with painted ornaments, ivory chowrees elaborately carved, chowrees made of the tail of the yak (Bos grunniens), beetle-nut wands with silver, handles, supple-jacks from St. Vincent, and whale's tooth sticks from Trinidad, are merely objects of curiosity. The same may be said of the sticks used for staffs carried before African chiefs, of the stained quina walking-sticks made at Groenkloof, of the too-roo-plam-rind canes, and of the staff of solid gold, set with carbuncles and diamonds, exhibited by the Rajah of Kisnaghur. None of these, however, can be considered as representing the art of stick-making in a commercial sense.

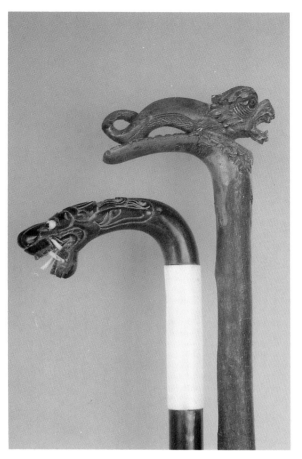

Two Oriental dragons: Left: top carved wood, bottom carved bone in alternating bands of black and white. 34" high. Right: all wood. 35" high.

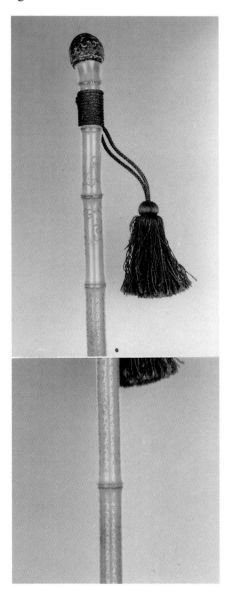

Highly ornamented and decorated sticks from the East and from Africa. Bamboo shaft with root handle, purple silk cord, signed oriental poem down the shaft, 36 1/2" high.

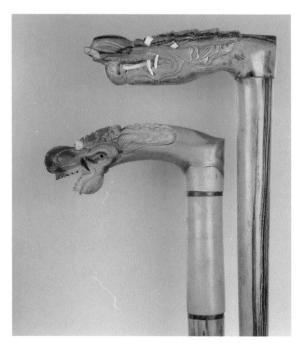

Two Oriental wood dragons. Right: with inlaid eyes, teeth & tongue, 36" high. Left: with inlaid eyes and a segmented shaft, 37" high.

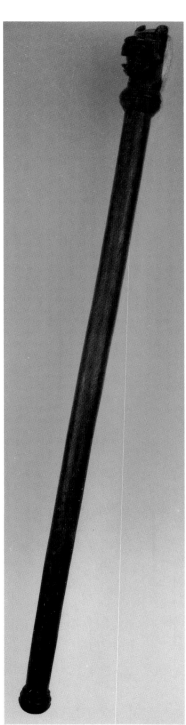

Small roaring lions head Oriental stick, 22" high.

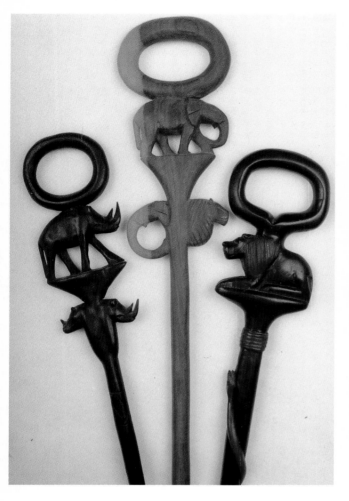

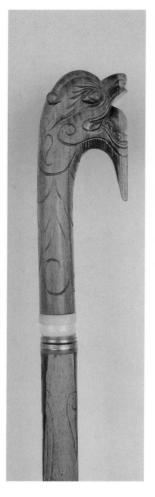

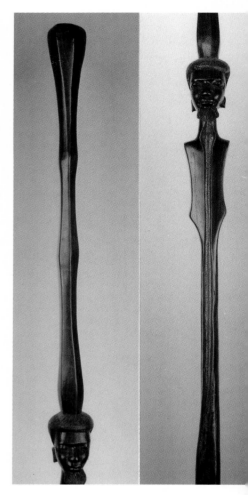

Three circular handled ebony canes with a rhino (left), elephant (center) and lion (right). Left: 37 3/4" high; center: 34 1/2" high; right: 36 1/4" high.

Chinese dragon, shaft in three segments, 34 1/2" high.

Goateed figure with snake attached and running down from goatee, black shaft, 33 1/4" high.

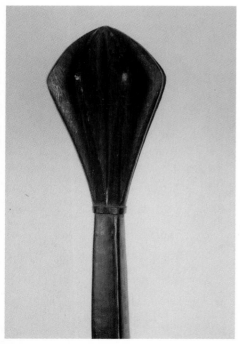

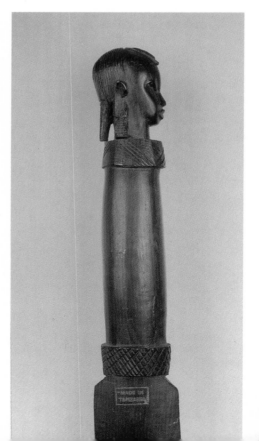

Wooden Tanzania blade ebony cane with figural handle, marked Made In Tanzania, 37 1/2" high.

Eight paneled handle, black cane, made by natives of Guadalcanal, 34" high.

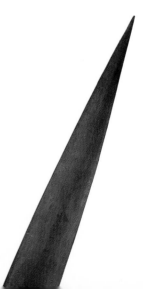

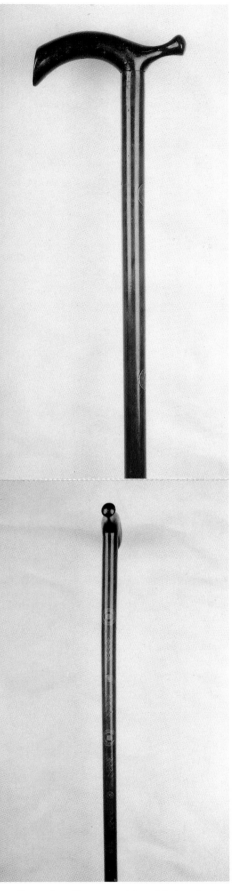

All that remains can be said in a word. Walking-sticks are in perpetual demand. While England supplies her home demand for the finished article, she exports raw material, both of native production and foreign growth, for more than a moiety of all the manufactures of the Continent. France to a great degree takes care of herself. Germany imports the raw materials only. The rest of the world, from Alexandria to Canton, and from New York around the Cape to Pacific ports of entry, depends for its walking-sticks upon those hives of industry, Hamburg, Berlin, and Vienna."

I must as a lawyer, however regretfully and blushingly, advise that in the Malay States there was a cane manufactured that was called a "Penang lawyer" because it was a local walking stick "of inferior quality." Similarly I ruefully recall that once while fishing with some clients in Tennessee or Kentucky, I caught the most awful looking, ugly and inedible fish I had ever seen. When I asked one of my companions what kind this fish was, he said with an ill-concealed smirk, "Down here, dems is called a lawyer!"

Ivory

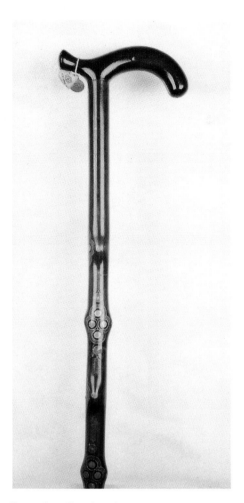

Opera handle with similar circular design and a tag MADE IN USSR, decoration in gold, 38" high.

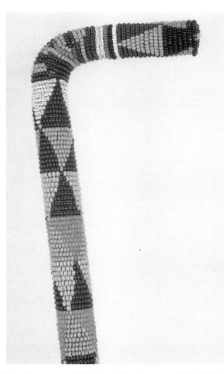

Bead covered L handled cane, 37 3/4" high. Purchased in Kenya, Africa.

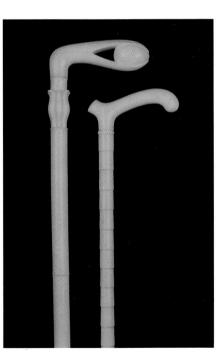

Two ivory canes with segmented shafts, c. 1870s. Left: L handle with egg, segments far apart, 36 3/4" high; right: opera handle with tapering segments close together, 34 3/8" high.

Opera handle cane with gold circular designs in the shaft, from Israel, 1974, 35 3/4" high.

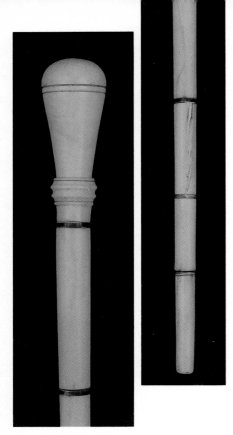

Straight knob elongated handled ivory cane with a segmented shaft, each section separated by washers, c. 1870. 33 3/4" high.

Ordinarily collectors choose the elephant ivory handle over the walrus ivory handle, believing it is more valuable. Walrus ivory is much harder than elephant ivory and is therefore more difficult to carve. In reality, it should be more valuable if the carving is very fine and detailed. In the 10th Century in India where elephants were plentiful, the ivory of a walrus tusk cost 200 times its original value. This could be due to the superstition that walrus ivory could detect the presence of poison and for this reason walrus ivory was in great demand for making spoons and vessels for containing food and drink. In India, walrus ivory was worth about 10 times as much as elephant ivory.

Elephant tusk has a great deal of oil in it which in dry weather and in a hot climate dries out. When this occurs, as in hot apartments with central heating, the ivory cracks. To some extent this can be remedied by soaking the ivory in water or even wrapping the ivory handle in a wet towel, as the ivory readily absorbs water. It is also a practice by owners of ivory objects to rub them with lanolin or some vegetable oil.

So readily does elephant ivory absorb water that even fairly large cracks may disappear as the edges come together when the ivory is soaked in water. Remember, if you have several valuable carved ivory sticks in a room, control the humidity to preserve your sticks. Also protect the ivory from the direct rays of the sun.

Charles Manghis, the scrimshander, ivory expert, and restorer from Massachusetts, says that the best preservative and restorer of dried out wood and ivory is Renaissance Wax made in England but obtainable from Woodcraft Supply, Montvale Avenue, Woburn, Massachusetts.

Ebony

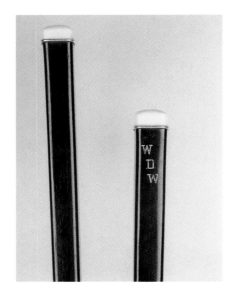

Two Tiffany canes with square ebony shafts. The cane on the right is marked "W D W." 35 3/4" and 36 3/4" high respectively.

This is one of the hardest woods and has been used since ancient times, hundreds of years before Christ, in ancient Egypt, Greece and Rome. In ancient Egypt ebony was so highly prized that it was accepted as tribute like gold from defeated countries.

It has an intense black color though there are some ebonies that are striped and some are pale, but the jet black ebony has always been most desired for canes. It is now a rare wood, and I will buy an ebony shaft even if its handle and ferrule are missing or worthless.

Ebony is an extremely heavy wood. Originally it was obtained from India and

Sri Lanka, but today it comes from tropical Africa. The texture of the black ebony is so fine and intense that it is impossible to finger-nail scratch it, which is how I test an alleged ebony stick. To test, scratch with the grain, and not cross-grain.

Ebony was particularly sought for use in physician's gold or silver handled canes and was always used by a gentleman with his formal evening attire.

The shaft of an ebony cane must be black all the way through. If you can dent an alleged black ebony shaft with your fingernail, it is not true ebony; if you can scrape off a black finish and it's white underneath, it is not true ebony. It may be "ebonized", which means treated by paint or chemicals to imitate the true ebony. True black ebony needs no paint or varnish as the bare wood will take on a wonderful glossy polish just by pressing it against a buffing wheel.

Although very much heavier in weight than malacca, ebony is preferred by some because of the aura of strength it exudes due to its weight as one strolls with it.

Ebony, malacca, and snakewood are the top three most desirable shafts of the cane connoisseurs.

Rhinoceros Horn

Two rhinoceros horn shaft swagger sticks with a rhino horn fashioned into a lighter. Left: silver handle with a rearing stag and the name Huntingdonshire on the handle, 26 1/2" high; right: Oriental scene on silver handle with three figures, a tree, and a house, 29 3/4" high.

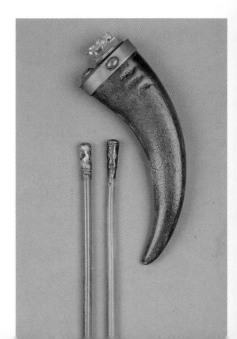

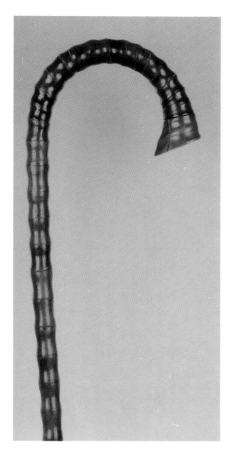

Very rare rhino disk crook handle cane, c. 1880, from Thailand, 36" high.

One of the rarest, costliest materials of which handles and even staffs of canes are made is rhinoceros horn. This is because the rhinoceros now is so rare that it is almost extinct. Once when in Kenya, Africa on a camera safari, my wife and I saw many elephants, but only one rhinoceros and as this was the rarest of all, being a so-called white rhino, it was protected by two armed native forestry guards. They followed the animal constantly to prevent poachers from killing it, cutting off its horn and abandoning the corpus to rot.

African rhino horn, according to U.S. Custom Authorities in November of 1988, will sell for $450.00 an ounce — roughly the price of gold — and as much as $1,000.00 an ounce elsewhere. At that time, the U.S. Fish and Wildlife Service in a sting operation agreed to buy seven rhino horns for $40,000.00 each. As this would be over forty times the yearly salary for an African poacher in any other occupation for which he qualified, it is easy to see why the rhino horn will soon become a legend.

Rhinoceros horn is made of densely packed fibers of keratin. Hair, hooves and fingernails are composed of keratin also.

Rhino horn, if accidentally knocked off, will grow back again just like a fingernail. The average length of a rhino horn is 1 foot, but I have seen rare 3 foot canes made of a single horn and I have several made of turned rhino horn washers threaded on steel cores to make beautiful, strong canes. Only by close inspection do the latter betray that they are not each made from a single piece.

The rhino is fast becoming extinct because sellers of the horn have an insatiable demand from Arabic countries where the horn is used for dagger handles and from Chinese and other Orientals who swear by the legendary aphrodisiac powers of pulverized rhino horn. Doctors have for years tried to establish that this is a myth without foundation in fact, but the dead bodies of rhinoceri are being constantly found rotting in the jungle with only the horn removed, the same destiny as the tusked elephants.

The hugh and cry is great today to save the rhino from complete extinction and we must sadly remember that the British slaughtered them by the thousands in the 1940s to encourage settlement in Kenya just as we in the late 1800s and early 1900s killed the noble buffalo by hundreds of thousands to conquer or destroy the Indians; we took only the tongue or hide and left the rest to rot. It is mostly the legendary aphrodisiac powers of the powdered rhino horn that destines the animals demise.

The tales of aphrodisiac food are many and varied, changing with the countries and the times and always of interest to males - and apparently only to males.

Once when giving a speech in Nashville to a large group of railroad trainmen, all prospective clients because of their hazardous occupation, I had heard and, therefore, told the story of a prominent railroader who had a large farm on the side where he raised fine cattle. Hoping to upgrade his herd, he purchased a very expensive thoroughbred bull from a long line of successful ancestors.

He was tearfully disappointed when his bull ignored the cows and merely munched and smelled the daises. He went to his veterinarian and told him the sad story. The vet said, "Don't worry, I'll make up a prescription for you. Give him one of these pills daily and I'll guarantee your bull will perform his duties lustfully."

A few weeks later, the trainman-farmer returned to the vet's office. The vet was on vacation and a young assistant was there in his place. The farmer told him about the pills he had been given and said it worked wonderfully and he would like another prescription for future use. The assistant said he never heard of such a pill, what was it called. The farmer said, "It didn't have name, the vet compounded it himself," and further said, "It was about so round (indicating the size of a half dollar), it was pink, and it tasted like peppermint!" This brought the house down. The farmer was in the audience and took it all very good naturedly.

In the fifties and sixties I had to go to Tennessee frequently on cases and trials. In between I would make the rounds of the antique shops in Nashville, Knoxville and Memphis. I found quite a few canes in Nashville, particularly in one shop. There I once saw a beautiful gun cane. The owner wanted $12.00 for it. I offered $8.00 and eventually came up to $10.00 but he stayed at $12.00 so I walked out — slowly — hoping he'd call me back. He didn't. The following week or two I had to go to Nashville again and even before going to my hotel to check in I went to the antique shop and offered the man $12.00 for the gun cane. He said it's $18.00 now. I came up to $15.00 unsuccessfully. I guess he was toying with me. I was in town a few days and decided I wanted the gun cane bad enough to pay the $18.00 so before leaving town I went to the shop and offered the $18.00. He said, "Sorry, I sold it the other day for $20.00!" I don't know if he really did - I guess he just hid it on me, but he seemed to enjoy my disappointment greatly. Next time in town I bought a nice sea captain's cane with compass, telescope and map compartments. There was no dickering this time. I paid his outrageous price for fear next time it would be higher.

At that time I was trying a most difficult case against a southern railroad and I had to have a new local associate. This is for local color, to help me get along with the judge and jury. The associate did nothing but sit there and act as though I wasn't from the north and if so, I was that rarity - a pretty decent northerner.

A very old lawyer was recommended to me. He was about 82 to 85. I phoned and met him at his office. He had a very primitive, bare office despite the fact that he was reputed to be a multimillionaire and owned farms and cattle all over the state. He sat at his desk in a corner as I outlined my case. He never said anything. He just looked at me. His secretary, who seemed to be at least 80, came in and he quickly excused himself and dictated a letter to her which she took down in longhand. I was beginning to think I was making a mistake. He then opened a drawer in his desk. I kept on talking and he appraised a number of knives, opening and closing them and testing their sharpness. I still kept on talking, faster now. He then reached over to a corner and picked out a branch of a tree, opening his knife and started cutting off shavings as I talked. Finally with a twinkle he said, "I'm a whittler." I said I see - what do you whittle (hoping it might be canes). He said I don't whittle anything, I just whittle and he did till he had a huge pile of shavings between his legs on the floor and quit. I told him I was a cane collector and asked if he had any. Yes, he had had some, but he said he whittled them all away trying to improve them.

At the trial, he said nothing as I put on and cross examined witnesses. He said he'd just make a closing argument. At the end of the case, I made an opening argument. My opponent replied and then my associate got up. He was about 5'2" all, straight as a soldier with bushy white brows and white hair. He stared at the jury quietly for a long time as he walked back and forth before the jury box and then stopped.

Suddenly, he let out a yell, jumped into the air and came down pounding the rail before the jury. In the loudest voice I ever heard in a courtroom, he screamed to the jury that they must not decide the case against me because I was from Chicago.

He fought the Civil War throughout his speech, but never mentioned even once all the fine points of the case; in fact, he never mentioned the case at all. All he continued saying was that they should abandon their natural hereditary southern prejudice and not hold it against me. And they didn't. He won the case for me and we got a very good verdict. But such inflammatory oratory I had never ever heard in all my years at the trial bar.

Now this old man was really a fine, gallant southern gentleman. I learned he had only one child - a daughter who was his pride and joy and lived with him as his wife was deceased. When the daughter married, it was a very glorious affair and all of Nashville's hierarchy was there. As a wedding present, the old man had a mansion built for his daughter and son-in-law. I understand he didn't care much for the latter, but his daughter really did. The old man even had a life-sized portrait of himself painted which he hung over the fireplace in the entrance foyer of the gift house.

The son-in-law persuaded his wife to take him on a safari to Africa and, upon their return, he mounted a prize elephant head over the fireplace and the old man's portrait disappeared. It is reported that when the old man visited his daughter and son-in-law, he looked quizzically at the elephant, stood up, never saying a word, walked around the room then went into another room glancing at the walls all newly decorated with animal trophies. Then, coming back to the fireplace, he looked up at the elephant head and said, "Hrump, who ever heard of anyone inheriting anything from an elephant," and he walked out of the room and out of the house. It is further alleged that the elephant head disappeared and in all his glory, the old man's portrait scowled down from the fireplace until his death. This was my taciturn associate - the whittler who came close to making a cane, but never stopped whittling in time.

I have a very fine ivory topped oriental cane that at first blush may seem to have also been owned by a whittler. The handle is umbrella shaped (crook) and is beautifully carved into the image of a roaring dragon with an open mouth in which there is a moveable ball that can be rolled around behind the gaping jaws. A fine silver band separates the handle from the staff that, as I say, at first blush could have been owned by a whittler. Closer examination reveals that it is entirely made of rhinoceros horn and has been shaved repeatedly along its length so that it is almost too thin in the middle to be used as a cane for support. It turns out that this whittler was really a fiddler and must have had great faith in the curative aphrodisiac powers of rhinoceros powder.

Snakewood, The Aristocrat of Canes

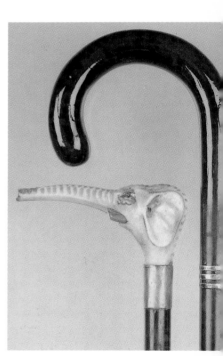

Two very rare snakewood shafts with bone ferrules. The elephant handle is carved from stag horn. Left: 36" high; right 35 1/2" high.

Chinese ivory dragon with an ivory floating ball in its open mouth and a silver collar intricately carved with two dragons supported on a shaved rhinoceros horn shaft, c. 1870. Owned by a "fiddler."

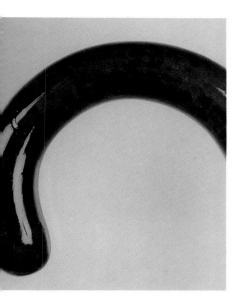

A closer look at the snakewood.

Even after I had been collecting canes for about 15 years, I rarely heard of snakewood. Finally, I had Theodore Fossel, the founder of the "British Stickmakers Guild" and president of the International Stick Society, as a house guest for about a week. It took us all that time to examine each of my 5,000 canes. As he was looking through a group of sticks in an elephant foot container, he picked up one and said this could be my most valuable stick. I was surprised as I had many that I thought far superior in beauty, heft and design. I asked why he thought this. He said because this is snakewood. I knew I must have some, but I didn't know how it looked. He explained that it is a very rare wood found only in Guyana in northeast South America and that it is so heavy that it sinks in water.

After Theo left, I found I had about four more snakewood canes. I became immediately interested and started studying the subject. I learned that in 1905 a shaft suitable to make a cane - that is a square blank - about 1 1/2" x 1 1/2" x 36" long cost $400.00. At that time this was about a year's wages for the average man. And that was the price of a stick that was not even tapered and had no handle or ferrule.

I learned the wood is called piratinera guianensis, but when I called all the dealers in exotic woods, many had never heard of it and others said they would refuse to handle it because it was so tough it would dull their tools and it had a tendency to start splitting as you were cutting it. It is found as isolated trees in the midst of heavy jungle and is obtained from native Indians in high mountainous territory.

As it is so very heavy, one is lucky to get a 3 foot log as it is carted out by hand labor. The trees grow up to 78 feet high and 3 feet in diameter but only the heart wood is desired, so all the sap wood surrounding it must be cut off by a machete. A tree 12 inches in diameter yields about 3 inches of heart wood. Snakewood weighs 75-85 pounds per cubic foot so you can see the struggle a native must go through to get this wood - first find it, then cut the tree down, then cut it into 3 foot to 4 foot lengths, cut off the sap wood and then haul it off the mountain, out of the jungle and to a lumber purchasing center.

As a consequence, the price is high even today. But I was a collector and had to have a really perfect piece. After many long distance calls, I located a small exotic wood dealer in California who knew a dealer in Guyana, but I was advised that I purchase at my own risk, and I had to buy a complete log 3 foot x 10 inches in diameter. The cost was about $450 not counting shipping. I ordered it and about 6 weeks later I received a very heavy package wrapped in bubble plastic sheets. It was so heavy I could hardly carry it into the house. I was luckier than a German collector of whom I read in Der Stocksammler. He had to buy a whole car load from another dealer.

It was wrapped like a treasure with multiple wrappings. Finally, the bare wood appeared, but it too was protected by a heavy coating of wax covering both ends and all the sides.

Now the quandary really arose. How would I get it cut? Every lumber yard that I called refused to cut it. They said that I would first have to cut it into boards, then staves, then have them rounded and finally have them tapered. But no one would even cut the log into boards because they said I would have to see a cutter who had a cradle on which the round log - all heartwood - could be secured as the cradle could be pushed back and forth to cut the logs into boards. This could not be done they said with an ordinary hand saw or circular saw and make exact and even surfaces by eye vision alone. The only cutters that had a cradle would not set up to cut one 3 foot log. They wanted a minimum of twenty 5 foot logs.

In desperation, I finally went to a factory owned by my son and demanded that the chief engineer cut it. He looked doubtful but finally agreed to try. We cut about 7 boards of various widths with fairly decent evenness, i.e., no wavy boards. But as we cut the log into boards, I could see cracks beginning at the top and running down the length of the board. So could the engineer and his helpers, so they refused to cut the boards into staves. If they cut the staves according to the grid I had drawn for them, they said many staves would have cracks down the center for the whole length. If they cut between the cracks, presuming no further cracks would appear, I might end up with only a few staves instead of about 24 that I had planned. You can now have a glimmer of why the snakewood cane costs so much. What do I do now?

Well, I took the boards home and made a brownish epoxy which I forced into every discernible crack. A few days later, I had about seven crack-free boards and found another cutter who cut them into about 25 staves. But I'm still only half way there. Now I must find a turner to make each stave round and then tapered.

After much inquiry, I heard of a man who was considered so knowledgeable in wood turning that he was called "The Wood Termite". I contacted him and he was willing to take a chance because he said, "I can do anything in wood," but I would have to pay by the hour. He was my last hope so I brought him the staves. He examined them and then, looking skeptical, said he would try but that he would not be responsible for the results.

We started lathing, but he kept stopping to resharpen his cutting tools. After about three hours we were only half way toward one finished stick. I quickly calculated that at this rate and at this price, I could not afford to have even one stick made. So I stopped him, paid for his time and took my staves home again.

I eventually heard of a man in Milwaukee who made risers for stairways. I phoned him and he said he saw no problem; whereupon, I drove to his place in Milwaukee with all my staves. He examined them and then turned them over to his Mexican wood turner who placed one in a lathe and in five minutes had it completed, completely round and tapered. And what beautiful wood! They had not seen that type before and just marveled at the coloration of the cane-shaped snakewood. They ran a wet rag over it and all the coloring became alive. Though I had seen snakewood, I had never seen such perfect coloration. It had black markings like a snake or like Cyrillic lettering, hence its name snakewood or letterwood. In an afternoon, we finished all but 5 or 6 staves. The latter the Mexican wouldn't put in the lathe. He had seen cracks in the wood and at the tremendous speed the lathe turned, it would, he said, splinter the wood so violently it would fly about and blind or kill us all. I was gradually learning why snakewood canes are so scarce.

I was overjoyed with the result so far, but I wanted the last five to be finished too. When I got home I again made my brownish epoxy and filled all the cracks I could find in these last five staves.

As a member of the British Stickmakers Guild, I had seen reference to a British man who made tools for the chair making industry. In England men make chairs as a hobby and he made their tools. Amongst these were "rounders" to make square staves round, and "taperers" to taper the round staves into tapered canes by a hand cranking method in a vice. I now ordered a set.

These are hand-held tools clamped over the stave and moved by hand as the stave is turned by the hand crank. I found this too slow for me so I used a metal lathe to turn the stave while I ran first the rounder and then the taperer (something like a child's old fashioned pencil sharpener) over the turning shaft.

It worked perfectly and I salvaged the last five staves.

I then sanded all the cane shafts and used maxi-cloth of about seven grades. The final grade could clean the lenses of your eyeglasses it was so fine. This gave a wonderful finish to the shafts. I also gave each cane shaft seven coats of a special marine varnish, sanding between each coat. I then applied handles and ferrules and I had real treasures.   All this work for snakewood canes. It took about 6 months and averaged about $500.00 a shaft. These, however, are far superior to anything I had ever previously seen because they are pure heart wood. The other

canes of snakewood that I have seen or own are usually sap wood on one side and heart wood on the other so you do not get the complete figuration all around the shaft. This is truly the aristocrat of canes.

Gutta Percha

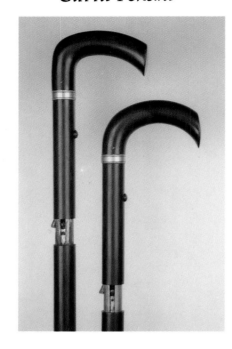

Two Remington gun canes with gutta percha shafts and button firing mechanisms. Left: 35" high; right: 37 3/4" high.

Canes are also made from sap of a tree. All the Remington gun canes were made of gutta percha. Gutta percha is a resinous gum of the Payena and Palaquinium genus of trees growing close to the equator and found only in Borneo, Sumatra, and Malacca.

Originally the gum was taken from the inner bark of this rare tree, thus destroying it. Later it was found that the leaves and twigs themselves had twice as much gum. It was also taken from the tree by tapping, much as maple syrup. By a chemical process, this was then made into moldings for American Civil War picture frames, surgical instruments, buttons, dental plates, golf ball covers, and canes. It is now so rare that it is a collectable in its own right. I once had such a collector call me, wanting a Remington gun cane because all Remington gun canes were made of gutta percha and he needed one for his gutta percha collection.

Bovine or Phallic Canes

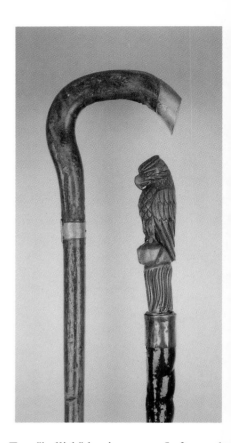

Two "bullish" bovine canes. Left: crook handle with silver end cap and collar in shape of a buckle, 35 1/2" high; right: wooden eagle handle on a twisted shaft, 34 1/2" high.

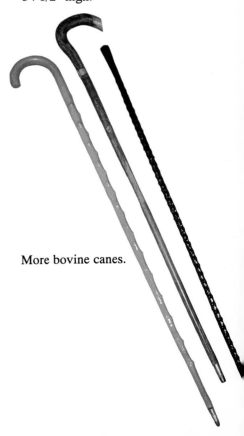

More bovine canes.

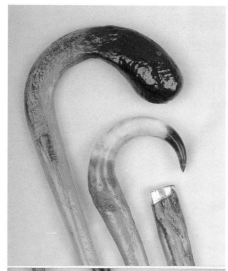

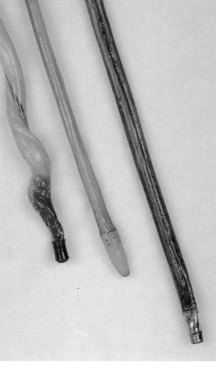

Three bovine canes. Left: red crook handle, 38 1/4" high; center: bull's penis with a horn handle, 35" high; right: silver end cap and ferrule, 36 1/4" high.

I have previously mentioned that canes were made of almost every conceivable material, organic and inorganic, from creatures flying in the sky, running on the ground, swimming in the sea and slithering underground. Similarly, speaking of animals that it butchered, in the Chicago Stockyards one packing house said, "We utilize everything but the squeal." This could be the motto of canes made from living organisms — the horns of all wild and domestic animals, vertebrae of many, and yes even the reproductive organs of the male species.

These are called phallic, penile, or bovine canes. Tribal kings of ancient times were probably the first to use such material — it started centuries ago and is still practiced. In Africa only the king was permitted to carry a cane or scepter made from the copulatory organ of a wild and ferocious animal, as it was hoped that the sexual powers of the involuntary donor would enhance the virility of the king so that he could fertilize as many of his harem as the bull of the species could impregnate his cows. Undoubtedly even Solomon with his thousand wives was no stranger to this custom.

In the Spanish countries where bull fighting was a national sport, an exemplary bull in the ring who fought bravely would very frequently, because of the tumultuous olés from the amphitheater, be spared from the death thrust as the cheering spectators cried for his survival so that he could propagate his genes of bravery to a very desired and needed progeny.

If, however, he had been so seriously wounded so that he could not survive, he was killed and honored by having his copulatory organ, dismembered and offered (after suitable preservative treatment) to the highest foreign dignitary present as a memento of this brave animal and his superlative action in the ring.

After the offer was made and appreciatively accepted, the object was taken to experts who would stretch, dry, varnish and embellish it with silver bands and ferrules — all suitably named, dated and engraved. The end product was shipped to the honorary guest in the form of a cane with either a straight or a crook handle. I have several such in my collection. This was an honored and universal custom for many decades in the Latin countries that enthusiastically favored the toreador and felt in all conscience some obligation to the toro victim.

Repugnant as this may seem to many people, we must be reminded that the enthusiasm of collectors for exotic canes to parade before fellow collectors, even in this country and in this century, went so far that canes were made of human skin of executed criminals and caused a scandal in Ohio.

As much mysticism and care is attached to the bovine canes as to the Irish blackthorn, especially in tribal and early rural areas. It was considered the ideal stick to reprimand a recalcitrant wife be-

cause it left no welts or scars from the beating. I quickly must add that I have no personal knowledge of the veracity of this folk tale and present it only as hearsay evidence.

In farming communities these bull-organ canes are seen in barns and are made by local farmers who, upon showing one, usually state, "Bet you don't know what this is." Just recently I attended a garden show in Lake Forest, Illinois, and at the northern outskirts of the town was a beautiful farm estate on the lake. We were shown all the beautiful gardens, ponds, and exotic barns of Spanish architecture. Before going through the main mansion, I eluded the crowd and went into one of the other barns and there I saw two bovine canes. As I was examining them, one of the farm hands came up and said, "Bet you can't tell me what that is." Later in going through the manor house, I saw a few canes and an oosick too, so I assume the owner is starting a cane collection.

The demand for the bovine canes must be great, for in this country there was and probably still is a company specializing in their manufacture. Not only does the bovine shaft make canes, but golf clubs and putters, gear shifts, judicial gavels, pool sticks and many other things. One can write to:

International Biologics, Inc.
531 Ninth Street, N.W.
New Brighton, MN 55112
Attention: Department of Genitalia
　　　　　Paraphernalia

A fulfilled order states:

In honor of that group of Minnesota's finest bovines that made these gift items possible, we offer the following:

ODE TO FERDINAND

The bulls a mighty, manly beast
And one with whom you'll trifle least,
He's lusty, crusty, mean and proud,
And some would say he's well endowed,
A bull could tell you many yarns,
Of exploits in the fields and barns,
His fertile days have come and went,
And now in his retirement,
I.B.I. now use that part,
That bulls use in their lusty art,

We make some nifty, gifty things,
Out of that part from which life
    springs,
We clean and stretch and trim and dry,
All so that we can beautify,
That part that folks will not consume,
When Fredinand has met doom.
I only hope that those who use,
That special gift that they did choose,
Will not forget from whence it came,
From Ferdinand of pasture fame.
He gave his thing so you could putt,
Or use a cane so you could strut.
We thank him as we use this stuff,
On city streets or in the rough
He gave beyond his duty's call,
We all agree he gave his ALL!

We show a grouping of bovine canes herein. Most have a steel rod running down the center which in itself is a subject of ribald and envious comment amongst the possessors of octogenarian age. All are about alike in appearance which phrase reminds me of the famous duckman in Chicago where I had my law office.

During the depression, this homeless beggar could be seen daily walking through the loop followed by his pet — not a dog but a duck. So beloved was this itinerant and his loyal duck that from time to time he was depicted in the newspapers.

The story is told, not in the newspapers but by the legal fraternity that on one very cold winter day, he tried to enter a cheap theater on Madison Avenue in the loop. His duck was waddling dutifully behind him and the ticket seller told him he could not take his duck into the theater. In a quandary he left but he and his duck were still cold so he went into the alley, picked up his duck, unbuttoned his shirt and put the duck inside where the duck was all buttoned up, cozy and warm.

As the duck nestled quietly and unobtrusively, the old man presented himself again at the ticket office and they sold him a ticket and he went inside and sat down in a seat in the dark theater.

After a while two old maids on their lunch hour, eating their popcorn, came in and in the darkness sat next to the old man. In the meantime he had unbuttoned his shirt and the duck stretched out his neck and eagerly watched the action on the screen. Suddenly, the old maid to his left nudged the one to her left and said, "Don't look right now but when you can, look to

my right. It's very dark and I think that a man there is exposing himself." The other lady said, "Oh, no, I needn't look. If you've seen one, you've seen them all. They're all alike." The first lady said, "Oh, no, they're not, this one's different as it's eating up all my popcorn!"

These bovine canes, though sometimes called phallic, do not resemble a phallus in any way, though made from one, and, therefore, are more properly called bovine canes. I have many of various different animals, mostly African, but I display only a few of these bovine canes in this book. While they are an important item in a collection, as the old maid said, if you've seen one, you've seen them all. They're all alike.

Cleverly similar to the bovine cane, though not a cane because of insufficient length is the oosick. This too is lamented by the elderly gentlemen who have one in their collections as further evidence of the lack of impartiality by nature in bestowing its favors more upon the males of the various animals than upon the human species. An oosick is generally found in collections of those who specialize in scrimshaw items.

I was once phoned in my office from the arctic circle by a lawyer friend who tried to persuade me to join him in the last legal hunt for polar bears. This is a prominent trial lawyer from Iowa, who had turned down several federal appointments to the judiciary.

We had once collaborated on a large case, and I had visited and worked in his office which he tried to design as early Lincolnesque, with wooden furniture and roll top desk, etc. He told me he wanted a polar bear standing upright in his reception room and now he was calling from the arctic circle for me to join him. He said he and some companions had a chartered private plane, which they would fly around until they saw a polar bear. Then they would fly ahead a mile or so, land behind a high ice or snow hummock and then wait for the bear to walk into shooting range. They would then kill and skin it, leaving the carcass behind, and get back into the plane to look for another bear.

I declined his kind invitation saying I couldn't waste such a beautiful animal just for its skin and leave all the rest behind. Then too, the license cost was $2,000 not counting all the expenses of getting to the arctic circle.

I did ask him, however, if he could get me an oosick from the Eskimos. I wanted one large enough to make into a walking stick. He said that would be difficult as the Eskimos cherish the oosick. What is an oosick? It is the penile bone in the reproductive organ of a male walrus. It is about 18 inches long, of an ivory-like bone and looks like a war club. My friend said the oosick is rare because the walrus does not give it up without a fight to the death. When the Eskimos get one, they engrave it with arctic scenes of a primitive Rabalaision type consistent with the material being used.

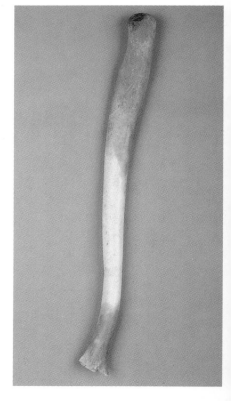

An oossic from the Eskimos, 21" high.

I understand that an oosick is possessed only by walruses (who have the largest) and raccoons. This lawyer being quite a raconteur, had a number of raccoon oosicks. They are about 5-6 inches long and he said he used them as swizzle sticks when he threw a cocktail party. The ladies drinks always contained one, and invariably one would ask what this was. He would nonchalantly say, "Oh, that's an oosick." This created more curiosity and when they persisted in questioning him, he would tell them what it was and watch the different shades of red that the ladies' faces turned. He was and is a brilliant lawyer with a robust sense of humor.

Well, he got his polar bear and I got my oosick. His polar bear was too large and my oosick too small for our intended purposes. His polar bear when stuffed and standing upright was so tall that he had to cut a 3 foot deep well in his reception room floor to stand up the bear so it would clear the ceiling. The walrus oosick I received was too small for me, but as my lawyer friend said, it should make a fine cane for a midget.

Kelp

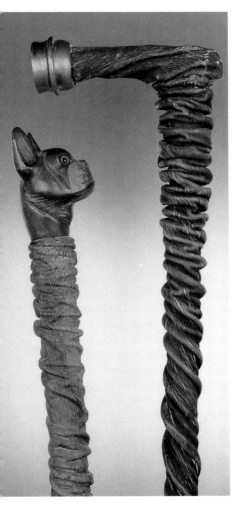

Kelp is a Seaweed that grows to great length in the shallower parts of the ocean. It has broad leaves and hollow shafts and in canes it is frequently confused with bovine tissue or considered an animal intestine. It is vegetable matter. Captain Thomas, a retired sea captain, settled near an Indian reservation near La Push — state of Washington — where he made and sold these canes for a living in the late 1890s. All have wooden shafts over which the kelp is threaded and allowed to dry, giving a wrinkled skin-like surface to the shaft.

What you may, as many do, consider as a bovine cane, on very close examination will be found to be kelp. One way of distinguishing between the two seems to be the old age cracks in a kelp cane which always go crosswise and never seems to occur in the bovine canes that I have.

Narwhal

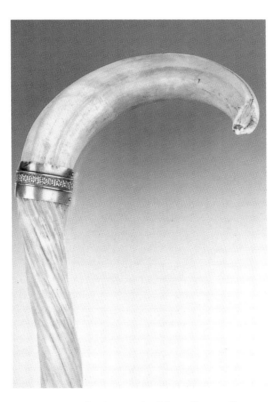

Tusk handle fastened with a silver collar to a narwhal tusk shaft, 36 1/2" high.

Rare Narwhal shafts are much in demand by advanced collectors. The entire cane may consist of just the shaft of narwhal with a silver cap. This shaft is a real ivory and spirals always counter-clockwise in a taper from top to bottom.

It allegedly was first discovered in July of 1577 when Martin Frobisher was seeking an Atlantic-to-Pacific passage on top of North America. At Baffin Island, his crew found a dead fish which he described as "roundlike to a porpoise being about 12 feet long — having a horn of two yards long growing out of the snout or nostrils." The horn was properly described as it is still that description — straight, spiraled and tapered. Frobisher thought it was the marine equivalent of the fabled land unicorn and called it the "sea unicorn." He brought it home to England and presented it to Queen Elizabeth. These mammals were hunted by arctic whalers for their horn which was worth its weight in gold. The horn was pounded and used as a prescription to alleviate epilepsy and heart disease into the 18th Century.

They still are found in the Northwest Territories, Canada and Greenland coastal waters but are rarely seen. We know only that they are mammals and that the adult male has two teeth and the one on the left upper jaw grows continuously, reaching as long as 8 feet. Narwhals are the only mammal in the world that produces a spiral tooth.

So fraught with mystery and superstition in the middle ages was the "sea unicorn" that it was reputed to counter the effects of poison. As a result, many emperors, kings, popes and aristocrats owned goblets carved from narwhal tusks. It makes a most desirable cane shaft but it is hard to find.

Shagreen

Shagreen (shark skin) and ivory crook handle, malacca shaft, and horn ferrule, 35 3/4" high.

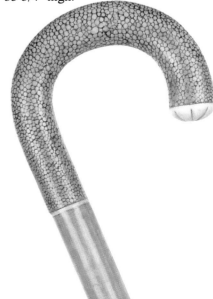

Two kelp canes with dog handle and silver end cap handle on an L shaft. Dog's head cane: 37" high; L handle: 34 1/2" high. Kelp, which is a hollow seaweed, grows to great lengths in the shallower parts of the ocean. These were made by a Captain Thomas in the 1890s. Captain Thomas was a retired sea captain living near Push, Washington in the 1890s.

A rare, long-forgotten hide called shagreen is taken in small batches from the bellies of stingray fish and sharks and was used to cover canes. A single shagreen skin is smaller than a sheet of typing paper. By the time it was treated, sanded, and dyed, it cost in 1986 about $50.00 and is rarer and more expensive now. I have a malacca cane with a shagreen handle and have seen a whole stick covered with shagreen but it was horribly expensive.

Sharkskin was used by the Turks in the 12th Century for inlay on their shields. Louis XIV was enamored of it and became a patron to shagreen workshops. The craft in this country died out during World War II. The labor was so demanding that clients had to wait 6 months or longer for a custom order. A cane of this material is consequently very old, rare and most desirable as a collectible.

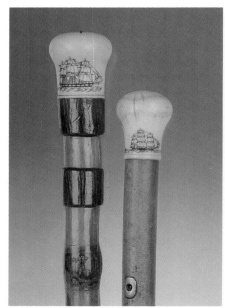
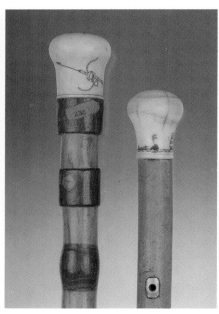

Two knob handled canes with whaling ships and whales. Left: 34 1/2" high; right: 33 3/4" high.

Scrimshaw

I have many scrimshaw canes. These were originally made by sailors on old sailing vessels that hunted the various types of whales for their oil and also their bone which was ground into fertilizer. Sometimes these poor men — many were kidnapped by the ship — were at sea and away from home for years at a time. To wile away their time, especially when in a lull with no wind for days, the sailors would cut and etch and turn out canes and other objects of whale bone. Particularly favored was the jaw bone of the sperm whale that looked so much like ivory it is called whale ivory. The teeth were also made into handles for canes and other artifacts. The etching was done with a sail needle and lamp black. Even whale blood was rubbed into the incised lines. This type of artistry is called scrimshaw.

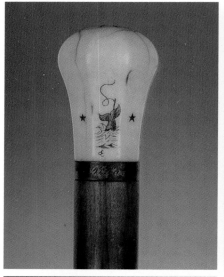
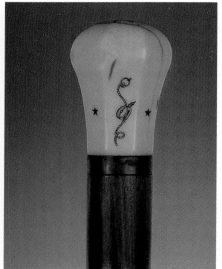
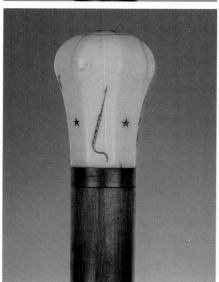
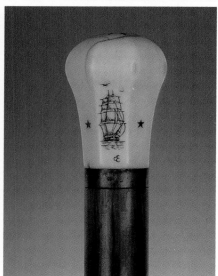

Old knob handle scrimshaw cane with panels inscribed with whaling tools, a whaling ship, and a whale's fluke. 36 1/2" high.

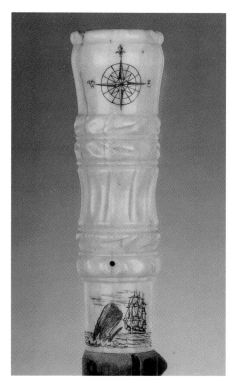

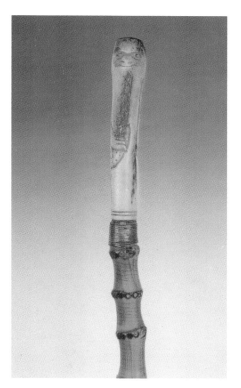

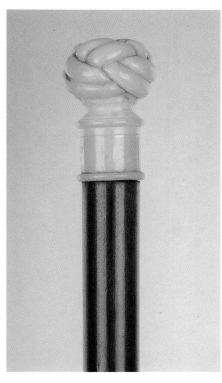

Long scrimshaw handle with ship and whale and compass bearings, 36 1/4" high.

Sailor's depiction of a lonely monkey taking matters into his own hands, 33 1/4" high.

Sailor's Turk's head knot of walrus ivory, 32 3/4" high.

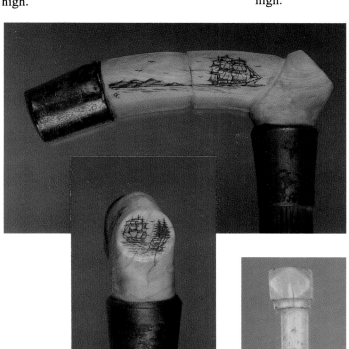

Two views of a whaling vessel, silver end cap and collar, 34 3/4" high.

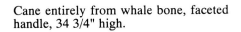

Cane entirely from whale bone, faceted handle, 34 3/4" high.

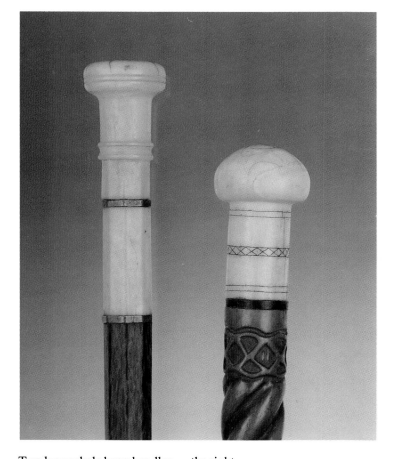

Two long whale bone handles — the right hand shaft is nicely carved with knots and spirals. Left: 35 1/4" high; right: 32 1/4" high.

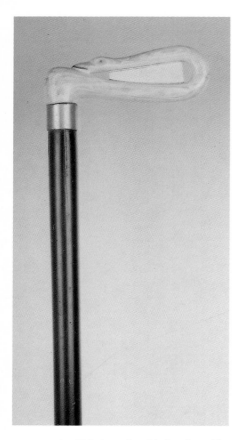

Long necked bird resting it's head on it's back, whale tooth ivory on an ebonized shaft, 34 1/4" high.

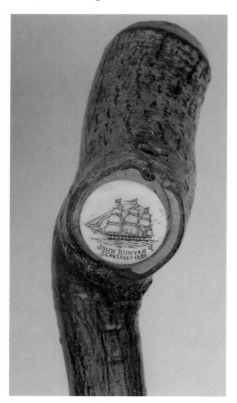

Wooden cane with inset whaling vessel and the legend "JOHN BUNYAN SEARSPORT 1850", 36 1/4" high. This is an example of modern scrimshaw.

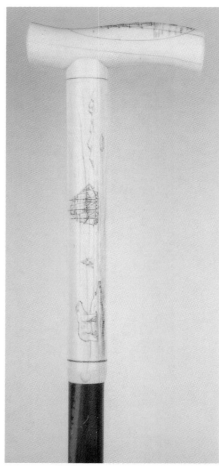

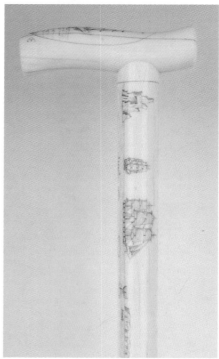

Old opera style handle and upper shaft of whale bone with modern engraving of a whaling ship and polar bear on one side and on the other the ship and a whale's fluke. The initials "FHM" are engraved on the end of the handle. 37" high. Carved for the author by a modern scrimshander.

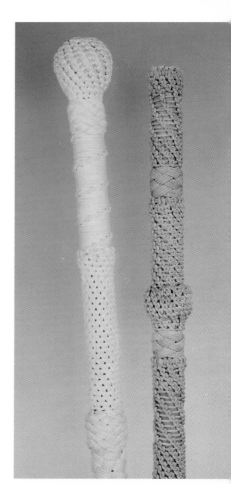

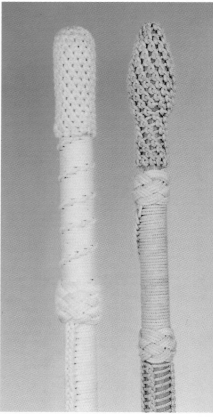

Two nautical canes covered with cord in sailors' knots from top to bottom. Left, white: 45" high; right, tan: 56 3/4" high.

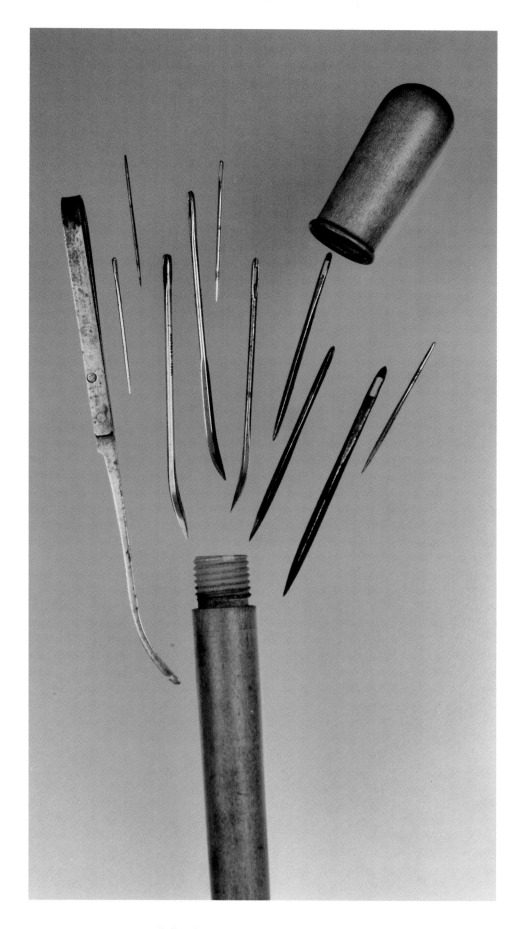

Sailmaker's cane with tools inside, 33 1/
4" high.

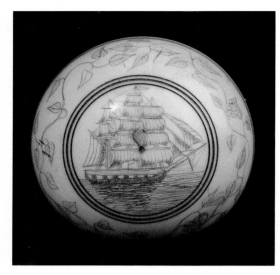

Scrimshaw, whaling ship carved in ivory knob, malacca shaft, silver collar marked with owners initials PLA, 37 3/4" high.

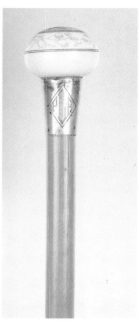

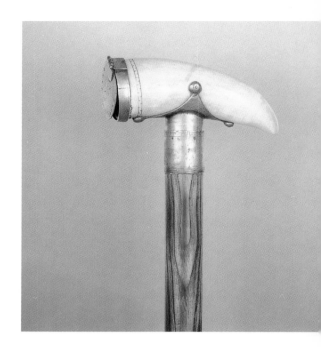

Whale's tooth with silver collar and a silver lid at the open end of the tooth which raises on a hinge to reveal a snuff container. The tooth pulls off to reveal a dagger. This cane dates to c. 1880 and measures 34 7/8" high.

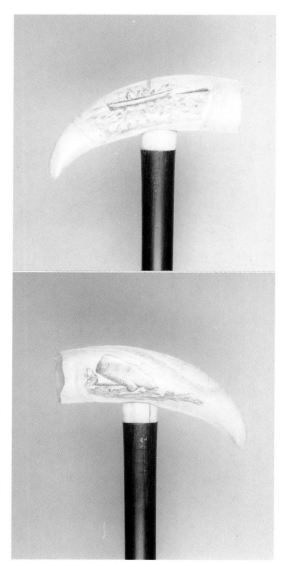

Whale's tooth on ebony shaft, scrimhander depicts whaling disaster on both sides of the handle, 36 3/4" high.

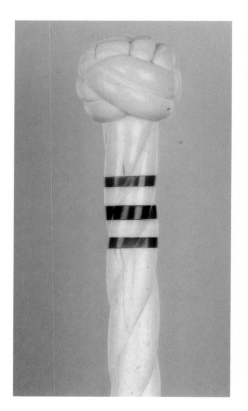

Whale tooth ivory handle in shape of a Turk's head knot, whale bone shaft, baleen rings in collar, 34 1/2" high.

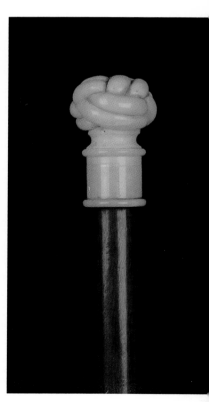

Scrimhander's Turk's Head knot in ivor or bone, bone ferrule, c. 1890. 32 1/ high.

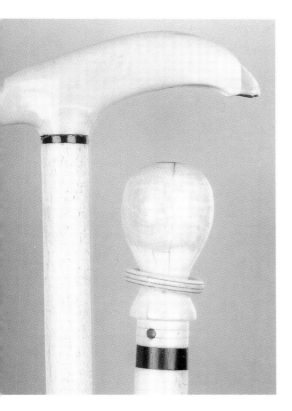

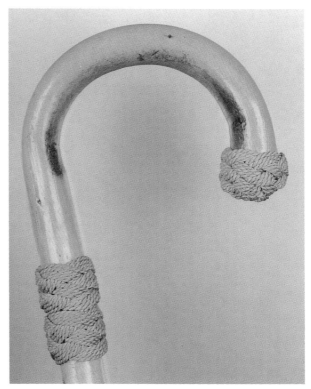

Two whale tooth ivory handled, whale bone shafted, scrimshaw canes, left: ivory tooth handle, baleen collar, c. 1870, 35" high; right: ivory knob handle, bone shaft, black baleen collar, and whimsy ring on the handle, 36 5/8" high.

Wooden crook handle sword cane with a sailor's knots tied at intervals down the shaft, 36" high.

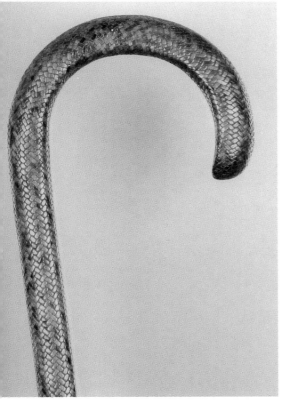

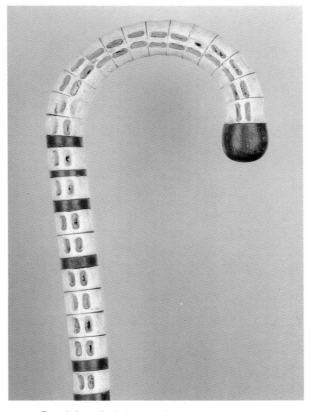

Woven Baleen cover for crook handle cane, c. 1900, 35 3/4" high.

Crook handled shark spine cane with baleen rings, c. 1880, 34 1/2" high.

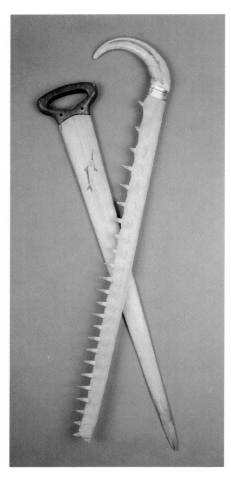

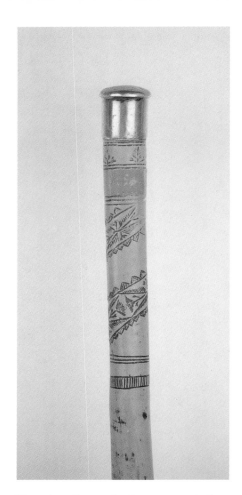

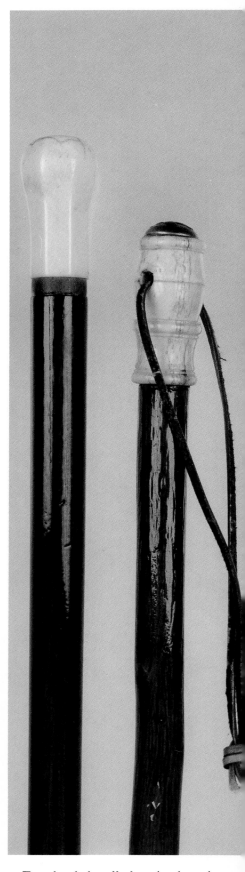

Two large scrimshaw canes. Left: sword fish cane shaft with a loop handle. The sword fish the shaft came from is depicted on the shaft, 35 1/4" high; right: has a tooth handle and a saw fish shaft, 36 3/4" high.

Unusual sting ray tail cane with faceted silver handle and initials "EWT" on top and the stinger held in place on the side of the shaft with a silver coil, 34 3/4" high.

Silver handle, scrimshaw presentation cane reading on top of the handle: "GE Gooch to Gen. M.M. Trumbull, Chicago, 1889." 33 3/4" high.

Two vertebrae canes. Left: snake vertebrae with young Napoleon's head (imago handle); right: dolphin vertebrae with knob handle of bone. Left: 33 1/4" high; right: 35 1/2" high.

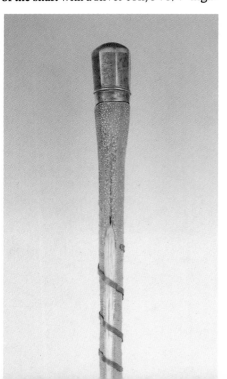

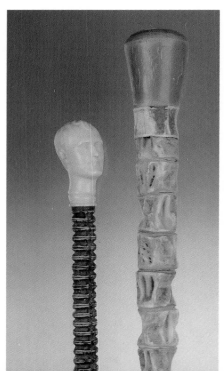

Two knob handled scrimshaw ivory canes. The right hand cane features an eyelet in the handle and a brass cap featuring an eagle. Left: 37" high; right: 37 1/4" high.

The modern method of scrimshawing is more advanced. One must first polish the ivory (whalebone or whaletooth) and then blacken the entire piece with black ink. Then the real artist etches thousands of hair thin lines on the ivory with a sharpened piece of piano wire. With this method the design will stand out, being white on a black background. Then the background is completely cleaned off and the object dried well. Finally, the now white object is again rubbed with black ink, so that it sinks into the scratches. When the object is now cleaned; the black ink remains in the scratches as a black design on a white surface. This is scrimshaw as done today. Of course, the fine work of the old masters is preferable to collectors, but the modern artistry will really be appreciated in a hundred years from now.

Many old canes having fine old whale ivory handles are made into a modern scrimshaw by having their ivory etched this way. I have many of these too and they make a beautiful collection in themselves, when the antique scrimshaw canes are unobtainable.

Scrimshaw is also applied in name to similar work done on non-ivory pieces such as bone or wood. It is found in inland areas where none of the requisite whale bone or ivory is obtainable. It is frequently used by folk artists to beautify wooden canes.

Since the ban on whale ivory, fossilized ivory from prehistoric animals was also turned to. Many houses are found in the frozen Siberian tundra made almost entirely from fossilized ivory and bone. This material is also found in the Pacific Northwest.

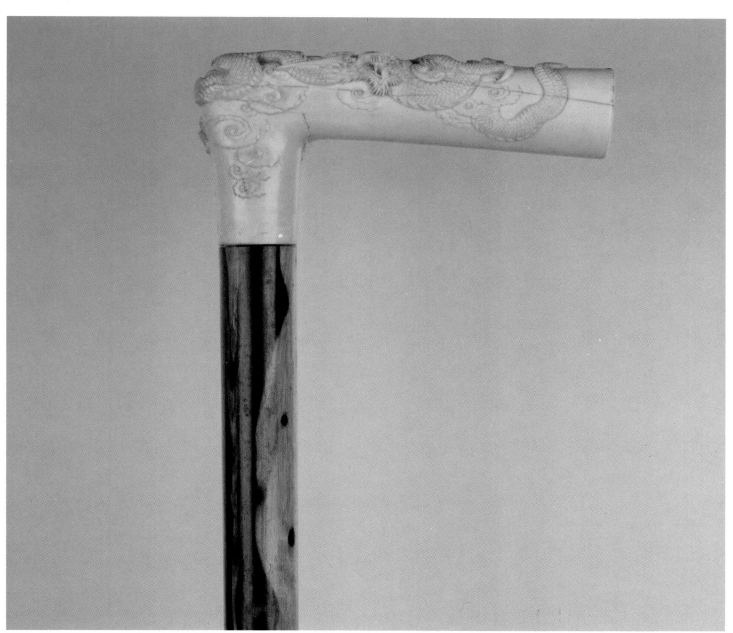

Intricately carved scrimshaw ivory dragon handle on lignum vitae shaft, 35 3/4" high.

127

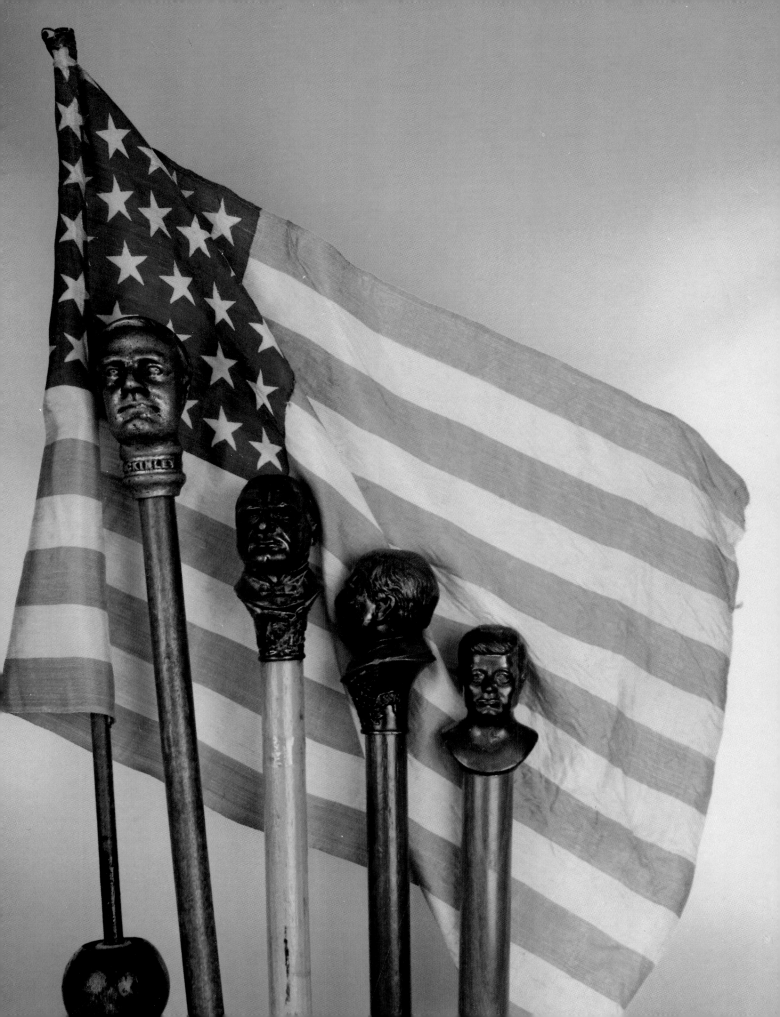

Chapter 5
Diversity in Canes

Royalty had long used the stick as a suitable gift, which custom was followed down almost to recent times by the "presentation cane." The costlier the cane, the higher the esteem in which the recipient was held. Is it then surprising that Catherine II gave King Gustavius a diamond-studded cane worth approximately $50,000?

Gold-headed canes, therefore, were especially selected as gifts from working men to their employers, from flock to minister, all suitably inscribed. It was a tacit recognition that the recipient was a man of culture and leisure—a gentleman.

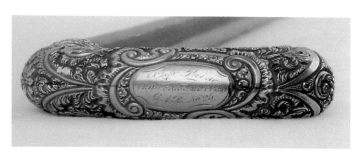

Top view of an L handle presentation cane to "CAPT. PAINE, FROM FARRAGUT POST, GAR NO. 25," c. 1885,

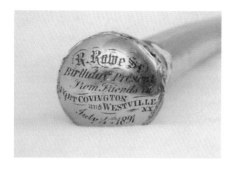

Top view of a gold knob handle presentation cane reading, "R. Rowe Sr. Birthday Present From Friends in Fort Covington and Westville, N.Y. July 4th, 1891."

Benjamin Franklin gave George Washington a cane with a gold knob in the shape of a "cap of liberty," which had been given to him by a European Countess.

George Washington had three gold-headed canes, and President Harrison owned more than 100. Andrew Jackson's gun cane can still be seen at his plantation Manor House called the Hermitage, just outside Nashville, Tennessee. J.P. Morgan, the financier, was always seen with a cane.

President Franklin Roosevelt was a cane collector whose collection may now be viewed in his library at Hyde Park.

At one time in America, many colleges had class canes, instead of the modern class ring, and in 1898, Dartmouth College had such a cane with a coat of arms of the school and graduates frequently had every classmate carve his nickname on the stick.

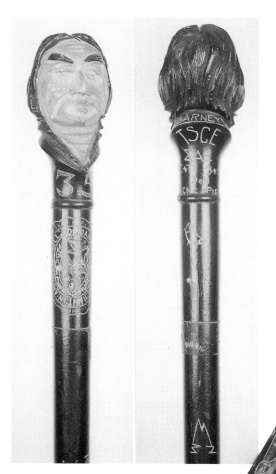

F.B. Tomlinson's Dartmouth college cane signed by his friends in 1935, 35 3/4" high.

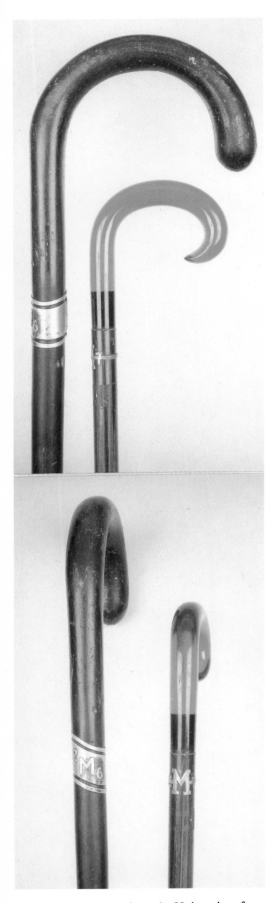

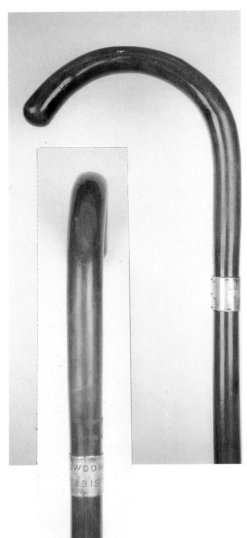

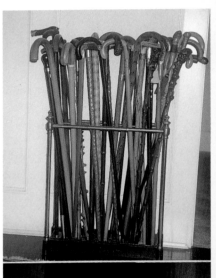

In the not too distant past, every home had a cane rack or umbrella stand or hall tree in which guests could place their canes for the duration of their visit.

I have read that in old churches, one can sometimes see a device near the hymnal rack for holding the worshipper's canes or umbrellas. Victorian ladies were said to have a container of gentlemen's canes near the front entrance so that intruders and unwelcome callers would think that there was a man in the house.

School cane "Bowdoin" 1915, University of Maine, 36" high.

School cane, M (for Maine) with a pine tree and 28 (for the year 1928) as silver collar, eyelets, 35 3/4" high.

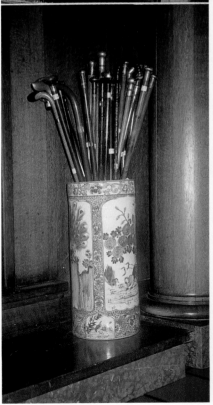

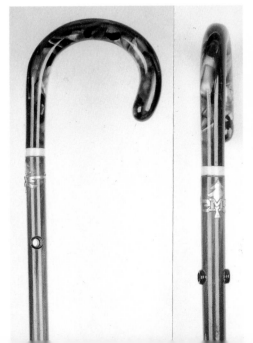

Two college canes from the University of Maine — left: 1926, 36 1/2" high; right: 1927, 35 1/4" high.

In the not too distant past, every home had a cane rack or umbrella stand or hall tree in which guests could place their canes during visits.

In America at the turn of the past century, it was customary to give each of the pall bearers at a funeral a suitable gift. What was, therefore, more proper than a black cane with silver eyelets and silver handle appropriately inscribed? I have one such reading:

Eli Lewis
1840
In Memory of
E.W.

Naturally, these came to be called funereal canes.

There is a saying— "one strolls with a walking stick and swaggers with a cane" and some differentiation is attempted to be made between the two. Generally, as I indicated above, a walking stick has a crook or umbrella-shaped handle, while the cane has a straight top.

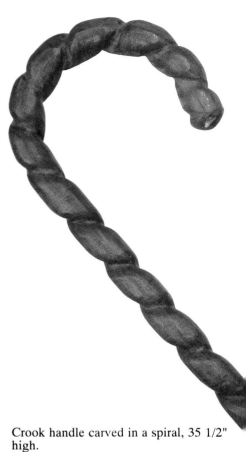

Crook handle carved in a spiral, 35 1/2" high.

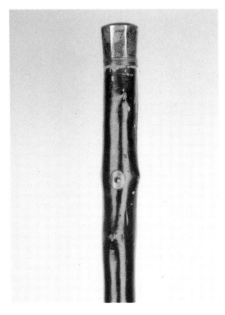

Funereal cane, given to pall bearers. On top of the faceted silver handle it reads "ELI LEWIS 1840, In Memory of E. W." 36" high.

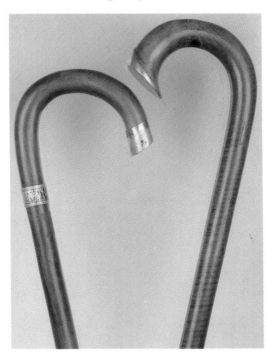

Two crook handles — lower: silver with gold trim and a signed band, c. 1890, 34 3/4" high; upper: gold with a rare wood shaft, c. 1890, 34 3/4" high.

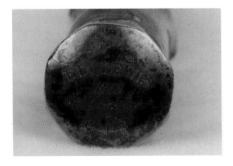

Eli Lewis inscription on top of the funereal cane.

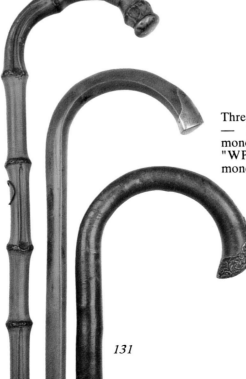

Three crook handles with silver end caps — left: 35 1/2" high; center: monogrammed on the silver with initials "WPB," 36 1/4" high; right: monogrammed "WHC 97," 35 1/4" high.

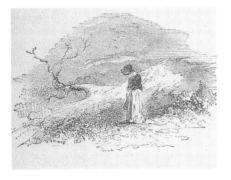

131

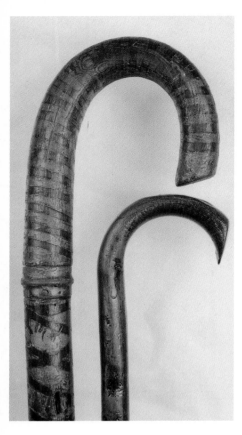

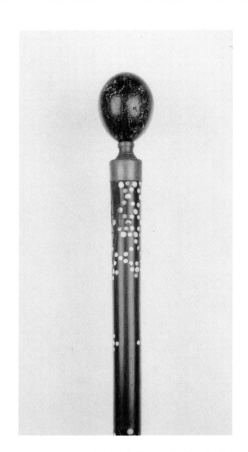

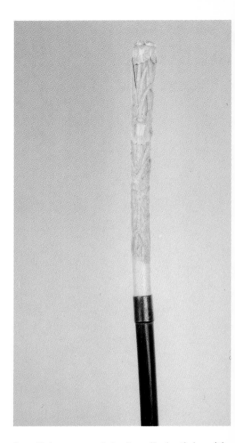

Two crook handles — left: painted with gold stripes and crosses, the handle is held to the shaft with a large brass collar and screws, 38" high; right: simple crook handle, 35 1/2" high.

Thunder egg with inlaid ivory in the shaft, 35 3/4" high.

Small ivory straight handled stick with foliate and iris design and oriental signature. 30 3/8" high.

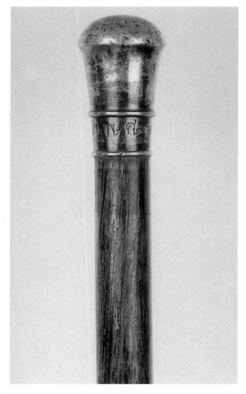

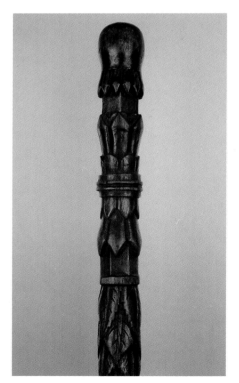

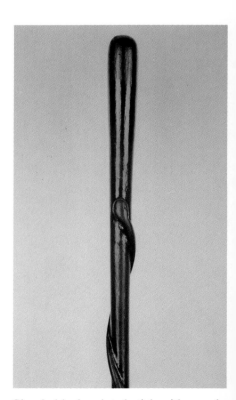

Thai Royal cane, signed, silver & rare wood, c. 1880, 37 1/2" high.

Elaborately carved folk art knob handle with leafs carved down the shaft, 34" high.

Simple black painted stick with a snake wrapping up the shaft, folk art, 33 1/2" high.

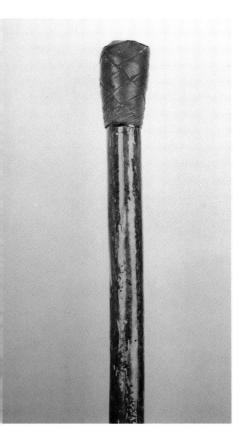

Leather wrapped handle and a bone ferrule on a laminated shaft, 35 1/2" high.

The carrying of a stick gives a peculiar feeling of power. As we have seen, men have become so attached to particular sticks that they have insisted upon being buried with them. I have a British newspaper clipping dated November 11, 1913, where the reverse was true. A Mr. Moberly Bell, Manager of the Times, lost a bone in his foot due to a railroad accident and had the bone fashioned into a handle for his cane so it would always remain with him.

What could be a more fertile field for collecting? And in company with such great historical figures as mentioned above. It is the writer's experience that most modern cane collectors are either doctors or bankers. Despite the fact that many, many millions of canes were made, surprisingly few have survived. Yet, enough remain to make the hunt exciting.

Some collectors, to more readily accommodate a collection to an apartment, had detached the handle from the cane and preserved only the handle. We see many of these now as the handle of fine large magnifying glasses.

Woods

Collectors can specialize in just collecting the hundreds of unique woods, or bone or ivory canes, or gold or silver handled canes. Many dedicate their efforts to regional canes, such as the Swiss alpenstocks, or the shillelaghs and Blackthorns of Ireland or the site-commemorative canes of travelers, or the Mexican walking sticks, which are gaily carved and painted and always show the flag and national eagle clutching a writhing serpent. The older of these canes make fine collecting due to their exquisite workmanship.

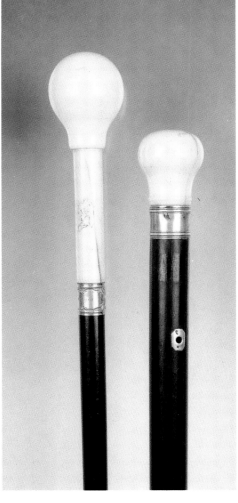

Two ivory knob handled canes with ebony shafts. Left: with gold collar signed J.A. Dyer, c. 1890, 35" high; right: has eyelets of silver and a silver collar, c. 1860. 36 1/2" high.

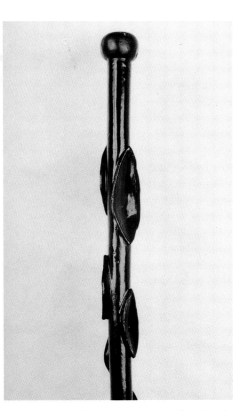

Diamond willow branch cane with a knob handle, painted black, 35" high.

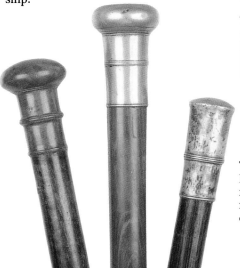

Three Thai Royal Canes, left with wooden knob handle and of rare wood, center and right with silver handles, center a knob, right more of a cap. Left: 38 1/2" high; center: 32 1/4" high; right: 33 1/2" high.

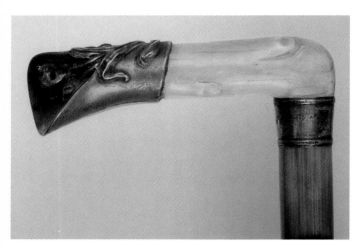

Bone L handle with silver end cap featuring Art Nouveau style flowers, silver collar, step partridge wood shaft, 35 3/4" high.

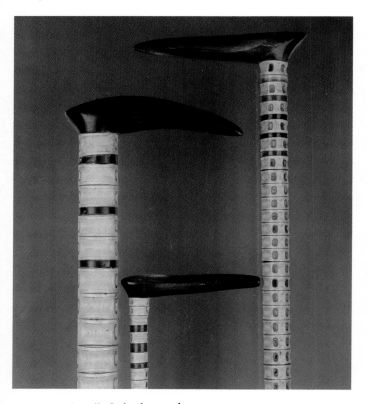

Three L handled shark vertebrae canes, ranging from 34 1/4" high to 35 1/2" high.

Two large knobbed presentation canes on ebony shafts, left with gold knob and uninscribed on top, right with silver knob inscribed: Presented by [name illegible] to John S. Webber, June 20, 1876. Left: 34 1/4" high; right: 35 1/4" high.

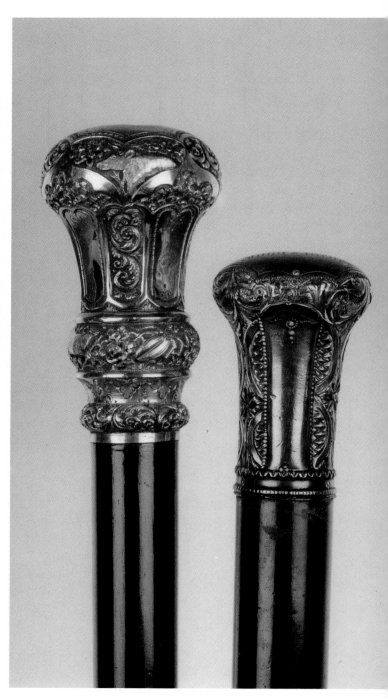

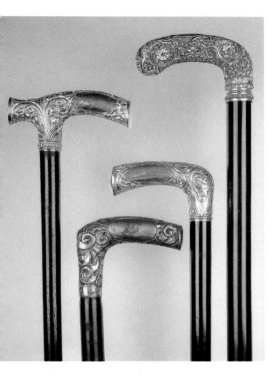

Four gold handled presentation canes, two uninscribed, one with initials JF and the far right reads on top, CAPT. PAINE, FROM FARRAGUT POST, GAR NO. 25, c. 1885, from 36" to 37 1/2" high.

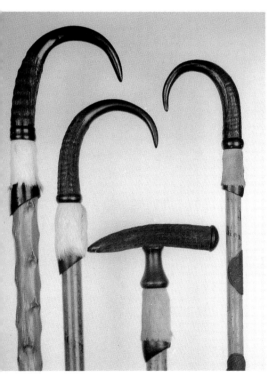

Four Swiss mountain canes of chamois goat: second from left marked JUNGFRAUBAHN; third from left marked MURREN; far left a woman's cane with metal town plates and Interlaken. Woman's cane 31 1/4" high. The rest range from 35 1/2" high to 37" high.

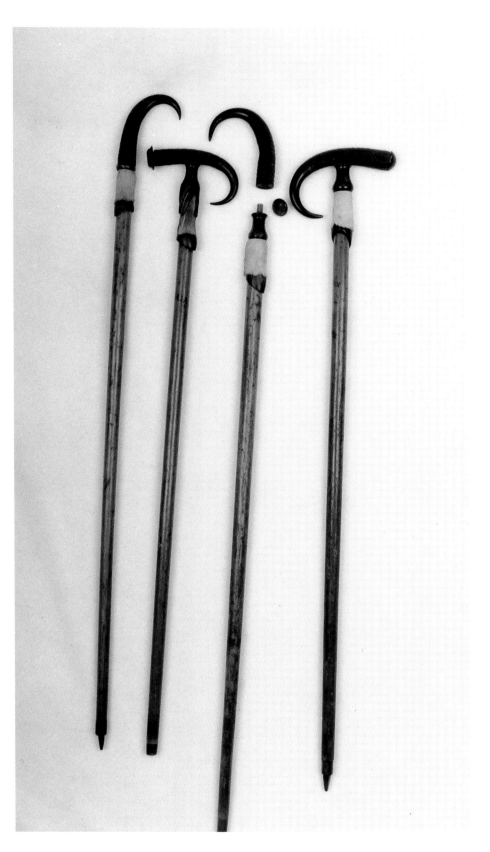

Four old mountain climbing canes, the handles change position depending on whether you have an uphill or downhill climb. Marked "Rigi Kulm;" "Ragaz;" (nothing); & "Chamonix." These four measure from 33 1/4" to 35 3/4" high.

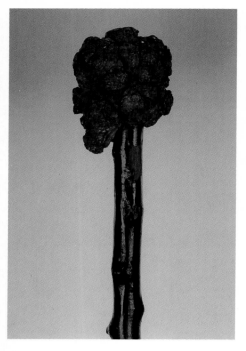

"The Leprechaun." Irish blackthorn with a natural burl in the shape of a face as the handle, 36 3/4" high.

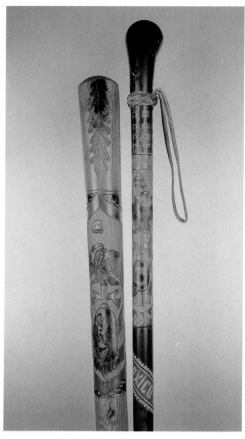

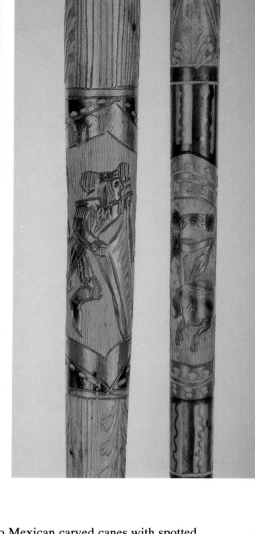

Mexican canes decorated with eagles and snakes along with bull fighters and bulls below. Left: 32 3/4" high; right: 35 1/2" high.

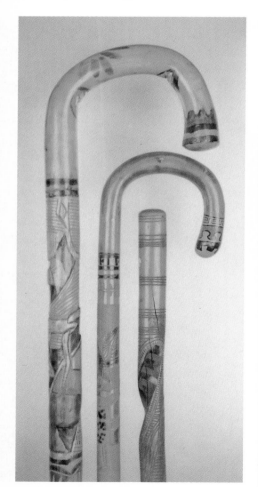

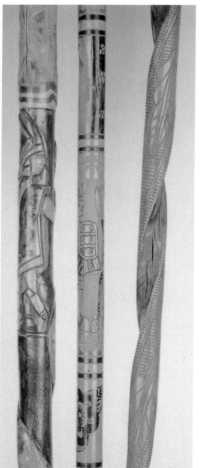

Three Mexican canes, polychrome paints on details, two crook handles, one straight, range from 36" to 38" high.

Two Mexican carved canes with spotted decoration, the left with a climbing snake, the right with a twisted shaft and the name "MEXICO" carved into the twist. Left: 35" high; right: 36 3/8" high.

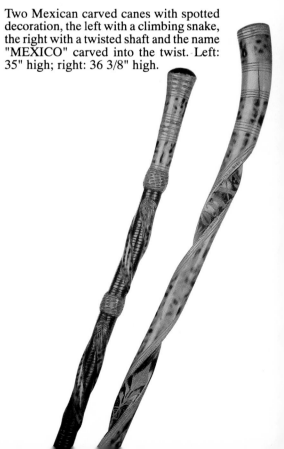

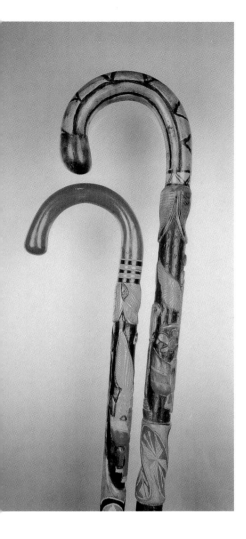

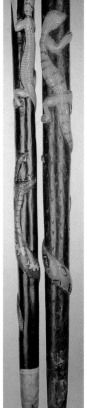

Three Mexican canes with snake heads at top and twining snakes or lizards, from 33 3/4" high to 37" high.

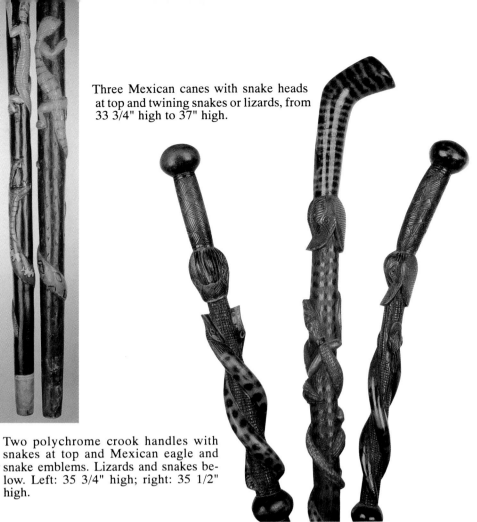

Two polychrome crook handles with snakes at top and Mexican eagle and snake emblems. Lizards and snakes below. Left: 35 3/4" high; right: 35 1/2" high.

Three Mexican canes with eagle and snake emblems. Below these emblems are snakes and men and women. These canes measure from 35 1/4" to 37 1/2" high.

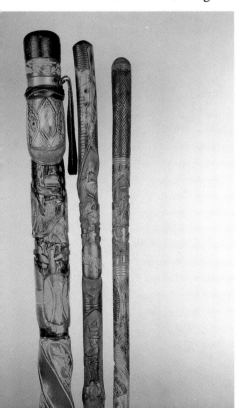

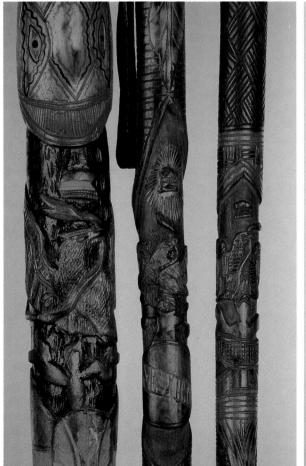

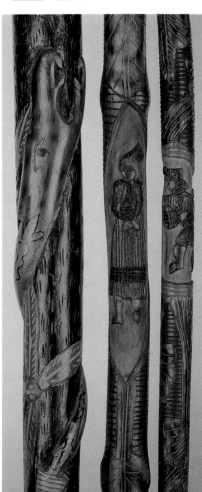

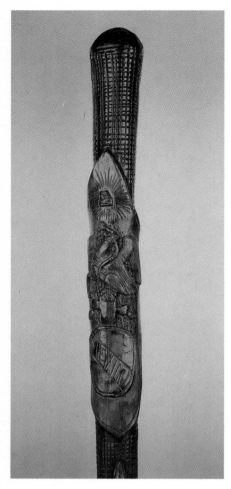

Mexican eagle and snake emblem along with the name "MEXICO" carved in the shaft above twining snakes, 36 3/4" high.

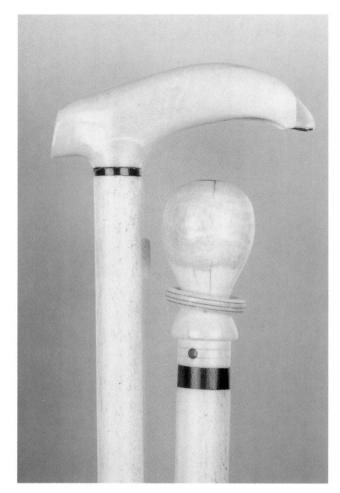

Two whale tooth ivory handled, whale bone shafted, scrimshaw canes — left: ivory tooth handle, baleen collar, c. 1870, 35" high; right: ivory knob handle, bone shaft, black baleen collar, and a free spinning whimsy ring on the handle, 36 5/8" high.

Scrimshaw, Folkart, and Gadget Canes

Happy collecting can be found in scrimshaw canes chair and stool canes of which many hundred different types have been patented, telescope canes, sword canes, primitive hand-carved canes, strange growth sticks, or canes connected with the sea, or owned by famous men.

Happy collecting can be found in scrimshaw canes.

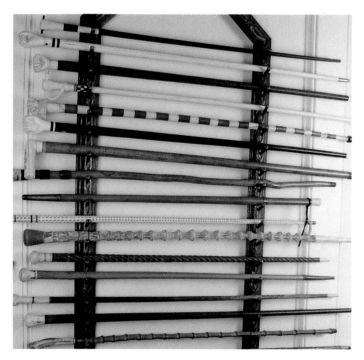

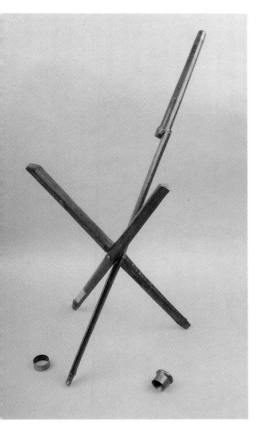

Unfolding seat cane — a tripod affair, 35 1/4" high. Canvas or leather seat rolls up and is carried in ones pocket.

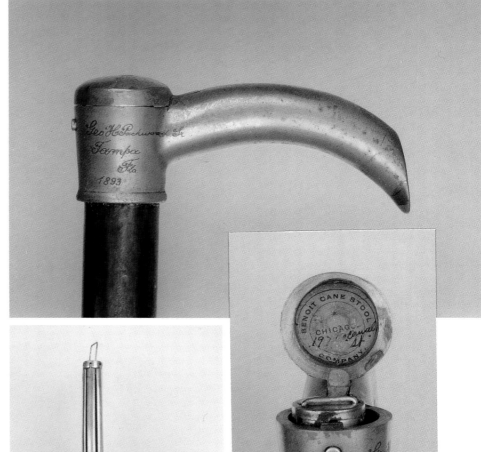

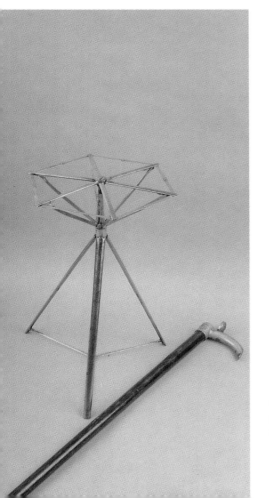

An innovative seat cane marked inside the lid "Benoit Cane Stool Company, Chicago," and engraved outside, "Geo. H. Packwood St., Tampa Fla. 1893." The seat is entirely encased in the hollow shaft. 33 1/4" high.

The fold away camp stool slides into the steel L handle shaft. It was made in Chicago, Illinois in 1905.

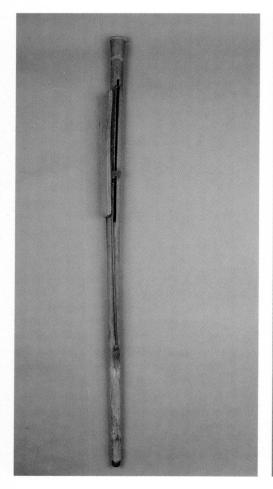

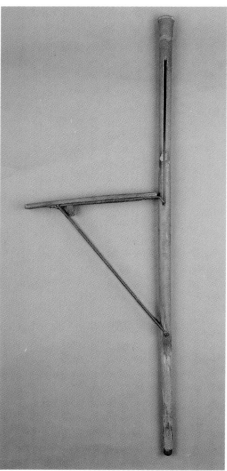

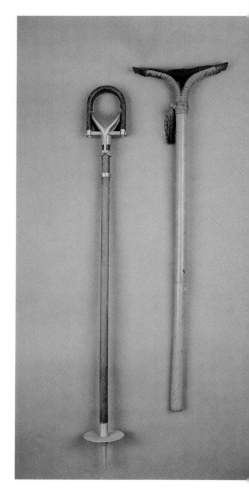

Seat cane. The seat folds out from the side. 37 3/4" high.

Two more seat canes. Left: folds out to be a one legged seat, 36 1/2" high folded shut, 32" high unfolded; right: always a seat, "ES-TIK Co. Hollywood" printed on bottom of the leather seat, 33" high.

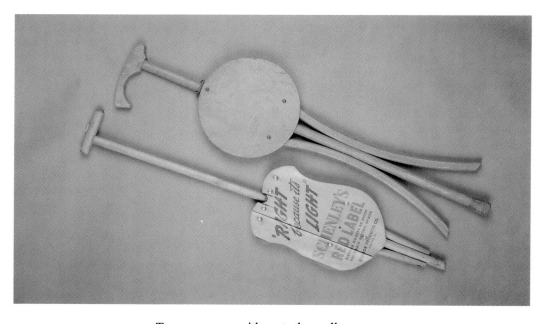

Two seat canes with seats that pull out to make three legged stools. Left: beer ad cane, 34 1/2" high; right: 35 1/4" high with a circular seat.

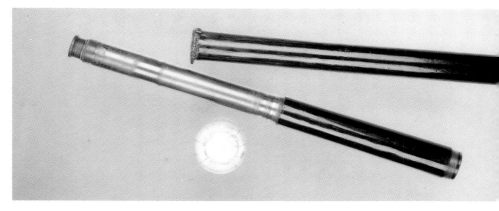

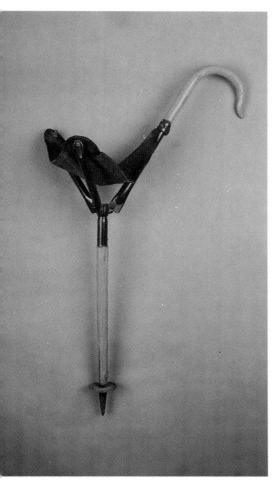

German seat cane folded out with a triangular seat and a crook handle, c. 1900, 36 1/2" high.

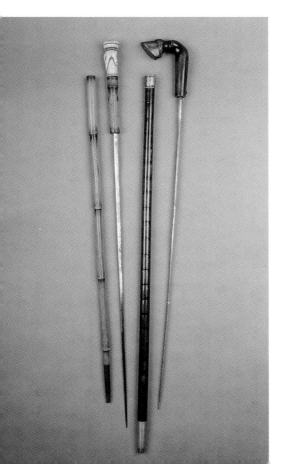

French telescope cane given to Isaac Hall by his friend Benjamin L. Swan in 1852. 36 3/4" high.

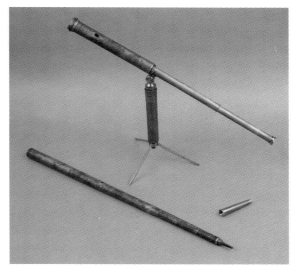

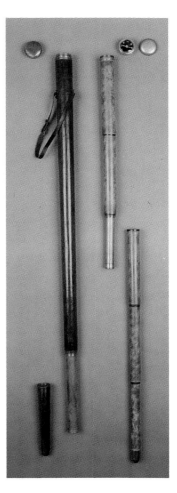

Very old seaman's telescope in brass. Inscribed on the tube is, "Davis Brothers opticians to HRH Prince Albert 33 New Bond Street London" ... and ... "Sold by Melling & Payne 39 S. Castle Street Liverpool." It has false eyelets, dates from c. 1750, and measures 36 1/2" high.

Two optical telescope canes. Left: the entire length of the shaft is the scope with a long brass ferrule, 33 1/2" high, 6 1/2" long ferrule; right: the scope takes up half of the shaft, a compass is hidden in the silver handle, and the bottom third of the shaft is hollow for the storage of maps, 36 1/4" high.

Ivory handle carved in the shape of a hand sporting a decorated triangular sword blade within, c. 1700, 35 3/8" high. Horse hoof handle with a decorated triangular blade, c. 1915, 37" high.

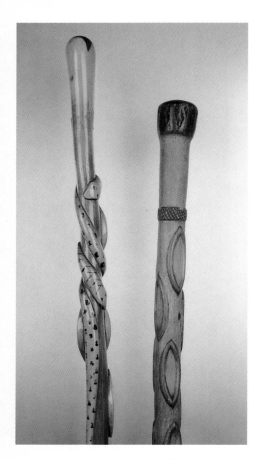

Two diamond willow wood canes — one with an entwined snakes: 35 3/4" high, and the other with a carved band: 34 1/2" high.

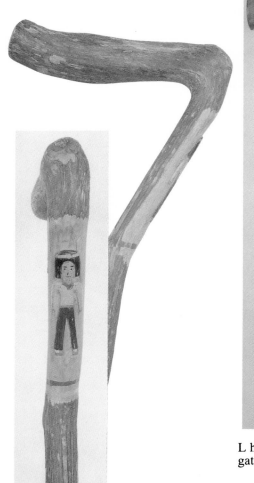

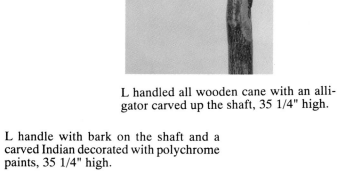

L handled all wooden cane with an alligator carved up the shaft, 35 1/4" high.

L handle with bark on the shaft and a carved Indian decorated with polychrome paints, 35 1/4" high.

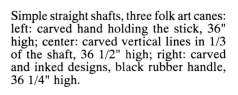

Simple straight shafts, three folk art canes: left: carved hand holding the stick, 36" high; center: carved vertical lines in 1/3 of the shaft, 36 1/2" high; right: carved and inked designs, black rubber handle, 36 1/4" high.

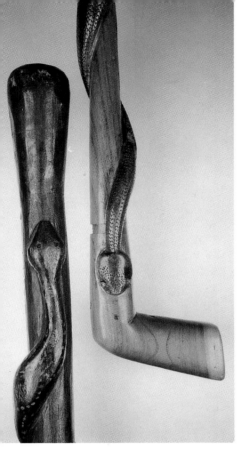

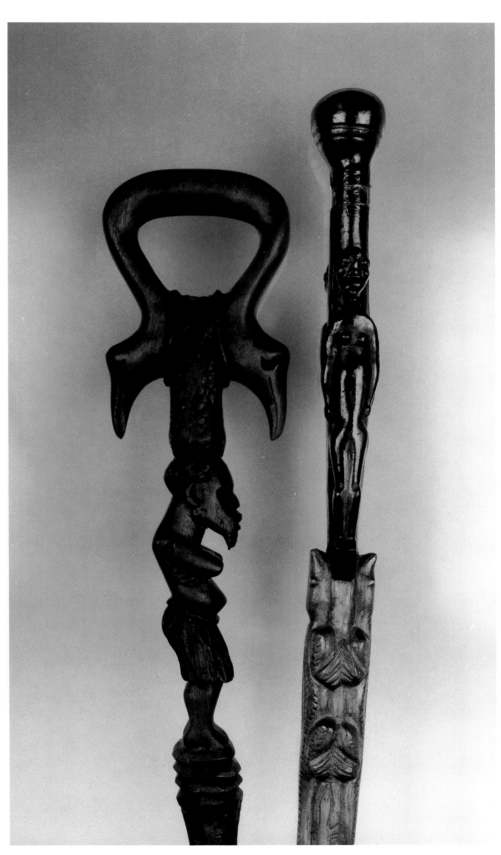

Knob and L handled canes with snakes winding up the shafts (the one on the right is a rattlesnake). L handle has wooden inlays forming the sun on the reverse. Polychrome designs. 33 1/4" high knob handle, 35" high L handle.

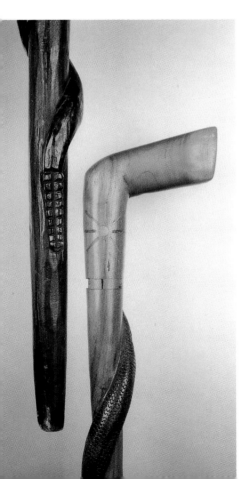

Two full figures on African canes, left with loop handle, right with knob. Left: 35; Right: 37" high.

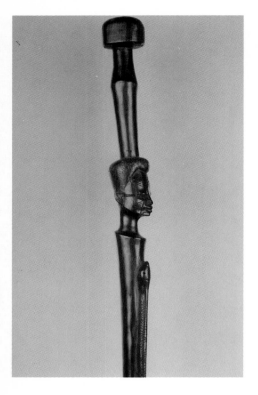

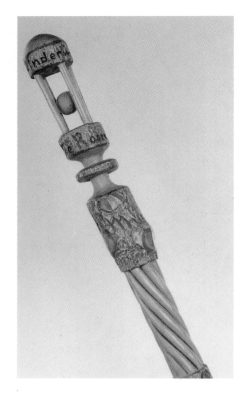

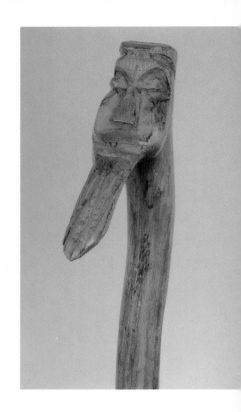

Smaller knob handle stick with a human head and a snake, 36" high.

Whimsy stick with caged ball and moving disk, bark remains on the shaft, inscribed Windermere, Lake Rosseau, Muskoka, 39 1/2" high.

Bearded man carved with puffy cheeks, folk art, 38 1/2" high.

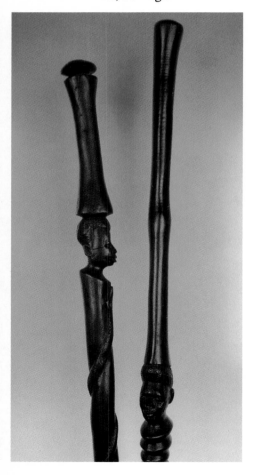

Two fish or snakes with carved and painted detail, 42 1/2" high, 39 1/4" high.

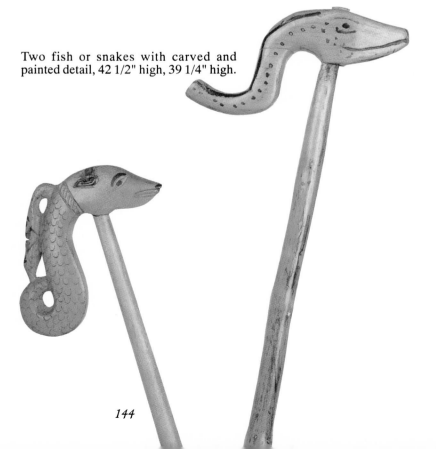

Two ebonized sticks with carved figures, left figure with snake, left: 40 3/4" high; right: 40" high.

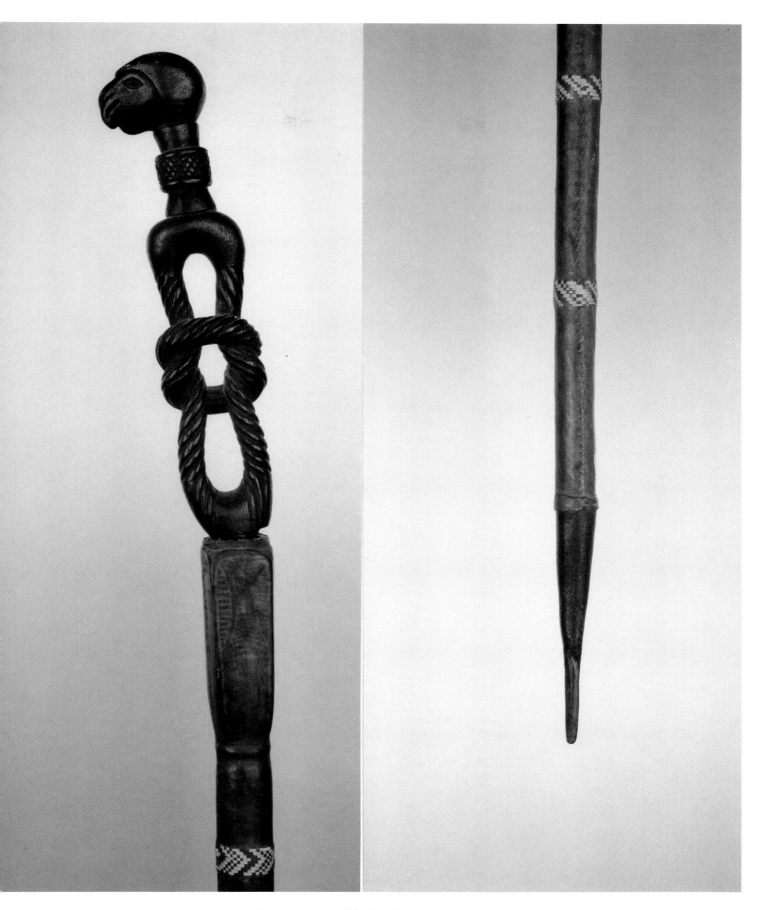

Carved knot and bird black handle on a
shaft covered with sewn leather, and
tipped with a pointed ferrule, 38 1/4" high.

145

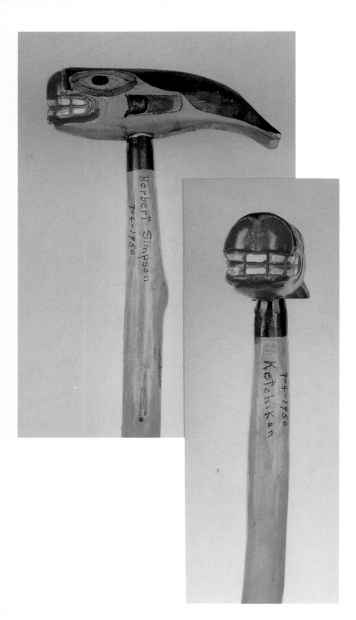

Opposite page:

Cane commemorating Thomas Jefferson and the University of Virginia, reads: "University VA" "Rotunda Burnt Oct. 27, 1895" "1821 Jefferson's Tomb" "Thomas Jefferson of VA Born Shadwell VA April 1743 Was President USA 1801 to 1809" "Wrote Declaration of Independence 1771 Founder University VA 1819" "Died July 4 1824 This Cane Was Cut Near Jefferson's Tomb Monticello VA" "Jefferson's Dying Words I Resign My Spirit To God My Daughter. To My Country." 35" high.

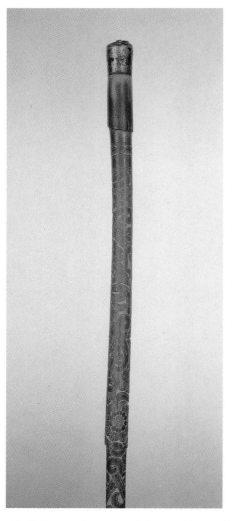

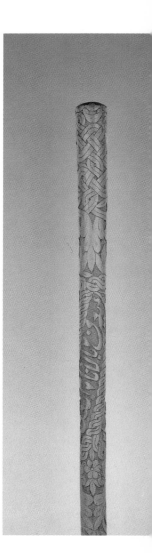

Carved and painted whale, signed by carver Herbert Simpson 7-4-1950 Ketchikan, 34 1/2" high.

Relief carved cane in a foliate pattern and silver handle, 35 1/2" high.

Carved Whitewood cane purchased in Paris. It dates from 1900 and is covered features Persian writing. 36 1/2" high.

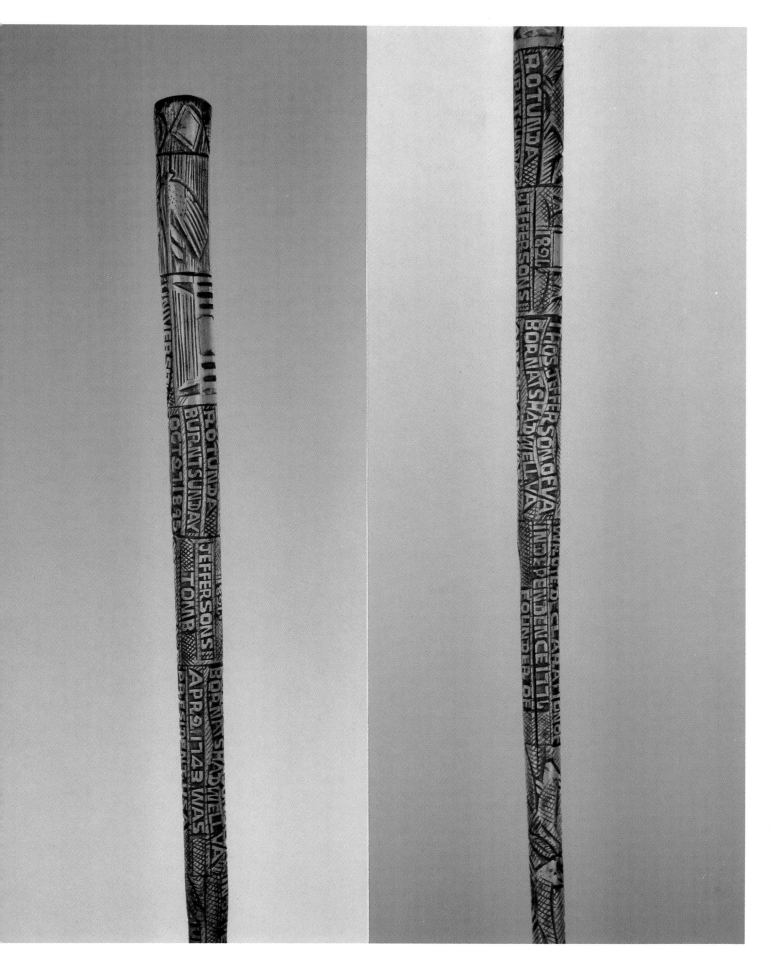

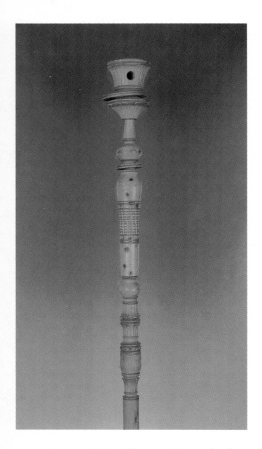

Whimsy stick with two free-spinning disks, 39 1/4" high.

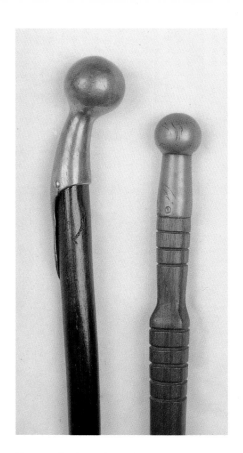

Two early American folk art brass knob handles made from buggy harnesses. 36 & 39 1/4" high.

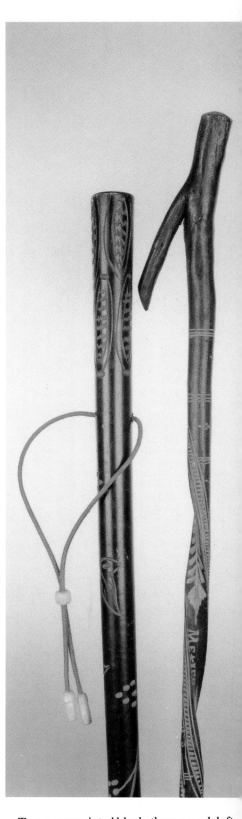

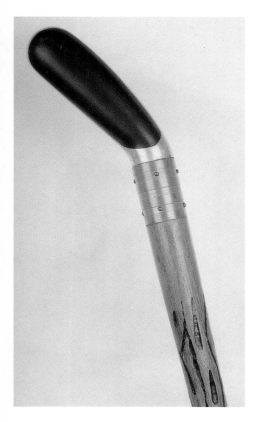

Pistol grip cane with brass collar from the Mideast or Orient, carved and painted shaft, 41 5/8" high.

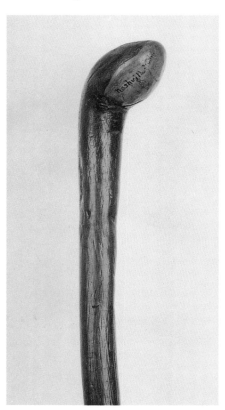

Simple pistol grip folk art cane with Nashville, Tenn. penned on the handle, 33" high.

Two canes painted black, then carved, left with eyelets and wrist cord, right with a branch at the handle. Left: 34 1/2" high; right: 33 3/4" high.

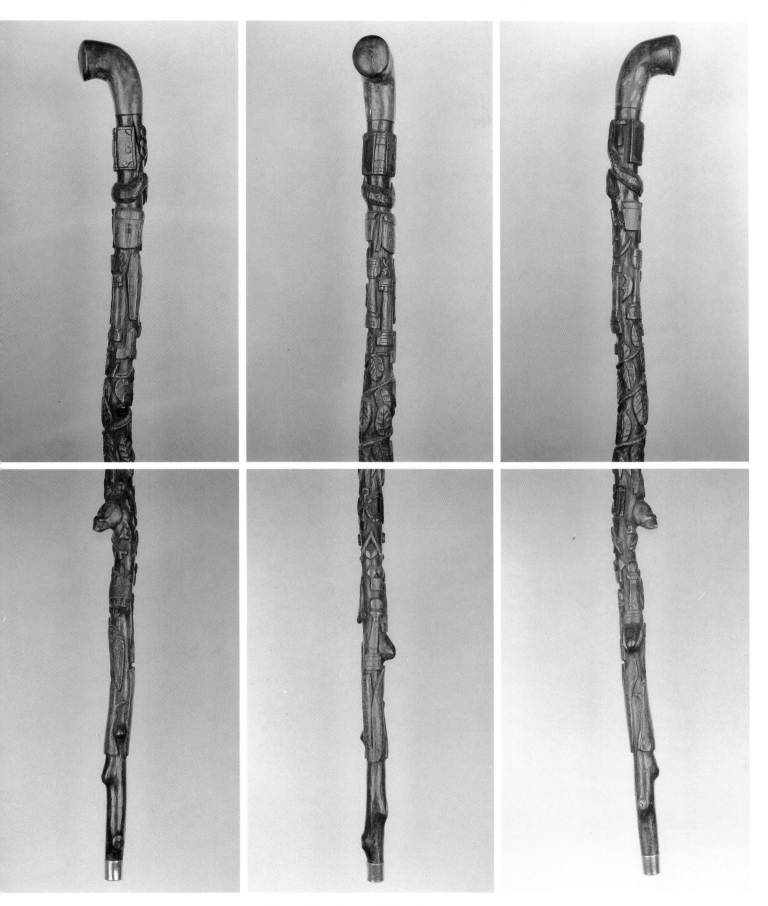

Masonic hand-carved folk art cane, covered with Masonic symbols from Bec de Corbin handle to ferrule, 35 1/8" high.

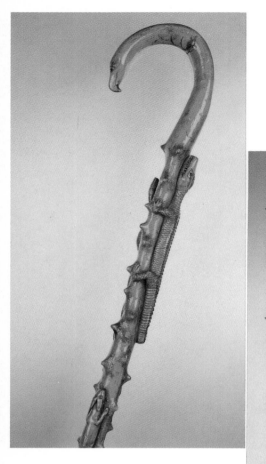

Folk art eagle's head handle with well carved animal menagerie climbing the shaft, 33 1/2" high.

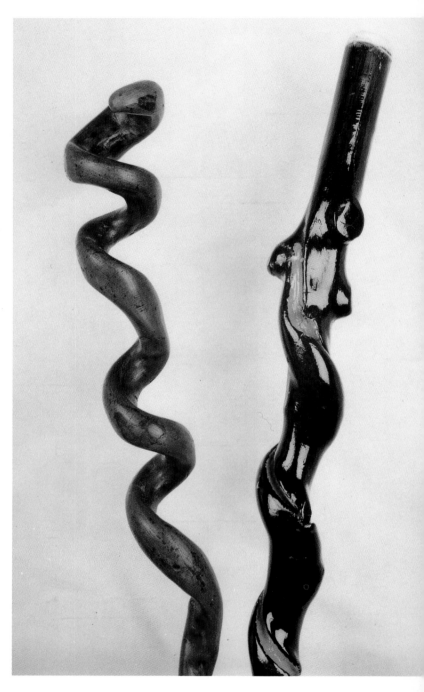

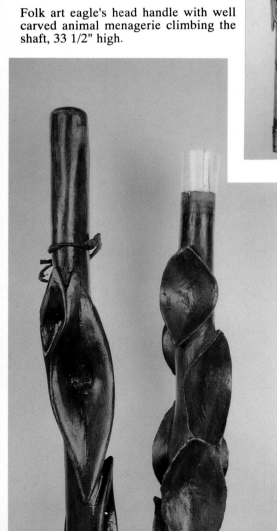

Two "twisties", naturally twisted shafts, the right hand shaft is painted white at the top and has gold paint down along the inside of the twist. Left: 35" high; right: 40 1/4" high.

Two diamond willow branch shaft canes. Left with unfinished eyelets, right with an bone handle. Left: 40 1/2" high; right: 34 1/2" high.

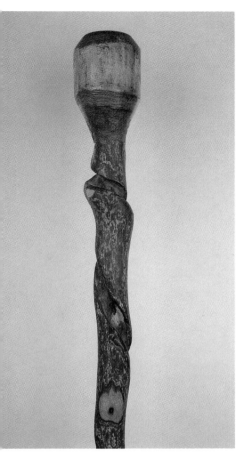

Knob handle with a naturally twisting shaft, 37 1/2" high.

Two diamond willow branches, left with a knob handle, 37 1/4" high; right curves, 37 1/2" high.

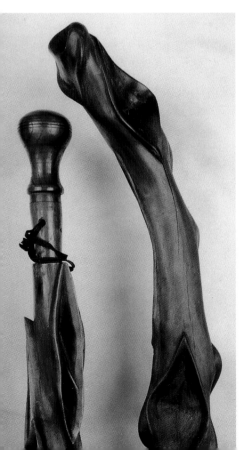

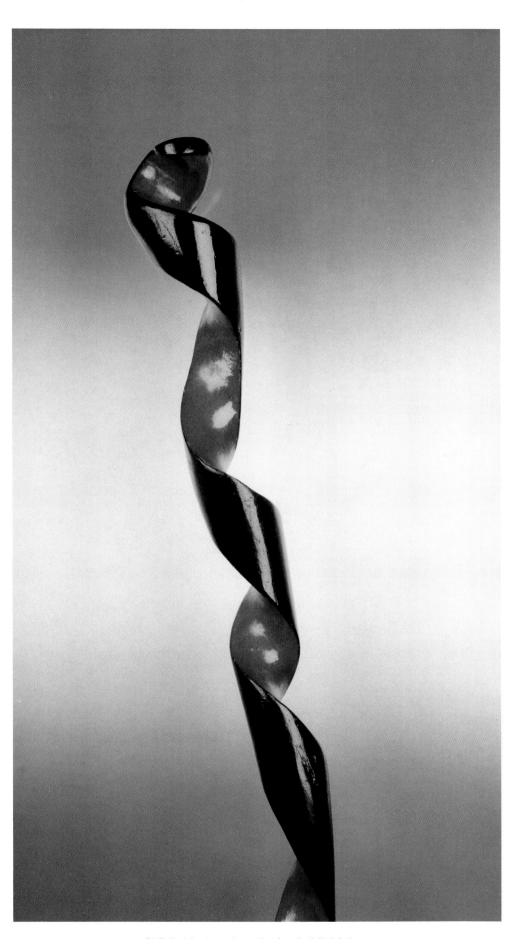

Child's black and tan "twisty", 35" high.

151

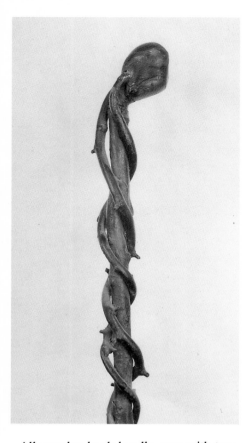

All wooden knob handle cane with two twined vines, 36" high.

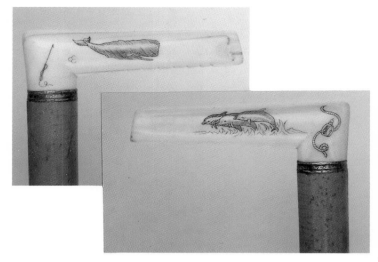

Whale bone handle with whale on one side and two dolphins on the other, malacca shaft, thin silver collar, 33 1/4" high.

Scrimshaw cane with a whale tooth handle featuring a fitted lid. The inside of the tooth is hollow and may have been used to store tobacco or snuff. Below the handle a dagger fits into the shaft. This canes dates to c. 1880.

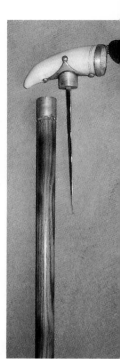

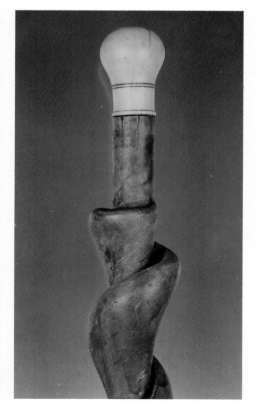

Old ivory knob on a naturally twisted shaft formed by a vine wrapped around a young tree, called a "twisty stick" in England. 35" high.

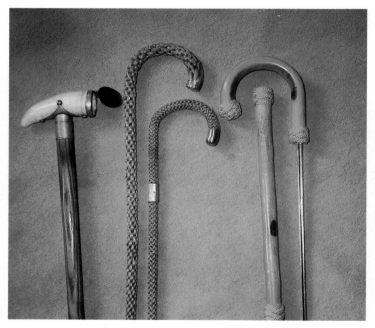

Scrimshaw canes. The canes at the left and right ends house a dagger and a sword respectively.

Silver straight handle, eyelets, and silver nail heads on knobs of shaft with one letter of Jackson on each head down the shaft. This cane belonged to General Andrew Jackson and was given to a Civil War soldier named George C De Zouche by Jackson himself. This cane was obtained by B.W. Cooke Sr. from the soldier's grandson Fred C. De Zouche in 1934. Thence it came into the hands of the author. 32 3/4" high.

Presidential, Political, and Presentation Canes

There are the presidential and political canes , and gold-headed presentation canes; canes made from wood of historical places such as old ships or old buildings. I have one fine gold-headed cane engraved on the top:

"Presented to James F. Henderson by his sons Charles & Wilbur 1865"

and on the side between the elaborate scroll it reads:

"A stick from the log cabin built by A. Lincoln in Macon Co. Illinois A.D. 1830"

I have another old presidential cane that has silver eyelets and a fine silver handle reading:

"James Lowden to Joel Manning, 1863"

surrounded by the legend:

"Tomb of Washington 1842"

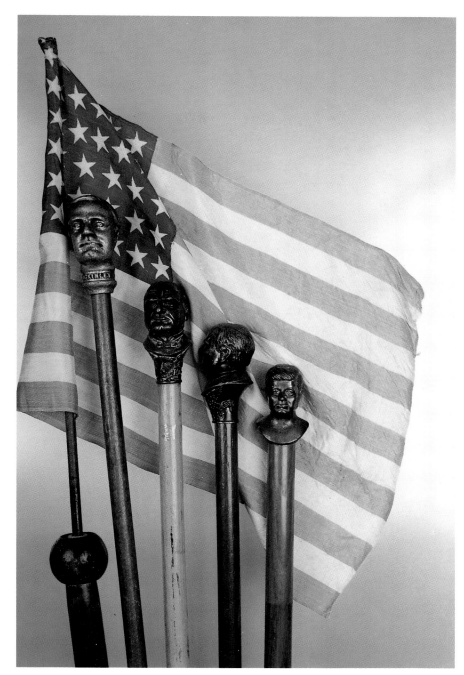

Red flag cane, 35" high; four campaign canes with busts: left McKinley 37 1/4" high; Two more McKinley's 35" high reading Protection on one side and 1896 on the other, John F. Kennedy bust, 33 1/2" high.

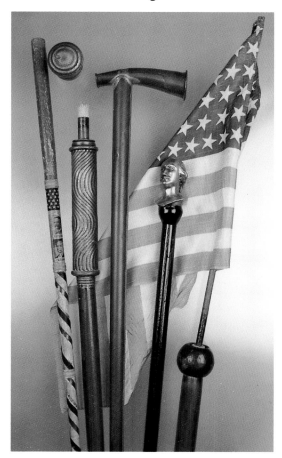

Five political campaign canes: left to right, Roosevelt and Fairbanks wood cane with paper decoration, 36" high; torch cane, sheet metal on a wooden shaft, 35 1/4" high; noisemaker horn cane with campaign slogan PATRIOTISM, PROTECTION, PROSPERITY, by the Winfield Manufacturing Company, 33" high; brass bust of George Washington on a black wood shaft, 36 1/4" high; red knob handled flag cane, 35" high.

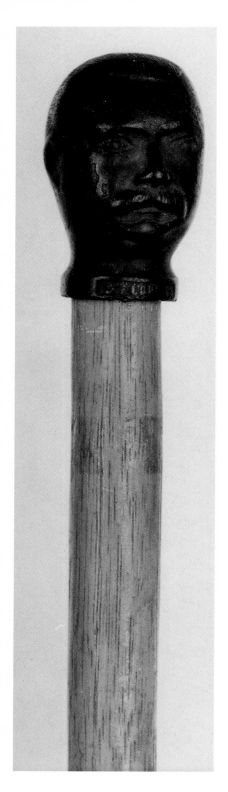

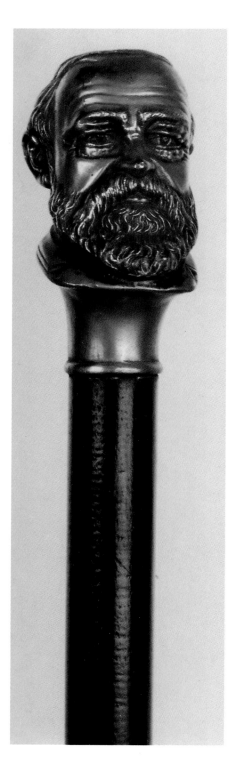

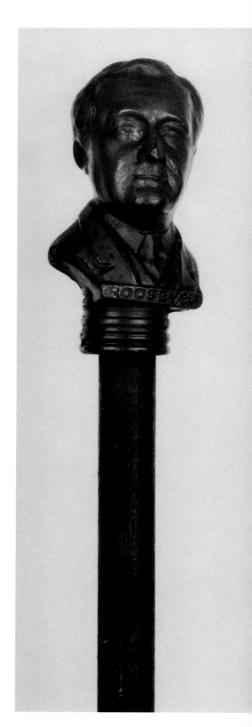

Bust of a man (possibly Cleveland) marked St. Louis below the head on the handle, 32 1/4" high.

A fancy William Henry Harrison campaign cane in silver plate, 34 1/4" high.

Roosevelt bust in bronze, on the back is printed CENTURY OF PROGRESS from the 1933 Worlds Fair. 32 3/4" high.

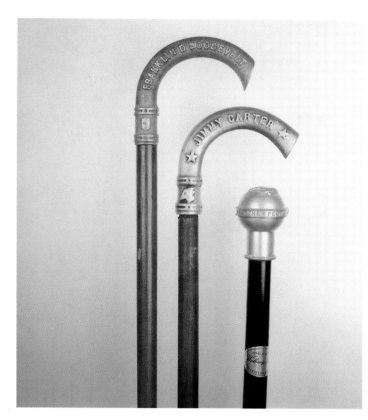
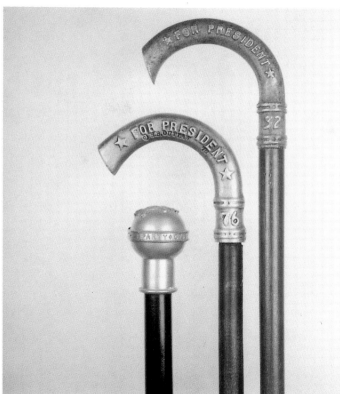

Crook handled Franklin D. Roosevelt and
Jimmy Carter canes with globe handled
The Party of the People of the Democratic
Party, both crook handles 35 1/2" high,
globe, 35 1/2" high.

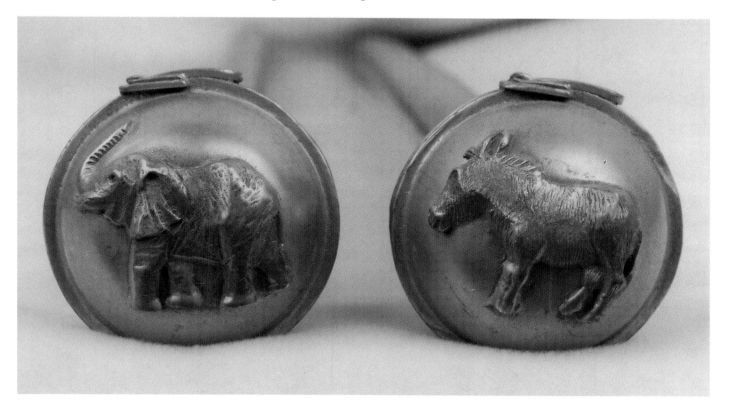

Political party globes, Republican elephant, Democratic donkey.

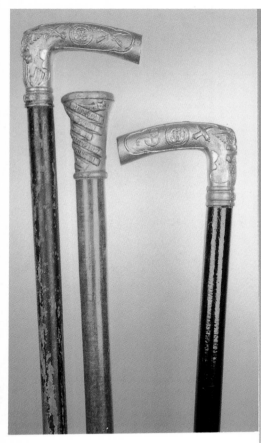

Three canes from Northern veterans of the Civil War, left and right marked GAR and with regimental symbology, center marked with Grant's portrait on top and on the side with 25TH ANNUAL EN-CAMPMENT G.A.R. SEPTEMBER 20TH 1892 WASHINGTON D.C. Left hand cane also has a flag in the ferrule with a cork attachment to hold it in the end of the cane for waving high. Left: 35 1/4" high; center: 33" high; right: 32 1/4" high.

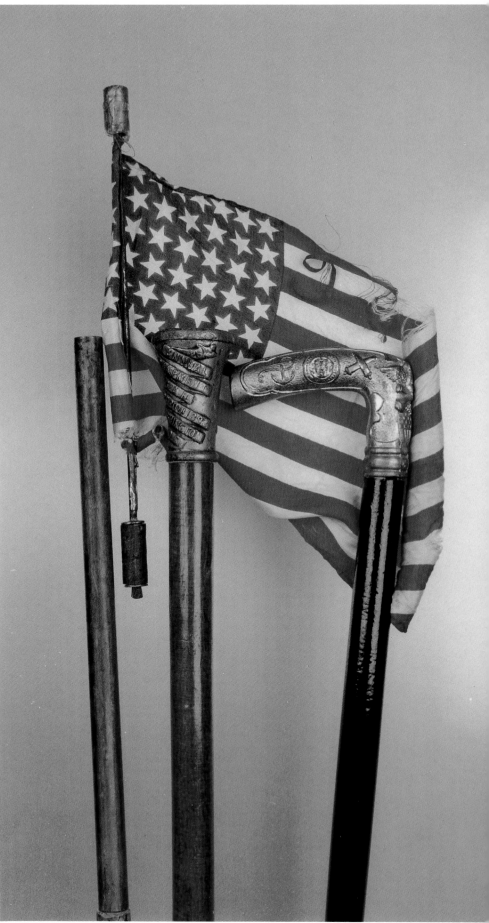

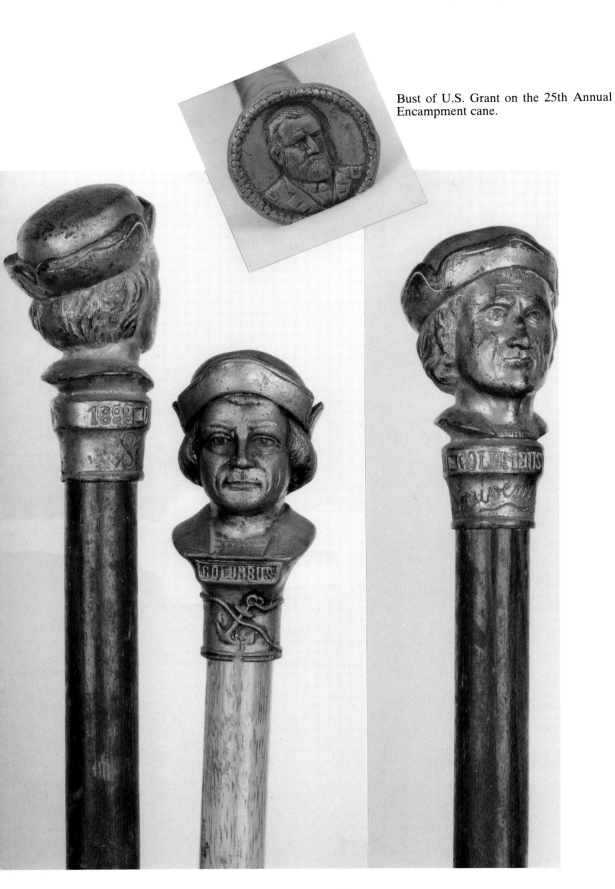

Bust of U.S. Grant on the 25th Annual Encampment cane.

Not exactly political or presentation canes, these two commemorate Christopher Columbus. The cane on the left is marked Souvenir, Chicago, 1893. Left: 33 3/4" high; right: 37 1/4" high.

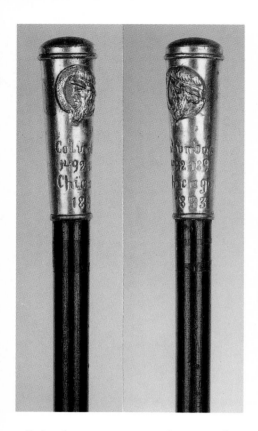

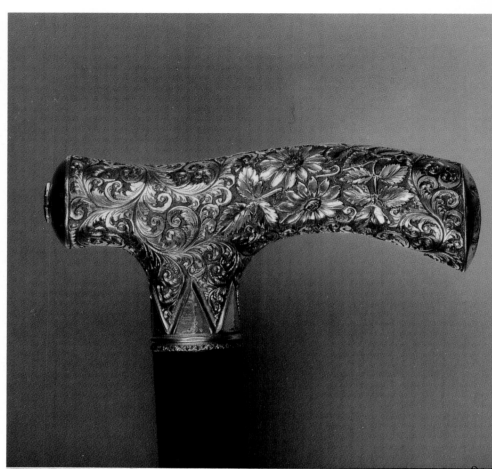

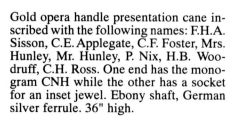

Columbus commemorative cane inscribed "Columbus 1492-1892 Chicago 1893," 36 1/8" high.

Gold opera handle presentation cane inscribed with the following names: F.H.A. Sisson, C.E. Applegate, C.F. Foster, Mrs. Hunley, Mr. Hunley, P. Nix, H.B. Woodruff, C.H. Ross. One end has the monogram CNH while the other has a socket for an inset jewel. Ebony shaft, German silver ferrule. 36" high.

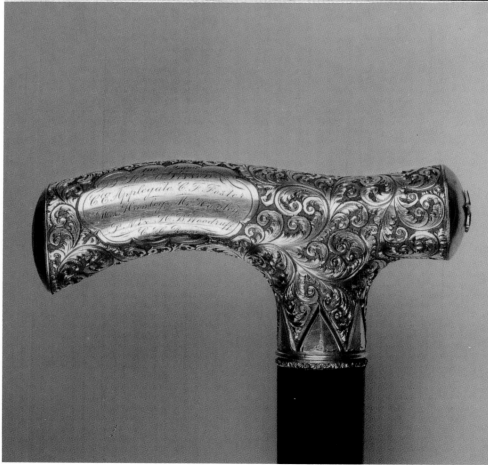

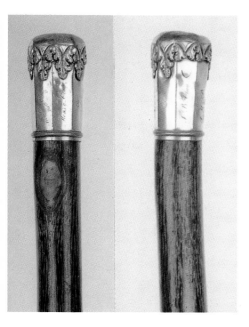

Small gold handled relic cane reading on the side panels From the Birth Place of Henry Clay. To J.B. Clay From J.W.B. (or just a souvenir), 34 3/4" high.

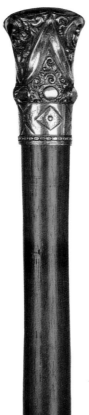

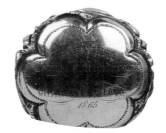

Presentation cane with a gold knob handle inscribed on top, "Presented to James F. Henderson by his sons Charles and Wilbur 1865," and on the side with, "A stick from the log cabin built by A. Lincoln in Macon County, Illinois, AD 1834." 35 1/8" high.

Presentation cane from the Abraham Lincoln log cabin.

Simple wooden cane with a deep relief portrait of Abraham Lincoln. 35 3/4" high.

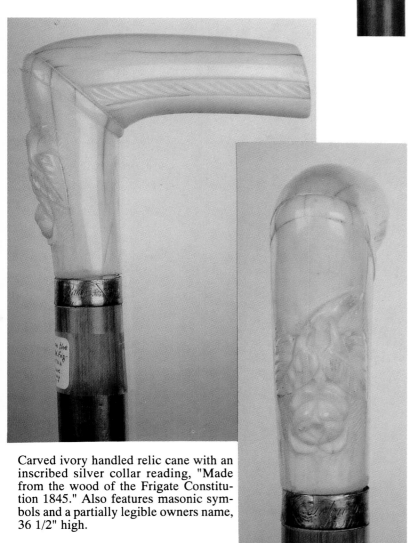

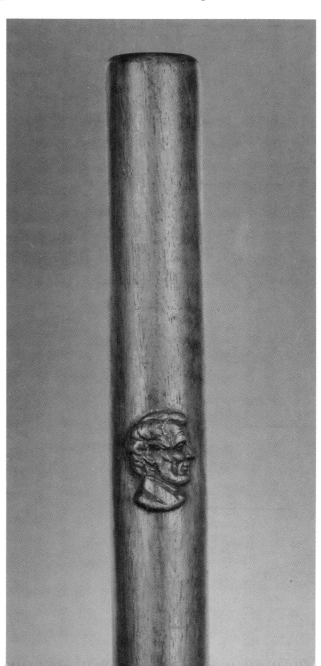

Carved ivory handled relic cane with an inscribed silver collar reading, "Made from the wood of the Frigate Constitution 1845." Also features masonic symbols and a partially legible owners name, 36 1/2" high.

Paired and Children's Canes

To some collectors the paired "his and her" canes have greater appeal , or the children's canes. It was quite the style at one time for children to have identical canes to their parents, much like modern Easter parade clothing. One is a child's gadget cane that opens up to conceal his pens and pencils.

His and hers walking sticks with pewter end caps. His measures 36" high; hers measures 35 1/8" high.

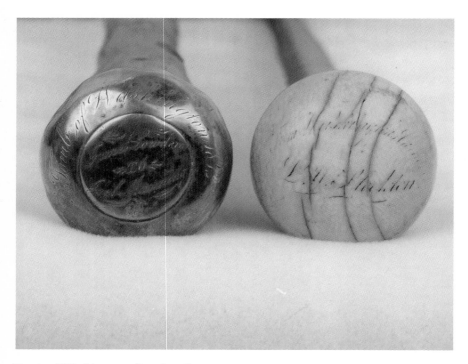

Political relic cane with a silver knob handle marked on top, "Tomb of Washington, 1842, James Sowder to Joel Manning 1962."

Tomb of Washington silver handle cane, engraved in center "James Lowden to Carl Manning 1863." Around the center is printed "Tomb of Washington, 1842." Knobby, light shaft with silver eyelets.

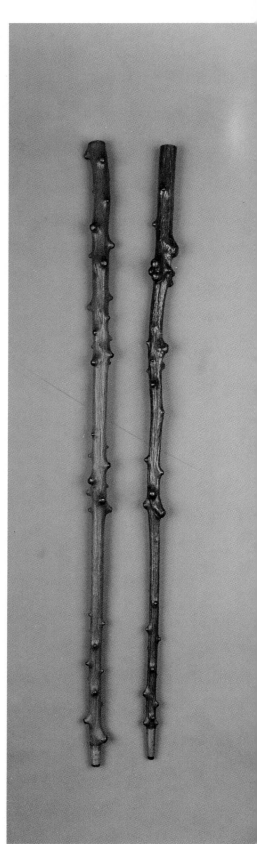

Weapon Canes

Pneumatic and cartridge gun canes and other weapon canes are all there for the hunter who can find them.

Animals

There are many canes with dog heads , horse heads or hooves , elephant heads , and bird's heads , that have a special appeal to some collectors.

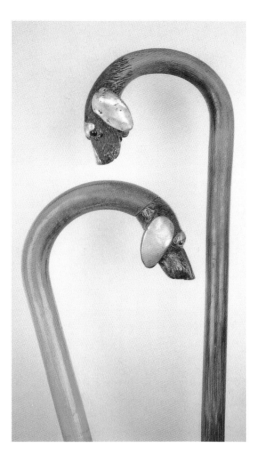

Two greyhounds carved in ivory with glass inset eyes and silver collars, c. 1910. Left: 33 1/4" high; right: 35" high.

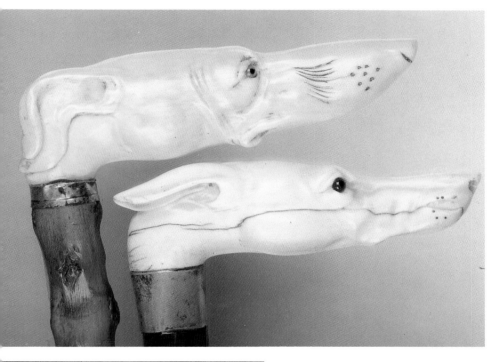

Two German crook handled dog's head canes with silver ears, eyebrows and noses, both 35" high.

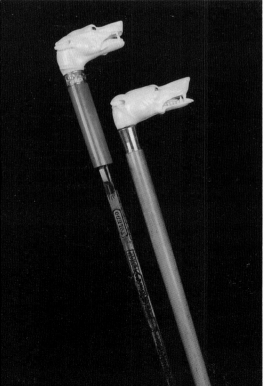

Ivory horse's head L-shaped handle with silver bridle and collar and inset glass eyes, 34 1/2" high.

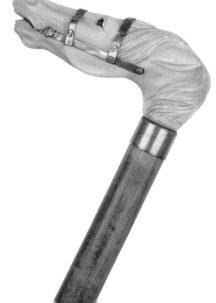

Two snarling hounds in ivory with silver and gold collars. The lower hound, with a twist of the wrist releases a fine Toledo sword blade. Malacca shafts. Produced in Europe and dating form c. 1870-1890. 35 3/4" high sword cane; 34 3/4" high for the silver collared cane.

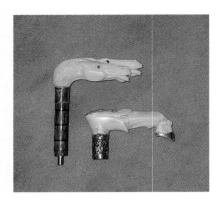

There are many canes with horses heads and hooves.

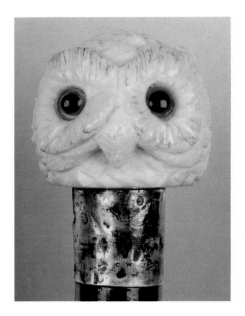

Two stag horn elephants with inset glass eyes and silver collars on malacca shafts, c. 1900. The right hand elephant is secured to a twisted shaft. Left: 34" high. Right: 34 1/2" high.

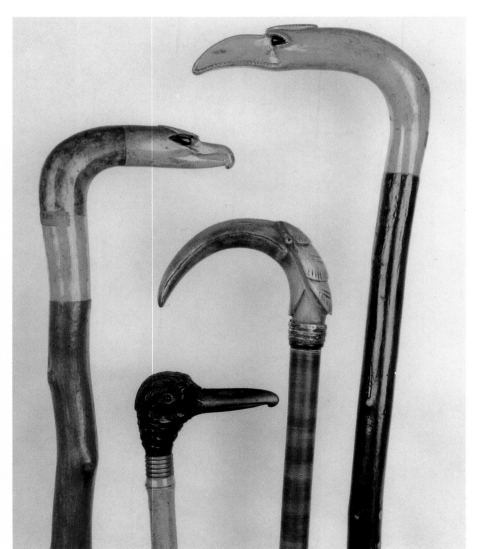

Four birds, polychrome detail, some with glass eyes, range from 33 3/4" to 35" high. Left to right: The first and fourth were made by Willard M. Chandler of the Old Soldiers Home in Togus, Maine. They were made prior to 1918. The third is a horn handle on a shaft of paper disks.

Ivory knob handle owl with glass eyes and a silver collar bearing hallmarks, c. 1890. 33 1/2" high, no ferrule.

Hands

One doctor in my town, specializing in hand surgery, wants to collect canes depicting hands. This is a rare field, but I have quite a few.

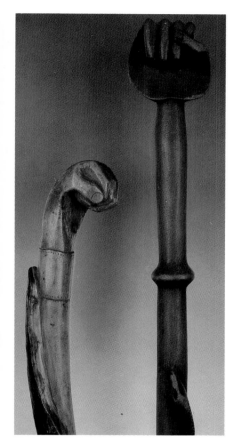

Six scrimshaw fists, one clasping a ball, two with batons, one a snake, three with shirt cuffs, from 31 3/4" to 35 3/4" high.

Two fists and snakes, the left fist is holding a heart shape, the right is simply clenched. Left: 36" high; right: 36 1/4" high.

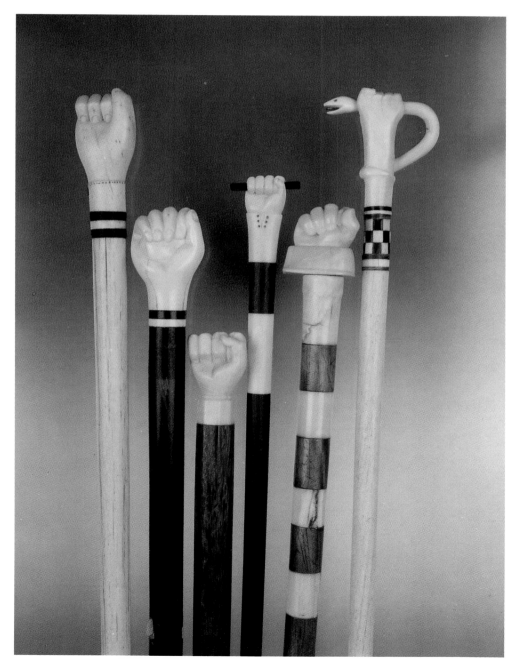

Bovine Canes

There are even commemorative canes honoring brave bulls who fought well in the ring, and the Spanish aficionados were wont to have walking sticks, suitably engraved, made of the copulatory organ of a famous Toro. In Africa, similar phallic canes of wild animals can be found that were the sole prerogative of the tribal chief to carry, for he was the one with the harem and it was felt the prowess of the animal would be endowed upon the man carrying the cane.

If these phallic canes are to be considered gauche, what about those canes made of human skin? And in America too! Until the abhorrent practice was stopped by publicity, convicts of the Ohio State Penitentiary who were hanged were skinned and their hide was made into canes and razor straps.

The Columbus Star for June 7, 1936, reported that in the 1880's convicts who were hanged at the Ohio State Penitentiary were skinned by workmen, and the hides were tanned and used for making razor straps and walking sticks. This precipitated a scandal in a gubernatorial campaign and the practice was stopped.

To me, however, of all the canes to be found, the greatest thrill is to discover a new gadget cane, for it is almost impossible to exhaust the wonders of these container canes.

Of all the canes to be found, I get the greatest thrill from discovering new gadget canes. It is almost impossible to exhaust the wonders of these container canes. Sterling silver handled shaving razor and brush, c. 1895, malacca shaft, razor marked "KEEN as is this razors edge invisible - Shakespeare Love's Labor Lost" and "George Sutler & Co. Trinity Works, Sheffield, England", 34 1/2" high.

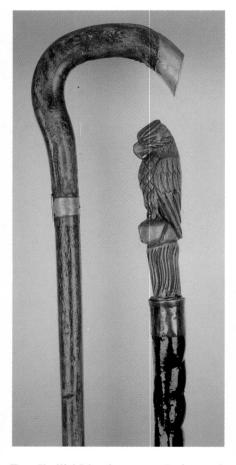

Two "bullish" bovine canes. Left: crook handle with silver end cap and collar in shape of a buckle, 35 1/2" high; right: wooden eagle handle on a twisted shaft, 34 1/2" high.

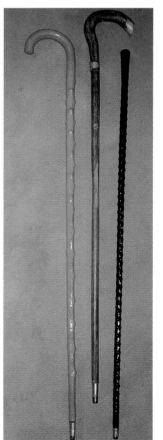

Three bovine canes.

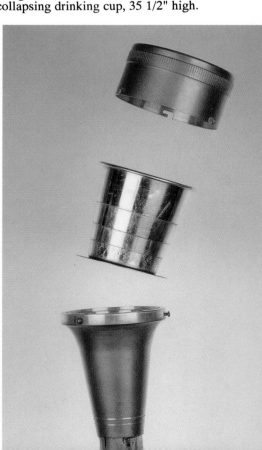

Gadget cane with a brass handle and a collapsing drinking cup, 35 1/2" high.

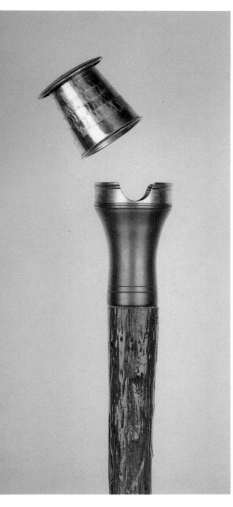

Silver collapsing drinking cup cane; pull the top of the handle off to free the cup, 35" high.

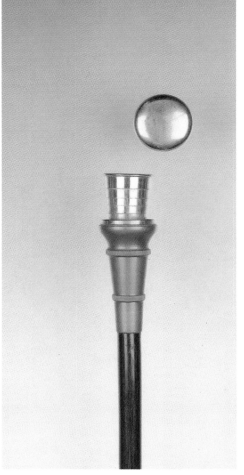

Yet another brass collapsible drinking cup cane, 36" high.

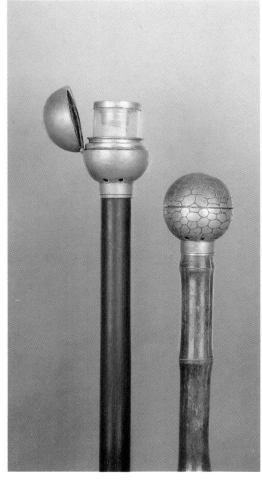

Two silver globular lantern canes with rising candle and glass lens within. Left: 35 1/4" high; right: 35 1/2" high.

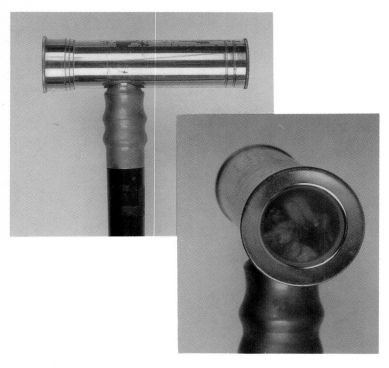

Brass kaleidoscope cane handle, 37 5/8"
high. Reads on top Van Cor[rest worn off]
Instrument makers.

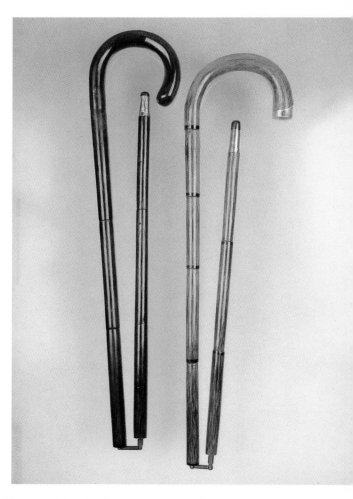

Two crook handled traveling canes. They
fold in half for convenient storage during
travel. Left: simple stepped wood only,
35 1/2" high; right: partridge wood shaft
with Sterling Silver end cap, 34 3/4" high.
Both c. 1910.

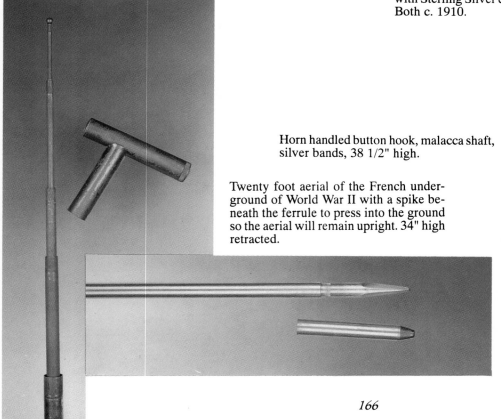

Horn handled button hook, malacca shaft,
silver bands, 38 1/2" high.

Twenty foot aerial of the French underground of World War II with a spike beneath the ferrule to press into the ground
so the aerial will remain upright. 34" high
retracted.

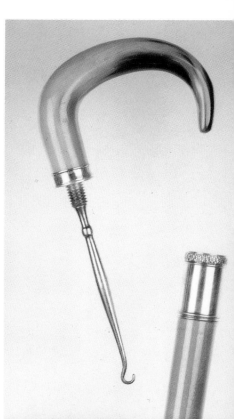

Chapter 6
Gadget Canes

There is a group of walking sticks called gadget canes. They are also known as container, trick or dual purpose canes. The English call them system sticks or patent canes. As the name implies, they are walking sticks that contain or do something other then merely hold one up as is the sole function of the orthopedic stick. As a concession to style, it was an attempt to make the walking stick useful as well as ornamental. They have existed from time immemorial, ever since man has tried to conceal something in his stick to give him an advantage over an unsuspecting fellow man (weapon cane), or to smuggle something in or out of the country, or to ease the carrying of more then one item at the same time (tradesmen's cane).

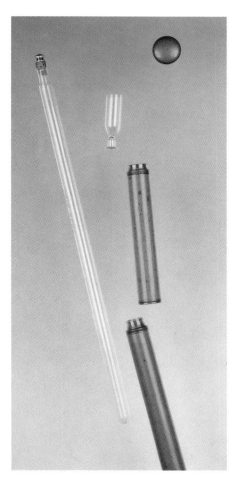

Toper's (or tippler's) cane used to carry an alcoholic beverage and a small glass in secret. Very popular during Prohibition in the United States.

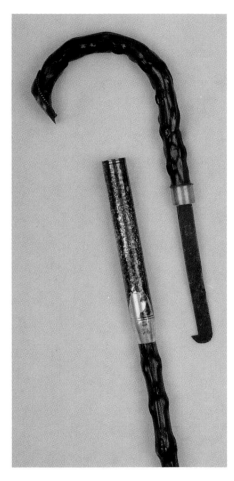

Lobsterman's old lobster measure, silver center and end cap, 33 1/2" high.

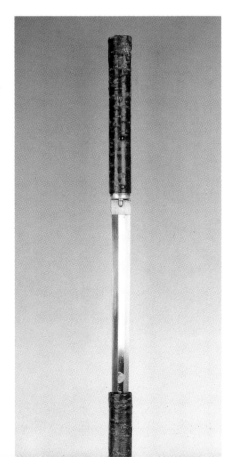

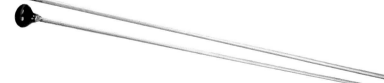

A Japanese sword cane with a push button release that reveals a very bright single edged blade, 34 1/2" high.

Angel Wing probe, c. 1950, 37 1/2" high.

Gadget canes evolved because of necessity. A man had need for and therefore made a gun cane, or a piano tuner in a cane - just to give an example of the thousand uses that have made a stick more than just a cane. All early canes of this type were first made by the individual requiring this particular device. It may thereafter have been patented, but just as many patented canes never found a market, so many a stick that was generally "homemade" and not factory produced became very popular. To decry the "homemade" dual purpose stick as a fraud is therefore foolish. It may be one of the finest collectibles except for the extra fastidious. Fifty years from now the "homemade" cane will be just as valuable as the patented canes and considerably rarer. I feel that any well-made stick that contains or does something to fulfill the double purpose definition is a good collectible, even if it was made only recently - such as the stainless steel angel-wing shell fish prober I display.

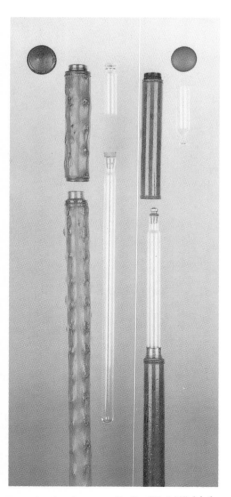

Two tipplers' canes. Left: 37 1/4" high; right: 35 3/4" high.

Certain needs may persist only at a certain time and then not last long. A stick supplying such a short-term need is even rarer than the modern stick, but if I as a collector were to find a reproduction, I would be happy to have it if I could not have the original. Frankly, at the present time, there are more sticks made and sold on Portobello Street and Bermondsey in London and other antique centers posing as antiques that were made only a week ago, than ever before due to the renaissance of the cane.

Some years back I was in the Bermondsey Market looking for sticks and a lady seller of sticks, when she saw me, recognized me and said she really had nothing that I would care for. Nevertheless, I looked through her collection and found a stick I had never seen before. It certainly looked old and when the handle was screwed off a fine folding scissors wrapped in chamois cloth could be extracted from a secret compartment. I bought it and was happy with it for about a year. Then one of my daughters went to England and came back with a stick for me. She was very proud of it and hoped I had never owned or seen one like it. It was the same scissors stick I had purchase the year before and she got it from the same lady who sold me mine. It's made of old parts — all of which are genuine — but it was assembled a few months before. Of course, I expressed surprise and appreciation and 10 years from now it will be an antique.

Once on Portobellow Street — the stupendous flea market street in London — I questioned the authenticity of a cane that had a brass measuring device for the contents of a barrel. The shaft showed no wear, the ferrule was obviously new. When I pointed this out to the seller, he told me he had the inner contents of many container sticks the shafts of which were worn and broken. He said, "should I therefore throw them away?" He said he had a new shaft constructed and drilled to contain the original insertion. Sort of like changing a worn tire on a new car. Is this fair and proper? You can find arguments on both sides, but I consider my barrel measuring stick as a real antique — at least for a collector who doesn't have one with a useless and broken shaft.

It's like buying a good reproduction item of furniture when one has no way of obtaining the original. They look the

same, feel the same, and are the same except in age — in fact, the repro may be much better because of its newness. Here again, we have two sides to the same question.

It is a different matter if a name or date were engraved on the renewal stick as this would be a real fraud.

There are still at least two companies that make very fine canes that are distributed world-wide. Both also make reproductions of popular gadget canes. These companies are:

France:
    Fabrique d'armes Barillet
    Cannes a Systemes
    B.P. 61-26600
    Tain-l' Hermitage-France

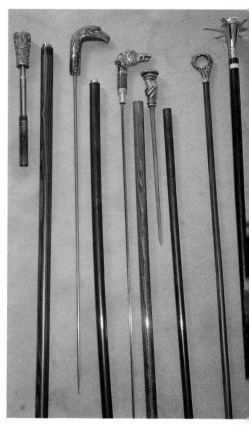

A grouping of modern defense canes produced by the French and Italian companies listed (Fabrique d'armes Barillet and Ravarini Castoldi & Company).

Italy:
    Ravarini Castoldi & Co.
    20139 Milano, via Gardonezo
    Milan, Italy
    phone: 560326/560497

Everyone has knowledge of at least one gadget cane though he may not know it as that. This is the simple rain umbrella. For surely it was originally a walking stick to which was added a sun shade or a rain shedder. Others have heard of the sword cane and some, remembering the days of prohibition, will recall the flask or liquor cane. But with these three, the umbrella, the sword cane, and the liquor cane, general common knowledge of dual purpose canes ends. As an attorney, I have searched the U.S. Patent office and have copies of more than 500 patents on walking sticks, dating from the inception of our present patent office in 1841. Similarly, I have searched the British patent office and have obtained copies of over 630 patents issued on canes since the year 1808. I also had a search made and have copies of all canes patented in Germany. This is over 1700 patents on canes — mostly dual purpose sticks and refinements of them. Inventive man really never ignored his most prized possession, his walking stick.

At one time every gentlemen "wore" a cane, just like until most recent days, every man wore a tie. A gentleman was a man with no visible means of support such as tools of trade or profession, and as every man wanted himself to be considered a gentleman, all men had canes as they did ties. And as with ties the more affluent the man, the more canes he had. They were not only of different woods, reeds, stalks, fibers, but also of different animal objects, such as bone, horn, ivory, muscles, skins, tendons, and the whole spectrum of metals and stones. It was but natural that with each man trying to out vie his neighbor in having a more unique cane, that the dual purpose cane should evolve, either of necessity, cupidity, or style. It is to be remembered that at one time it was the man who was the peacock in dress and his cane as his most prized object exemplified this.

It is reported that the Chinese so protected their silk trade that they decreed death to anyone who would smuggle out silkworm larvae. Wasn't it natural that the silkworm should find its way to the western world - Italy - by way of Constantinpole in a hollowed out cane of two traveling monks. In the same manner saffron came out of Greece and asparagus came to England in the hollowed cane of a Knight Templar, and the first

tulip found its way to Holland. The seeds of the melon, apricot, tomato, onion, cauliflower and quince were all brought from oriental countries to the west in the hollowed staffs of pilgrims.

Tradesmen and others wanting to appear as gentlemen on the street carried the tools of their trades hidden in their canes. So with the piano tuner, who had his hammer and wrenches in his cane, the musician who had his violin, guitar, chakan, flute, fife, even his music stand in his walking stick; the doctor who had his stethoscope, tweezers, pills and vials of medicine all in his cane; the army officer when traveling as a civilian had his swagger stick or sword blade (the handle he carried in his suitcase) in a walking stick. Railroad trackmen had track gauges concealed in a walking stick, to determine the gauge of a rail, or the distance apart of rails.

Traveling butter buyers used canes that had semi-cylindrical blades in a shaft which, upon visiting a farmer, they would pull out, plunge into a butter vat, twist and withdraw a sample for inspection, to insure that there wasn't lard at the bottom of the vat.

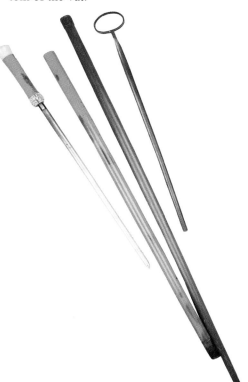

Two canes with scoops inside for checking butter and coffee bean quality. Left: Chinese designs in ivory, for checking coffee beans, 36" high; right: with loop handle for checking butter (or cheese), 38" high. Both date to c. 1890.

Similarly, grain buyers had grain-thiefs in their walking sticks to determine that the grain at the bottom of the barrel wasn't rotten or consisting solely of pebbles. Even the undertaker when walking about and masquerading as a gentleman had his specially patented (1886) cane designed for "closing the lids of outside burial cases after the cases are lowered in the grave."

As varied as the inventive genius of man are the items that have been inserted into his walking stick. Only with the rise of the bicycle and the auto age circumventing the need of walking, and the adaptation of the new status symbol of the brief case, has the use of the cane and with it the dual purpose cane disappeared. It is the hunt for these forgotten, and in most cases unknown, items that a wonderful collecting urge can be amply rewarded.

Would you believe that I have a very elegant cane, the silver top of which opens surreptitiously to drop a few grains of snuff, like out of a salt shaker, into a pan beneath, so that a fine lady could sniff her snuff without detection. Or that I have a spittoon cane with a hollowed shaft and a beautifully carved dog's-head handle, the nostrils of which are bored through so that a gentleman addicted to chewing tobacco could spit through them into the cane while at a concert or church. The 1881 U.S. patent specification on this is most amusing in declaring:

"It is perhaps, deplorable, but nonetheless true that many men who are addicted to the habit of chewing tobacco cannot be happy or contented without it during the continuance of a religious service, a lecture, or other entertainment, and those who are too well bred to spit upon the floor must have much of their enjoyment spoiled or stay away altogether.

A spittoon - cane from which the cover would have to be removed every time it was used would be very objectionable, as the movements of the user would attract attention; but owing to the construction of my cane it can be used anywhere and on any occasion without attracting the least attention or revealing its use, as the user has only to carelessly insert the projection (dog's snout) between his lips - a motion very common among the users of ordinary canes, especially when sitting, etc."

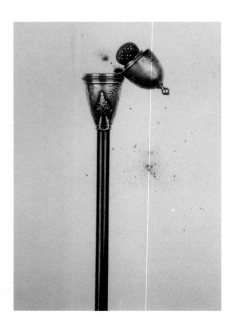

Ladies snuff cane, small silver handle, c. 1900, 36 1/2" high.

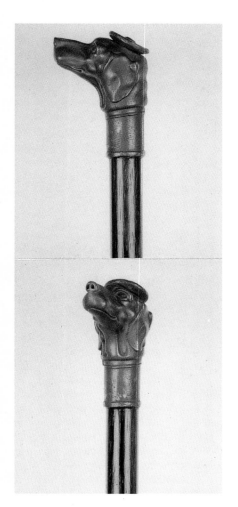

A very rare patented tobacco chewer's spittoon cane for spitting into the nostrils of the dog. The beret unscrews for cleaning the spittoon which runs the entire length of the cane. This cane measures 37" high.

You need not pity the deaf gentleman when you hail him on the street as there are a number of canes with hearing aids in them. The smoker has innumerable canes to carry not only his cigars, cigarettes, tobacco, matches, or pipe but combinations of these. Before the advent of matches, his flint and striker were also to be found in a cane that embodies a pill box, a cab whistle, and a cigar cutter.

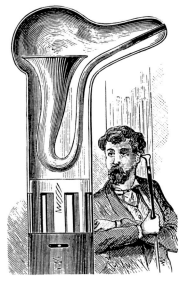

EAR TRUMPET AND CANE HANDLE.

Figure 50. Hearing aid gadget cane depicted in the September, 1883 issue of Scientific American.

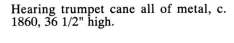

Hearing trumpet cane all of metal, c. 1860, 36 1/2" high.

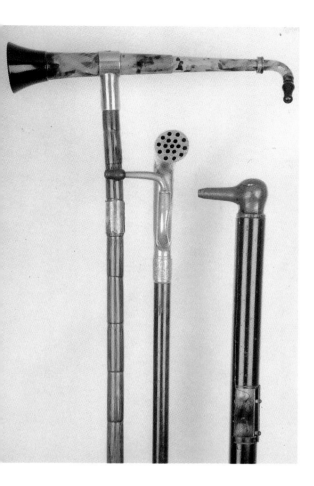

Three hearing aid canes: left: tortoise shell on partridge wood, c. 1870, 36 1/2" high; center: cast iron handle with swiveling ear piece, snakewood shaft, c. 1880, 35 3/4" high; right: battery powered hearing aid, iron handle marked Pat. Jan. 27th 1885, 34 1/2" high.

The smoker has innumerable canes to carry not only his cigars, cigarettes, tobacco, matches or pipes but combinations of these items as well. Left: cigar humidor cane engraved Paris with initials and the date 1900, 34 1/2" high; right: cigarette humidor, Pat. 1887, 35" high.

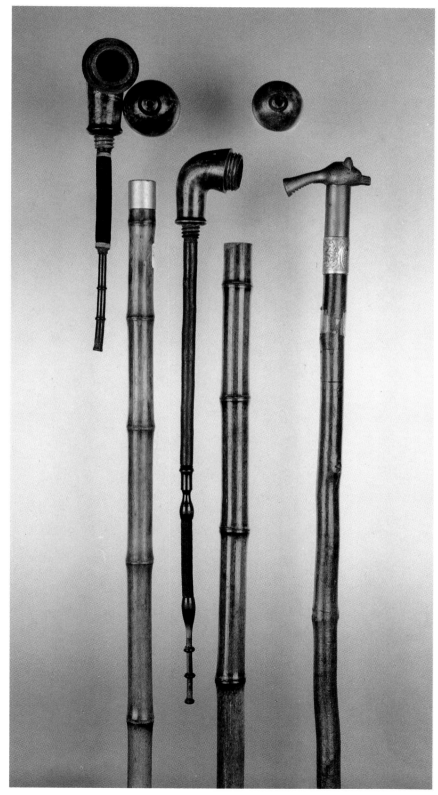

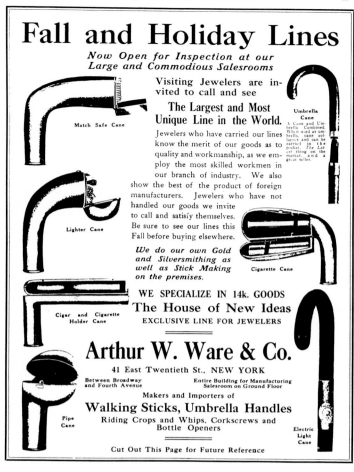

Figure 51. Smokers' gadget canes, umbrella cane and an "electric light cane" advertised by Arthur W. Ware & Company of New York in 1911.

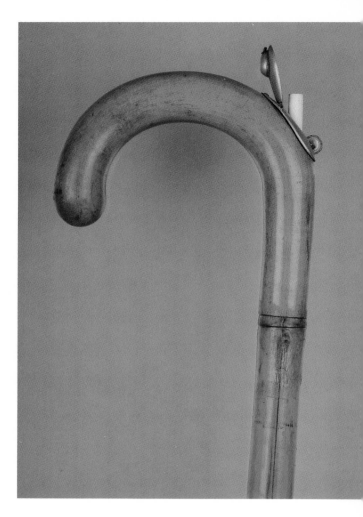

Automatic cigarette humidor cane. Turn the wheel and smokes rise. Lift the cap with your right hand, turn the wheel, and up pops a cigarette. 36" high.

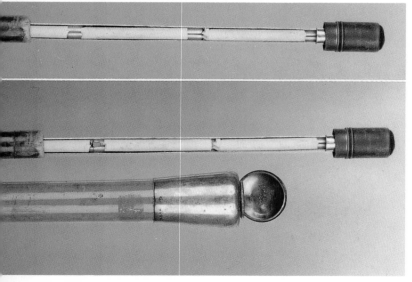

Two cigarette canes, left pulls up handle to reveal cigarettes, 36" high; right: smokes drawn up from within malacca shaft, English Pat. Feb. 10, 1888, 35 1/4" high.

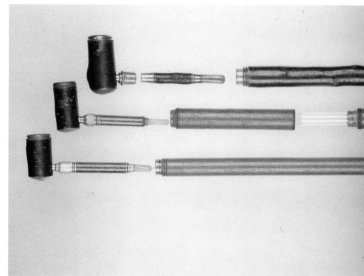

Three pipe and cigarette canes, center includes a glass for tippling, ranging from 35 1/4" to 37 3/4" high.

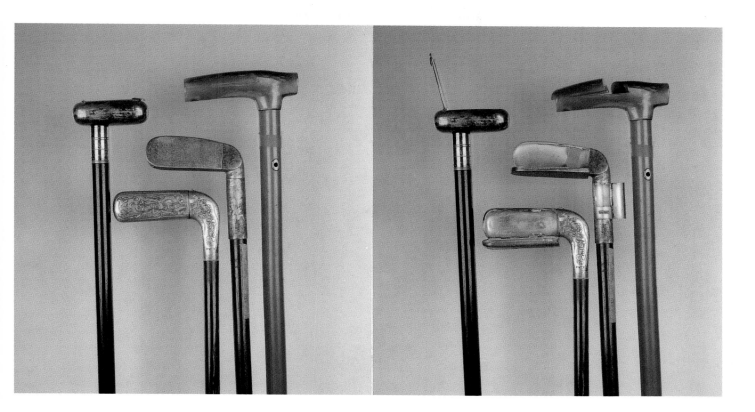

Four container canes: left is a snuff box and opens on top, silver handle, 36 1/4" high; putter shaped handle with foliate design, hinges open whole side when button pressed and reveals a cigarette case, c. 1860, 35 1/2" high; another putter shaped handle, plain silver, side opening, two elastic straps to hold cigarettes in place, and the neck of the handle has a match box and striking surface, c. 1890, 39 3/4" high; antler handled snuff box cane with malacca shaft and eyelets, c. 1870 - 1920, 34 3/4" high.

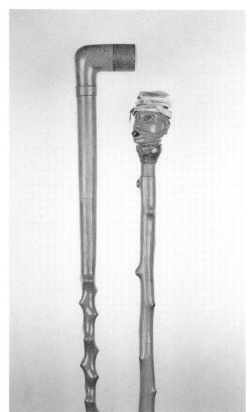

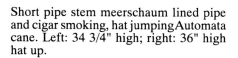

Short pipe stem meerschaum lined pipe and cigar smoking, hat jumping Automata cane. Left: 34 3/4" high; right: 36" high hat up.

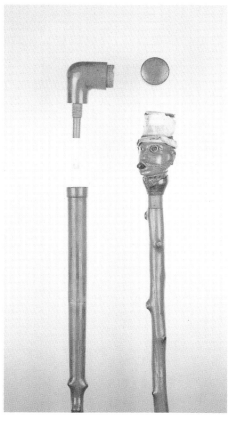

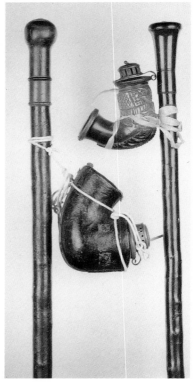

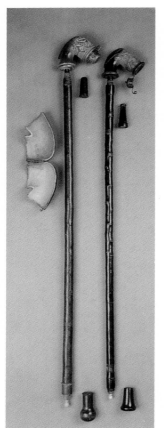

Two German pipe canes, the shaft of each cane is hollow. The smoke passes from the pipe bowl at the cane's ferrule, up the hollow shaft, and through the mouthpiece hidden beneath the cane handle. Left: 34 1/2" high; right: 36" high.

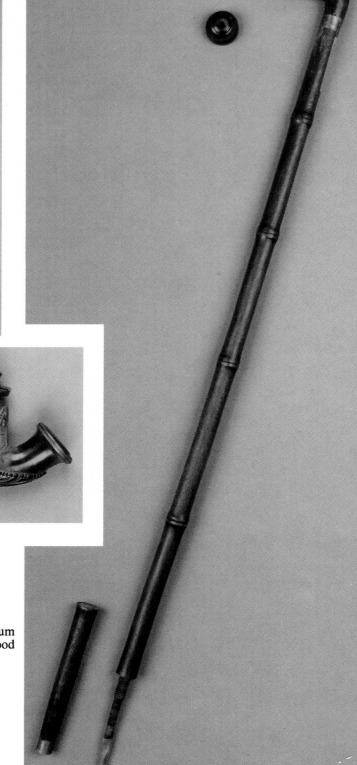

Another smoking pipe with meerschaum bowl and mouthpiece under ferrule, wood to bowl, 34 1/2" high.

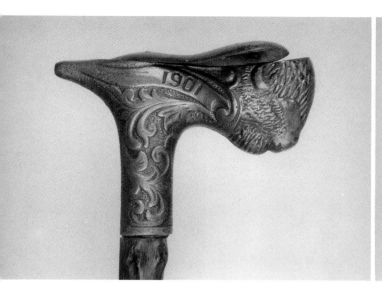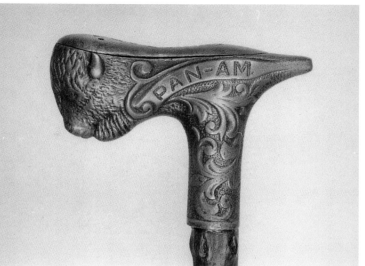

Cane with an aluminum smoking pipe in the handle marked PAN AM, NIAGRA, 1901, with buffalo on bowl, 34 1/4" high. This is a rare cane from the Pan American Exhibition at Niagara in 1901. The top slides aside to fill the bowl and is smoked through the narrow tip.

Two English fire pistons dating from c. 1880 — left: silver handle with a Spanish Reale in the top, 35 1/2" high; right: wood handle, 37 3/4" high. This is an early method for lighting tinder. Place tinder in the end of the plunder and quickly force down the tight shaft. The friction heat causes tinder ignition.

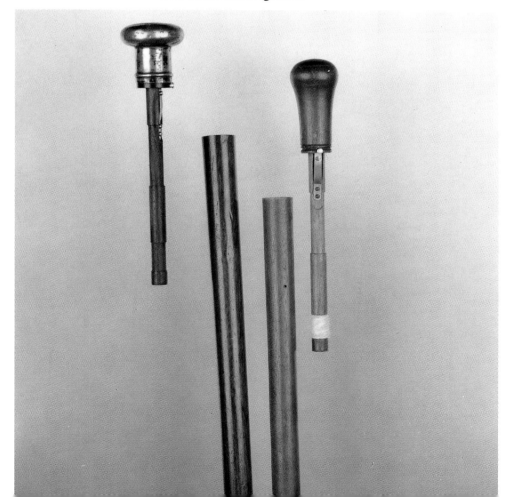

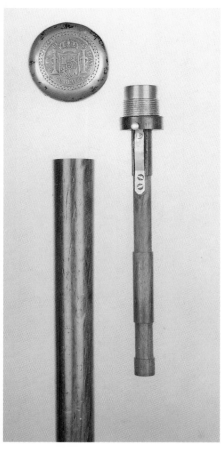

English fire piston decorated with a Spanish Reale coin.

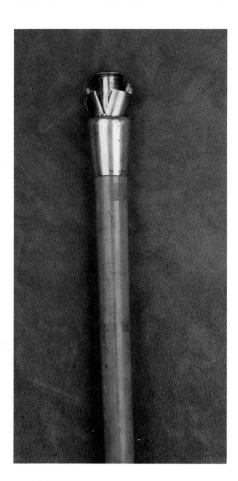

Match holding cane. Lift up on the top of the handle and matches are raised in two angled holders.

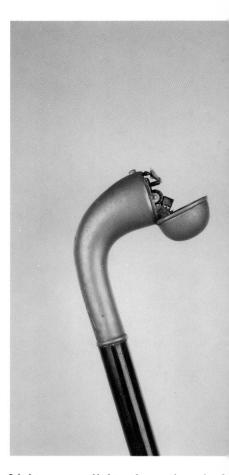

Lighter cane, lighter beneath end of handle, hinges open with press of button, 36" high.

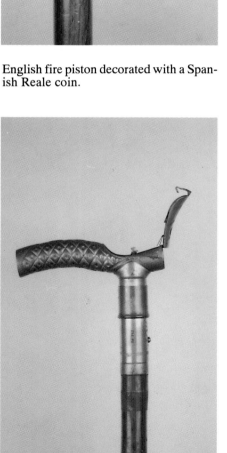

German Patented lighting cane with oil and a wick beneath a button released lid in the handle, c. 1890, 34 3/4" high.

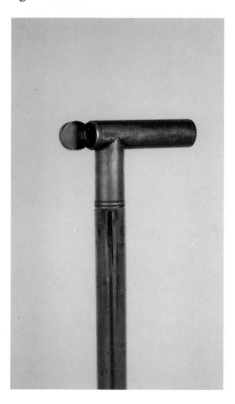

Match holding cane with swinging end cap, malacca shaft, c. 1880, 35 1/2" high.

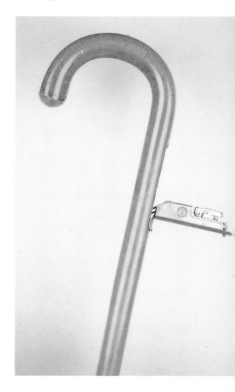

Crook handle with Ronson De Light Lighter with a fine malacca shaft, 36" high.

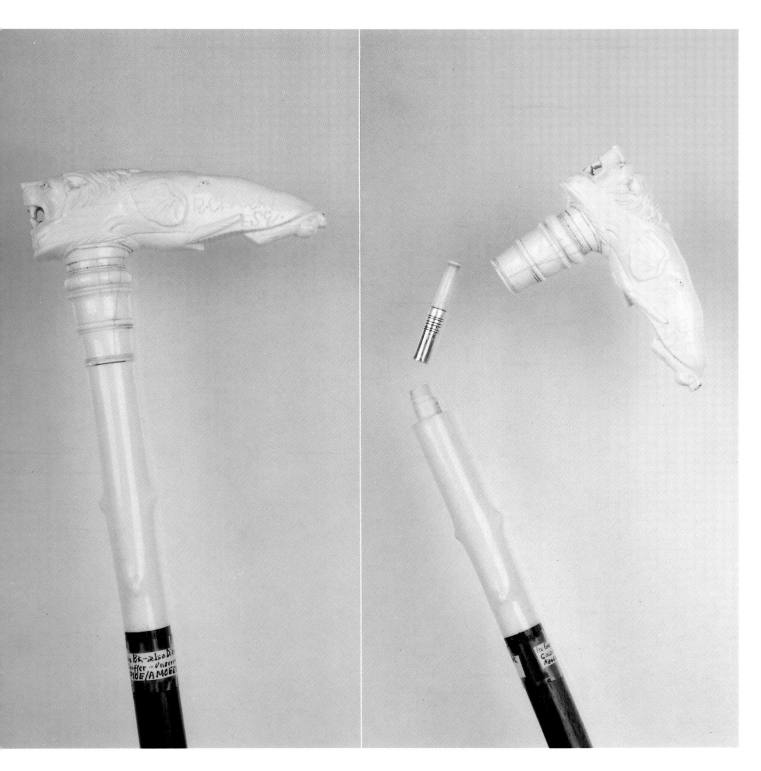

Ivory lion and elephant system stick, remove the ivory handle to find a silver and
ivory cocaine sniffer. Handle inscribed R.
Clarke Esq., c. 1890. 35 1/4" high.

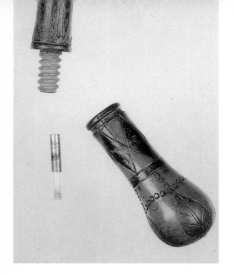

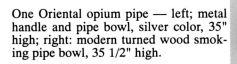

One Oriental opium pipe — left; metal handle and pipe bowl, silver color, 35" high; right: modern turned wood smoking pipe bowl, 35 1/2" high.

Middle Eastern cocaine smoker's cane, wood knob, c. 1910, 37 1/4" high.

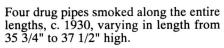

Four drug pipes smoked along the entire lengths, c. 1930, varying in length from 35 3/4" to 37 1/2" high.

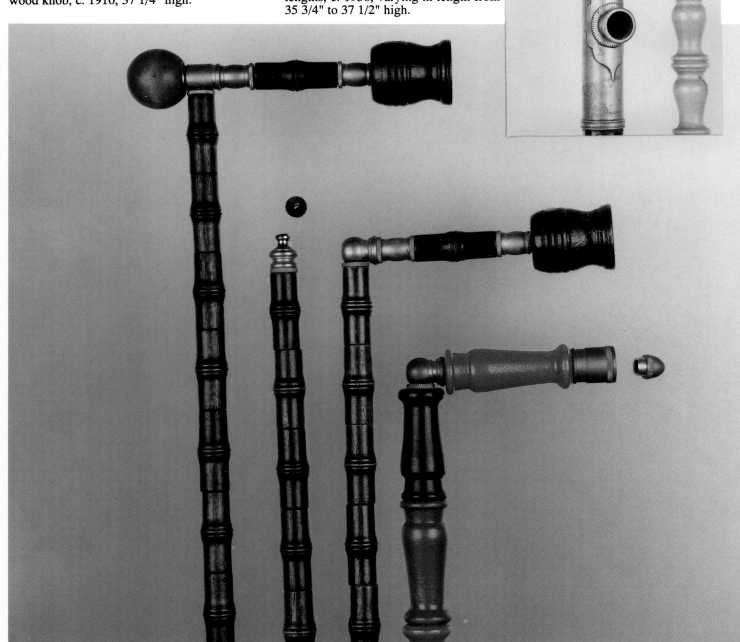

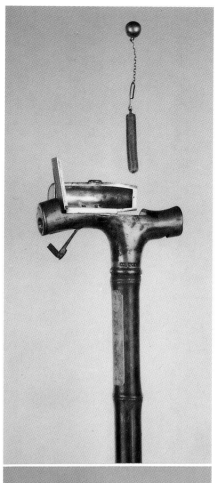

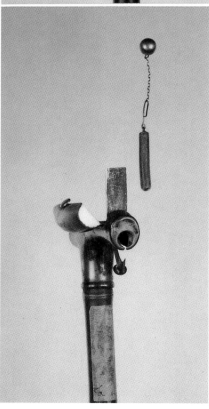

Our dandy who really was more interested in sneaking off fishing had his fish pole in his cane and some of these are precision instruments with fly rods well concealed in the stick. For years in the Orient, in the last century, carved and hollowed out bamboo sticks concealed telescopic fly rods that were sold to tourists.

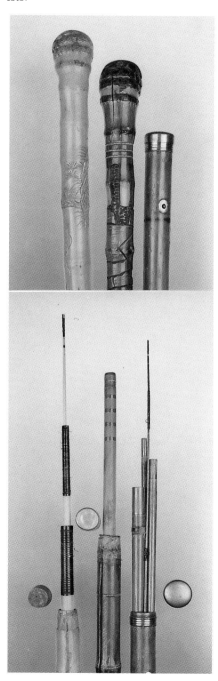

Even the man who picked up the paper in the parks and lawns carried his paper spear concealed in his cane as he walked to and from his work so he appeared as a gentleman twirling his cane specially manufactured for him in India.

Let us not forget that real gentleman - the professional gambler. His 18th century walking stick opened into a fine silken table and from his sash belt next to his derringer he extracted his cards to play The Three-Card Monte (now you see it, now you don't) with the country bumpkins.

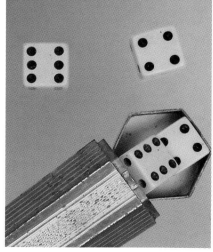

Multi-purpose cane with flint lighter, pill box, cigar cutter, and whistle, marked "BJA from WP, Feb. 6th 1886," 35 1/2" high.

Three fishing pole canes. Left and center: oriental bamboo with poles telescoping out of ferrule; right: bamboo with silver handle, eyelets, and fishing pole in sections within. Respectively, 36" high, 35" high, and 36 1/4" high.

Gold plated gambler's cane with dice beneath the lid, 36 1/2" high. Purchased in Cannes, France.

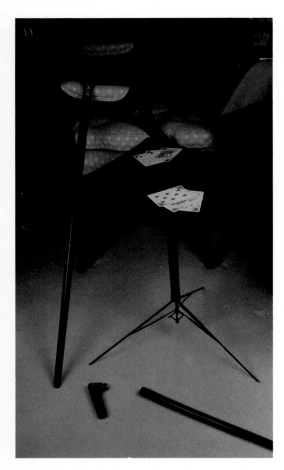

His 18th century walking stick opened into a fine silken table and from his sash belt, next to his derringer, he extracts his cards to play The Three-Card Monte with the country bumpkins.

Ladies were not to be forgotten apart from our elegant snuff sniffer. Down to the end of World War I, they had compact canes containing powder, rouge and mirror; ladies had beautiful walking sticks with bottles of perfume in the handles or shafts; with watches in the handle or on the shaft. Even gun canes were made by the famous American Firearms Company - Remington - in 22 caliber for ladies in the middle 1800s. These are both in cap and ball and cartridge. One of the most wicked and yet most rare and intricate ladies walking sticks I have is a thin flexible wooden shaft with an innocent appearing metal head that becomes a mace (the clobberer, not the modern atomizer). By the mere touch of a button our lady could eject six (6) sharp spikes that instantly locked in place on the head of her cane to dissuade any aggressive man.

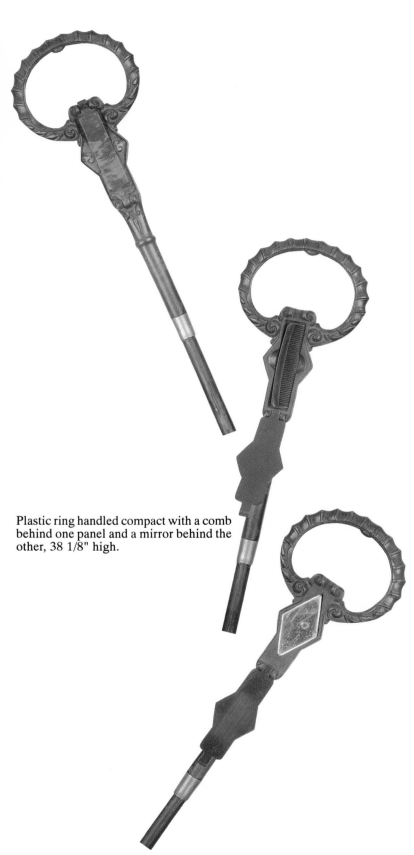

Plastic ring handled compact with a comb behind one panel and a mirror behind the other, 38 1/8" high.

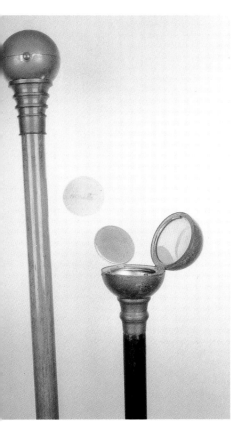

Two knob handled cane which hinge open at the mid point to reveal mirrors and powder puffs, 35 1/4" high and 35" high.

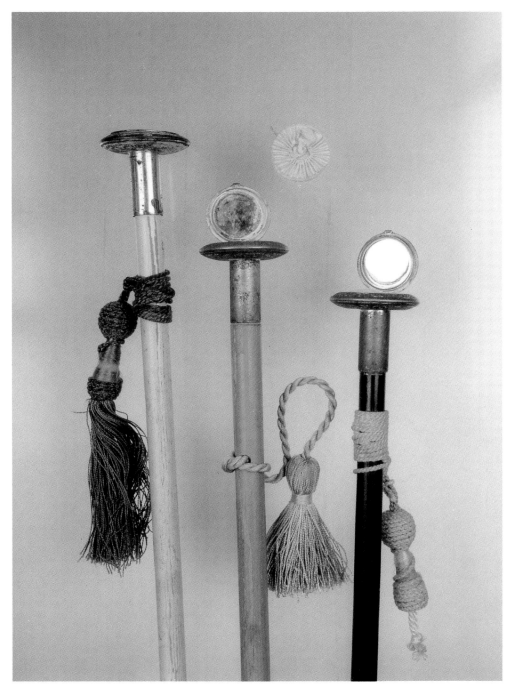

Three flat silver plated handles which open on top to reveal small mirrors and powder puffs inside, ranging from 37 1/2" high to 39 3/4" high.

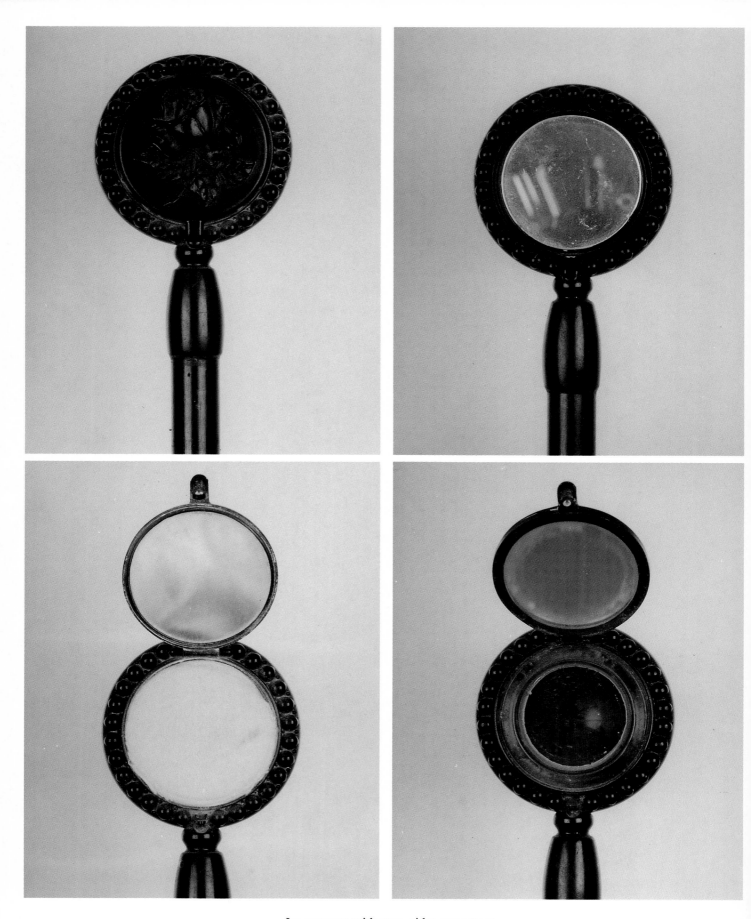

Jet compact with rose, sides open to reveal two mirrors and two powder holders, 36 3/4" high.

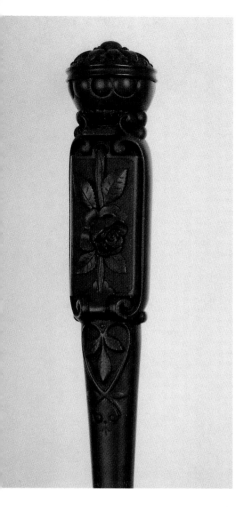

Gutta-percha handle with powder puff beneath unscrewing lid and a mirror behind the hinged side panel, 39" high.

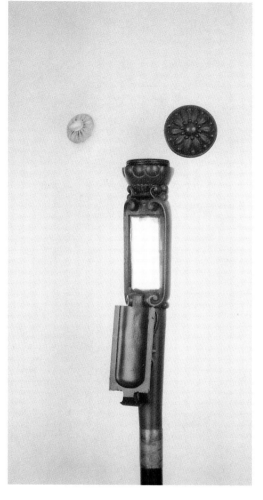

Large compact cane dating from c. 1920, featuring an engraved pine cone design. When opened, the top reveals a mirror. 36 1/4" high.

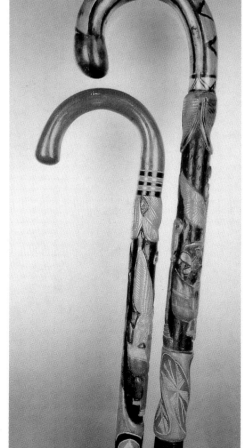

Two crook handled Mexican canes with carved and polychromed decorations.

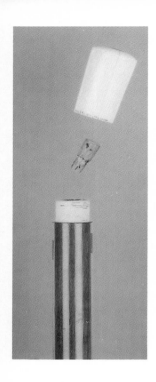

Ivory handled perfume or scent cane,
knob marked Swaine & Adeney, London,
malacca shaft, c. 1910, 36" high.

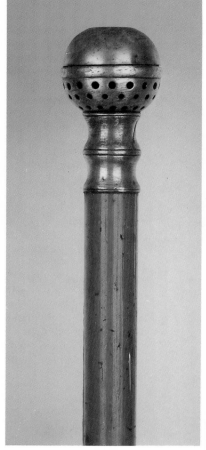

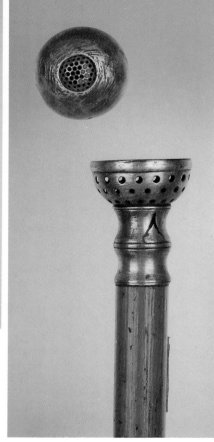

Perfume handle in silver, malacca shaft,
35 1/4" high.

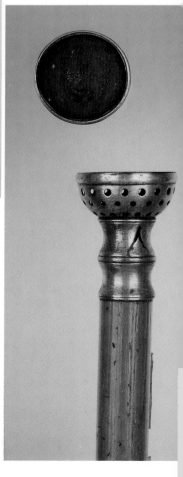

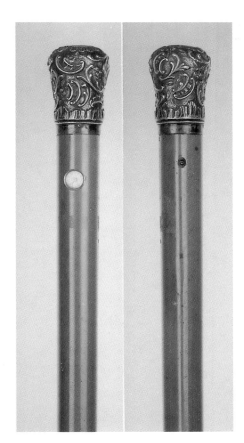

Silver and malacca watch cane, wind by turning handle, set with small set screw in back, 34 3/8" high.

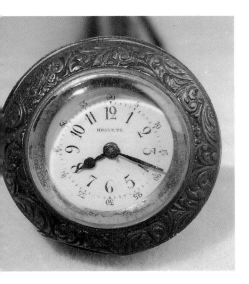

Umbrella cane with silver handle and watch, c. 1895, 37 3/4" high.

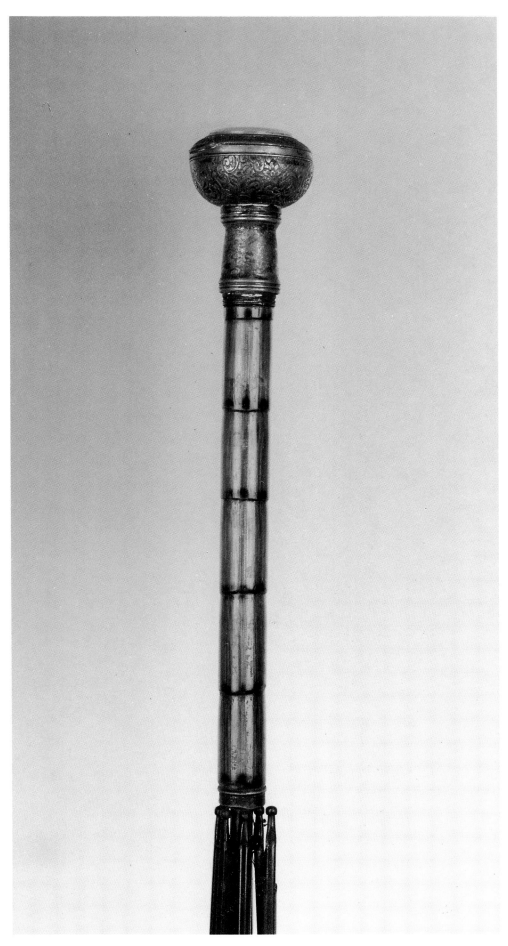

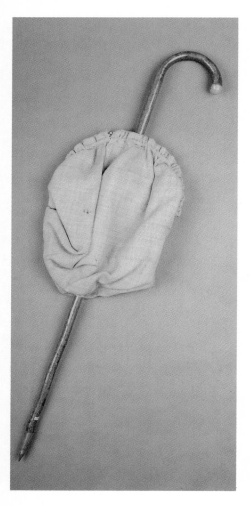

Crook handled cane with a shopping bag or a purse holder, 37 1/2" high.

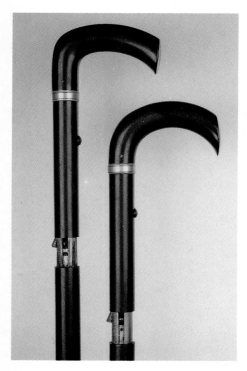

Two Remington gun canes with gutta percha shafts. Button firing mechanisms. Left: 35" high; right: 37 3/4" high.

Two ladies' weapon canes — the example on the left is old and the model on the right is modern made in France, both become 6 spike maces with the push of a button or pull on the collar. 34 3/4" high and 35 3/4" high respectively. The first was designed by Napoleon's engineers in Egypt for the protection of their ladies.

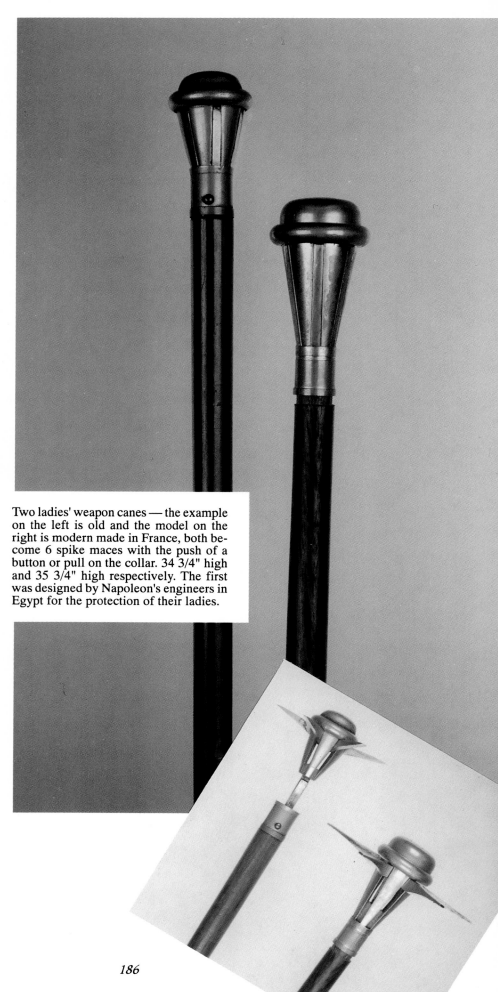

One retiring lady not given to idling away her time had a cane with a darning ball handle with needle and thread inside.

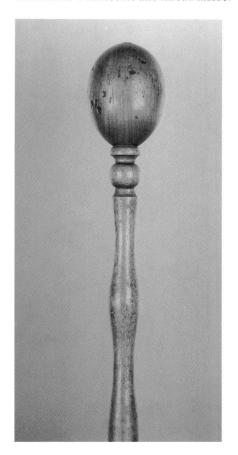

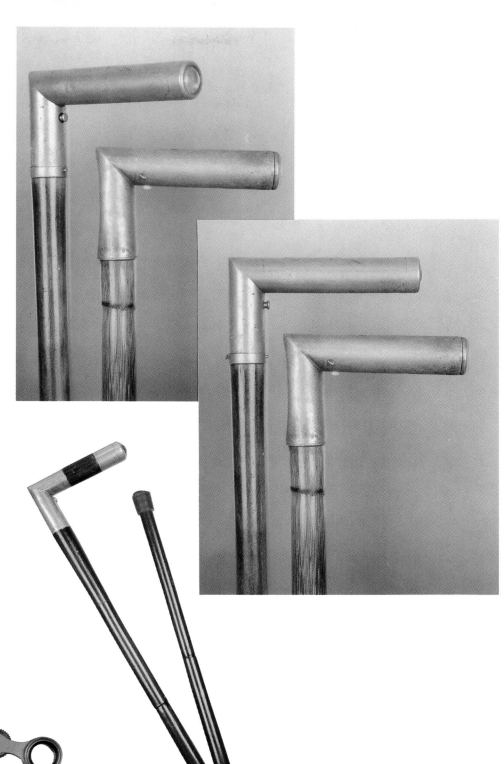

Ladies darning cane from the European mountains, designed to contain a needle and a ball of wool, c. 1890, 32 1/2" high.

The play or opera devotee had his walking stick containing his opera glasses, or his flashlight in the handle to read his libretto or playbill or his whistle to toot his disapproval, if it were a bad play, as was wont to be done in merry old England over a century ago.

Opera glass cane, focusing binoculars for handle, brass on black shaft, c. 1900, 36 1/4" high.

Two L handle flashlight canes, also called key-hole finders, or libretto readers, with lens in the end of the handle, the left hand model is a traveling cane that unscrews in the middle and folds in half. Left: 35 1/4" high; right: 36 3/8" high.

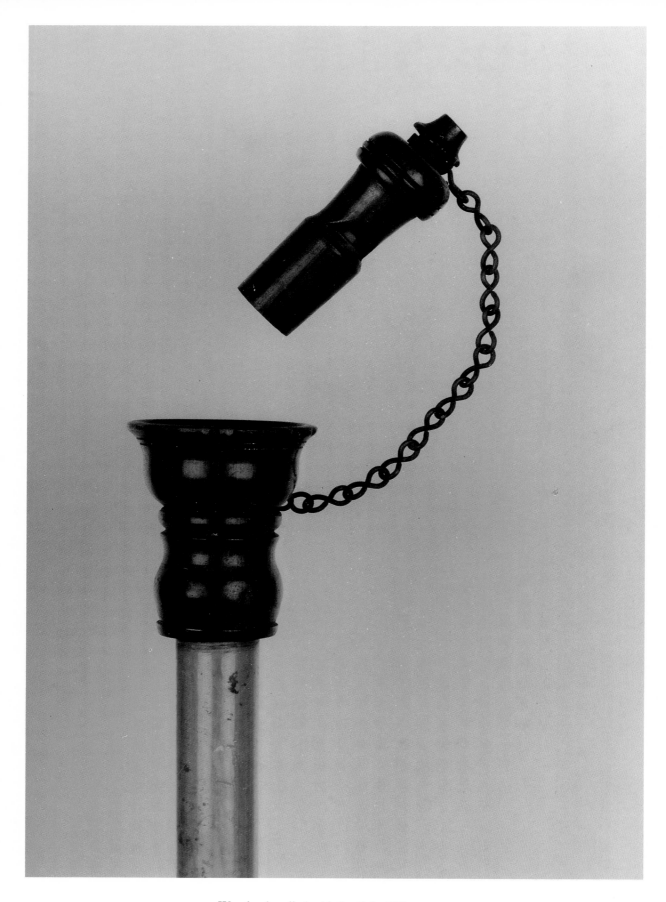

Wooden handled whistle stick, 19th century, malacca shaft, 35" high. Used at theaters in the 1700s and 1800s to show displeasure with performance on stage.

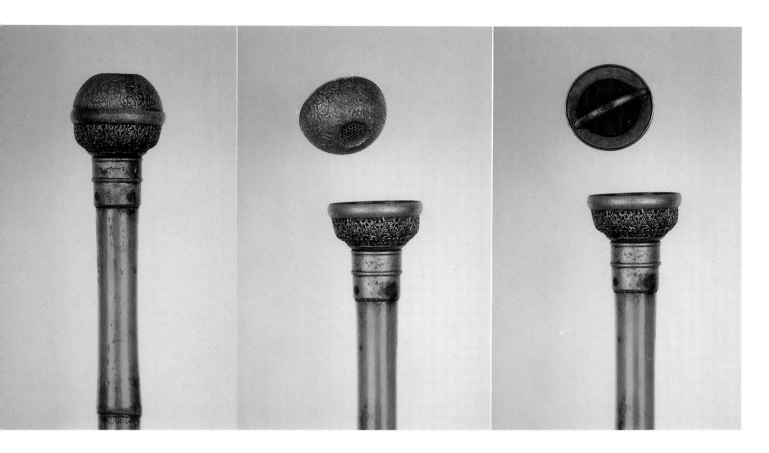

Silver noise maker siren handle on a bamboo shaft, 37" high.

The sailor and the voyeur had his telescope or spy glass in his cane ; the wine master had his measuring rod in his walking stick if thumping on the outer barrel did not satisfy his curiosity as to the fullness of the vat ; his superior even had a long auger in his cane to drill through the bungs of the unopened barrels to test the contents.

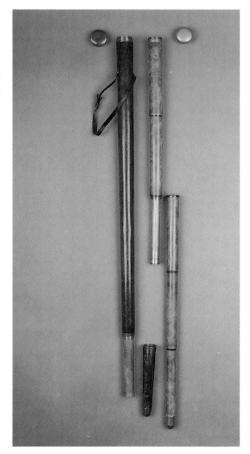

Two optical telescope canes. Left: the entire length of the shaft is the scope with a long brass ferrule, 33 1/2" high, 6 1/2" ferrule; right: scope takes up half the shaft, a compass is hidden in the silver handle and the bottom third of the shaft is hollow for the storage of maps, 36 1/4" high.

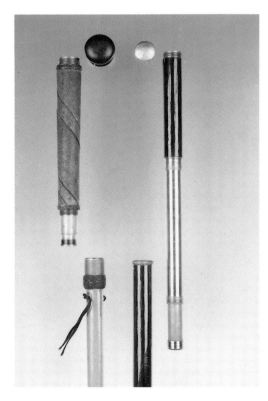

Two telescope canes. Left: shark skin on the upper third of the shaft, 35" high; right: gold handle, wood covering the scope, 34 1/4" high.

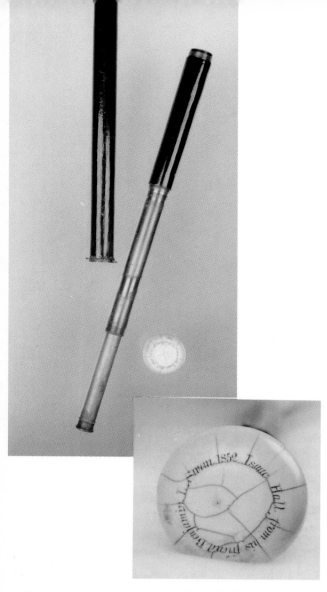

French telescope cane given to Isaac Hall from his friend Benjamin L. Swan 1852, 36 3/4" high.

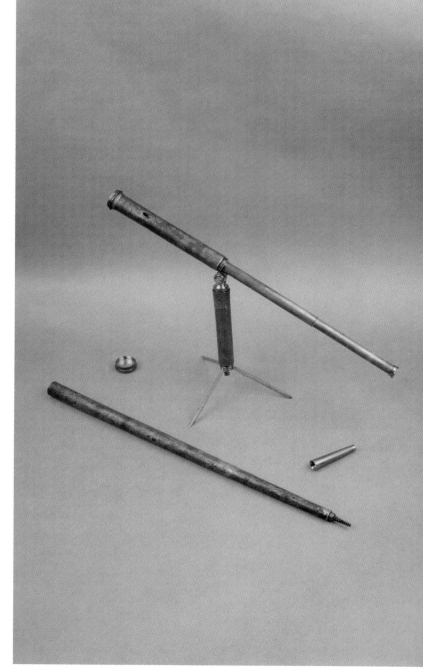

Very old seaman's telescope, brass, on tube inscribed, "Davis Brothers opticians to HRH Prince Albert 33 New Bond Street London ... and ... Sold by Melling & Payne 39 S. Castle Street Liverpool." Has false eyelets, c. 1750, 36 1/2" high.

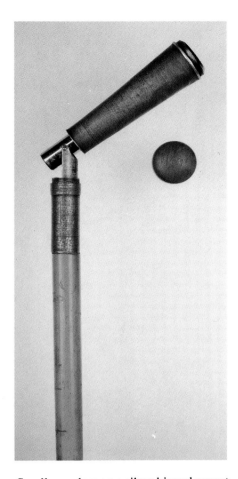

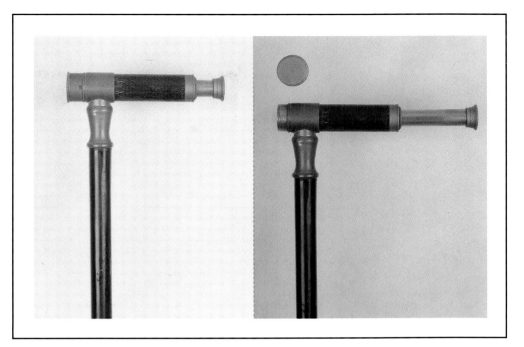

Brass telescope mounted as L handle on cane, wood veneer over brass scope shaft, 37 1/2" high.

Small spy glass on a silver hinged mount, upper third of cane, malacca shaft, 34 3/4" high.

Five foot ruler cane, the crook handle twists off and the double folded measure is removed from within the shaft, 36 1/4" high. This cane was to be used by carpenters, interior designers and others.

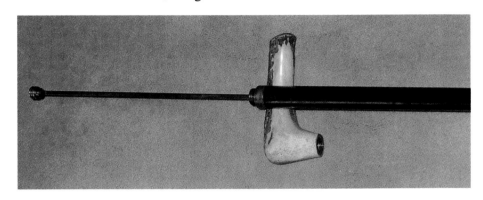

Barrel measuring cane.

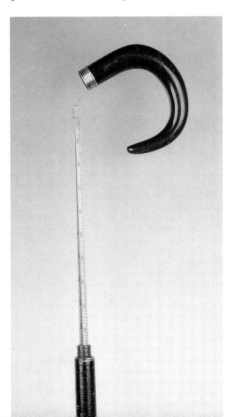

The horse auctioneer or fancier had his cane that would open at the handle to reveal a measuring rod with brass bar and spirit level that could be pulled out of the shaft and placed over the withers of a horse to calibrate its size in hands or in feet and inches. So prominent were these at one time that they even had one cunningly contrived to measure the extraordinary extra large horses of the British Isles.

Horse measuring canes, marked in hands. Left: red, 37" high; right: covered with leather along the shaft, c. 1870s, 36 3/4" high.

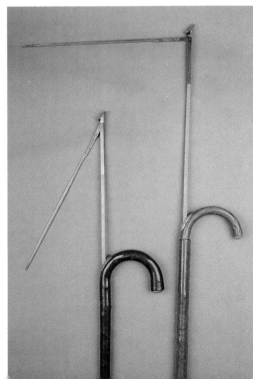

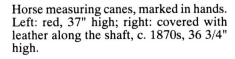

The day of the cane and walking stick was the heyday of the old fashioned political campaigns with the street marchers carrying canes, the handles of which depicted their favorite candidate and the ferrules so arranged as to receive a large poster. The heads are of Lincoln, Grant, Tilden, Hayes, Harrison, Cleveland, Blaine, McKinley, Bryan, T. Roosevelt, Taft and Wilson. Others in the parade carried flag canes or torch canes. The oldest flag cane in my collection has 36 stars. The torch canes were either hollowed tin staffs for whale oil with a wick under the cap handle, or kerosene containers and wicks with staffs. Noisier campaigners carried tin walking sticks with horns in the handle or staff. The two illustrated say on the handle: "Patriotism, Protection and Prosperity."

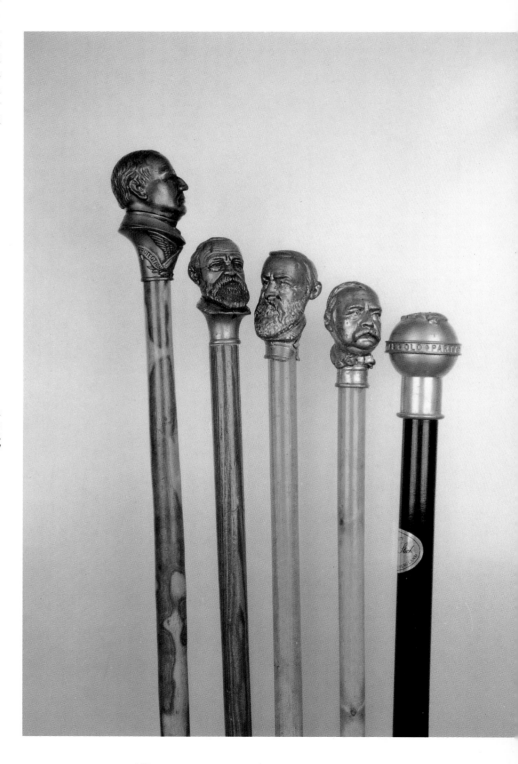

Four campaign busts and Republican globe reading The Grand Old Party. Left: McKinley, 34 1/4" high; two Harrison's of varying quality, 35 1/2" high & 36 1/2" high; Cleveland, 36 1/4" high.

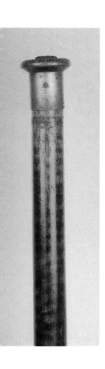
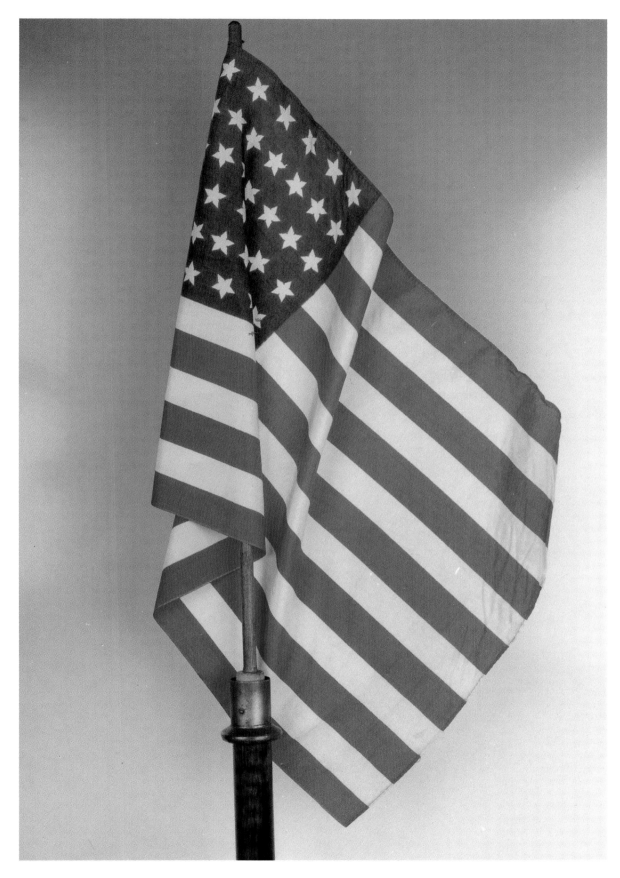

Flag cane, remove handle, reverse to reveal flag, and socket into cane shaft, 34
1/4" high.

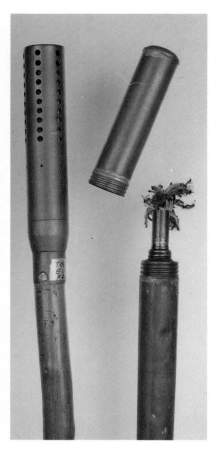

Two campaign torch canes, left with gas, right with wick. Left: 39 1/2" high; right: 33 1/4" high.

With the political canes must be mentioned the prankster canes which would surreptitiously squirt water from near its ferrule up a girl's leg when the top was pressed against the floor by her innocent-appearing charmer. Also in this group are the various whistling canes working in the same manner, and the naughty picture cane, the handle of which a man pressed hard against his eye to see better, not knowing that it left a tell-tale black smudge.

The day of the cane was the day of the horse and carriage and many a carriage driver, when walking as a gentleman, had his carriage key in his stick. In that day, as now, urchins would steal buggy whips that were left in the whip holder just as hub caps are stolen off automobile wheels today. Was it surprising that a company was formed to manufacture and sell the most practical of the various U.S. patents issued on buggy whips? The illustrated walking stick buggy whip is made by the Patent Cane Whip Co., Springfield, Ohio.

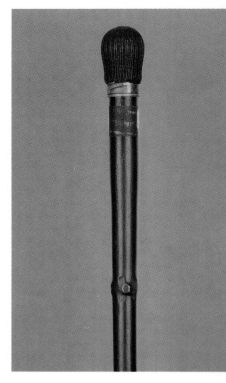

Cherry shaft buggy whip with woven mesh handle, c. 1870, 36 1/4" high.

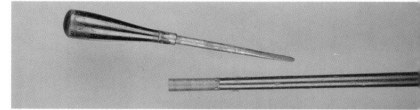

Horse carriage key cane, c. 1850, 35 1/4" high.

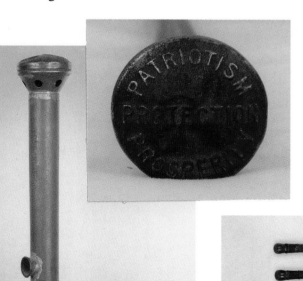

Top of campaign noisemaker cane marked "Patriotism, Prosperity, Protection."

Noise-maker campaign cane, blow in hole in side, tin, 33 3/4" high, marked PATRIOTISM PROTECTION PROPERTY on top.

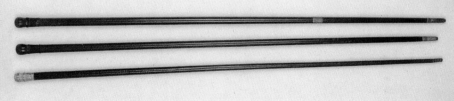

Three buggy whip canes. Left: flexible shaft with silver handle reading The Patent Canewhip Co., Springfield, Ohio, 36" high; center and right: gutta-percha buggy whip canes; center: 35 1/2" high; right: 36 1/4" high. The whip was half concealed in the shaft and pulls out and attached to the ferrule.

This ingenious walking stick comes in two portions with a woven and flexible innermost portion pulling out of, and inserting onto, the end of the outer — also flexible — shell to make a 6 1/2 foot springy buggy whip. These buggy whip canes are scarce, yet when found, can be purchased reasonably as the seller rarely knows its inner secret.

Photographers had walking sticks that instantly converted into camera tripods or unipods. One particularly rare and much sought after cane is the one with a complete camera designed as the handle of the stick (See Illustration.)

It seems that the British were the most reluctant to give up the cane. To perpetuate its memory, it is said they daily carried an umbrella which between showers they used as a walking stick.

The infinite variety and materials of canes assure one that his collection can really never be complete.

German camera tripod mount with hinged crook handle, c. 1910, 38" high.

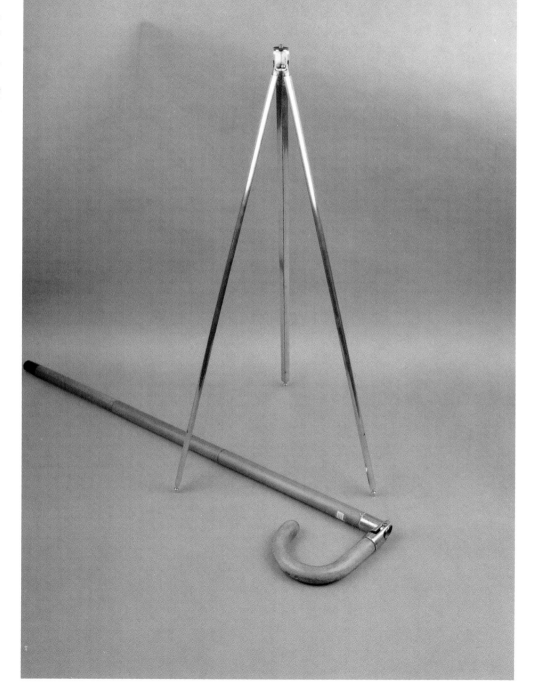

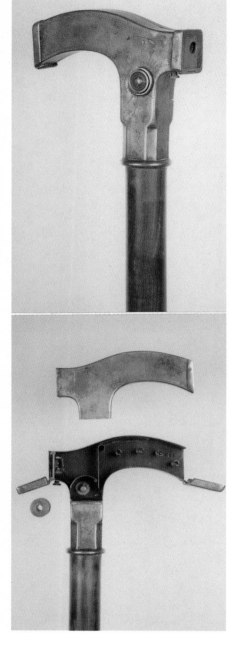

Very rare camera cane, camera hidden in the handle of the cane, holds five rolls of film, 1880s, 38 3/8" high.

How to Discover a Gadget Cane

How can one tell if the cane he is examining is just a regular walking stick or a more valuable gadget cane or container stick, also known as a dual purpose cane? Here is my method after 45 years of buying sticks all over the world.

I have purchased many a gadget stick from an unsuspecting owner, even from some knowledgeable collectors and presumably experienced dealers. They never really knew what they had. Few collectors who do know these tricks will divulge them to competitors.

If a close perusal of the stick indicates no telltale joint, perhaps the joint is hidden under a silver or horn band. It may even be the very edge of one of many natural rings encircling the stick and spaced serially a few inches apart. This could be a site where the cane may come apart and one should gently try to pull the cane apart at this location. If this fails, grasp the cane with two hands - each placed on opposite sides of the suspected line. Now gently twist in opposite directions and if there is any turning of the two sections, further examination is warranted. Many sword canes have not only a concealed joint, but one that has a locking device which is opened by making a half turn on the handle - usually clockwise. An internal mechanism, therefore, depresses a lock and the sword can be pulled out. Similarly travelers canes, i.e. sticks that fold up for carrying in one's luggage, also unscrew in the center or in two places to make the stick into 1/3 its original size for transporting. Many, many gadget canes are perfectly concealed in this manner and knowing how to detect the mechanism will more than repay the cost of this book in the long run. Finally, if none of the above methods produce any results, just very surreptitiously slap the cane against your thigh or the palm of your other hand. If you hear a rattle there may be a concealed blade or other device in the shaft. The rattle can also be produced by a loose ferrule. If further inspection shows this is the case, grasp the cane by the ferrule and, holding it in such a manner that your grip overlaps the cane and the bottom of the shaft, slap the upper part of the cane against the palm of your other hand. If again you hear a rattle, you're onto something.

All this must be done in such a way that it does not arouse the suspicion of the vendor.

I remember being in Madrid, Spain looking for canes in a large antique store that had quite a quantity of them. They prided themselves on their collection. I examined each and found one that looked prospectively suspicious. The dealer quoted a very high price and as we talked, I went through all of the motions cited above. It was a possible sword cane and well concealed. Going to the window — ostensibly to check the wooden shaft — and while my back was turned to the clerk, I pulled out a fair blade which I closed up before the clerk could see what I was doing.

We then started negotiating on the price, but he remained too high in his demand. In exasperation, I said the cane was not worth his evaluation as it was nothing but a "cheap sword cane". He said, "No, no, just a fine cane." I then operated the device and showed him the cheap blade. His eyes bugged. He took the cane away from me and ran into a back office. I heard an excited conversation followed by the clerk and the owner coming out to tell me that a big mistake had been made, etc., etc., and that they were now asking four times the original price as it seemed to be their only sword cane. Luckily, I hadn't wanted it in the first place.

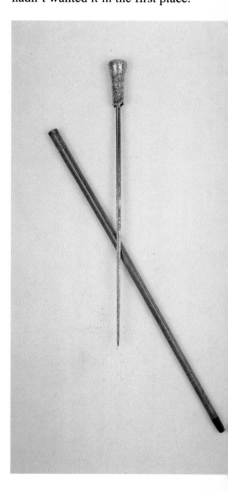

Sterling silver knob handled sword cane with cruciform blade, turn handle to release the blade, 32 1/2" high.

Gun Canes

While women frequently prefer more decorative canes, men seem to be the most ardent collectors of weapon sticks. They invariable search out the sinister and lethal canes that conceal swords, guns, daggers and devices for poisoning, blinding and mauling.

When I was a young collector, my very first acquisition was a sword cane. After its novelty decreased — it never quite ceases — I just had to have a gun cane. These two are the first types someone outside the field will inquire about upon learning that you collect sticks.

After I'd acquired my first gun cane, I enthusiastically searched for more. There are so many varieties of firing mechanisms that each was a new wonder. Anyone with a mechanical bent will be fascinated by the infinite number of detonating devices applied to ɔ hollow shaft that activate a lethal bullet. In my collection of over 100 gun canes, I have over 25 such mechanisms.

It now seems appalling that, in earlier times, so many wanted the advantage over a possible aggressor by possessing a secret weapon. What could be more secret or lethal than an innocuous-looking gun cane? By necessity, therefore, a gun cane must not be fancy or designed to attract admiration or attention. It must appear to be an ordinary stick. It should be noted that, after the Kennedy assassinations, gun canes of a particular type were outlawed as they were considered assassin's weapons. In some countries they had been used as such, but anyone who attempts to shoot one of these antiques today risks injuring himself far more than his intended victim. At one time a gunsmith who was repairing a gun cane for me became so fascinated by it that, in my absence, he fired it and blew up the whole end of the barrel. He had forgotten to remove the bottom tampion, an extension of the ferrule. He subsequently spent a week trying to repair it to conceal what had happened.

Nevertheless, the ownership of some gun canes (cartridge-types using readily available cartridges) is prohibited by law. Penalties for possession of such weapons can be as high as a $10,000 fine or ten years in prison or both, unless the weapon is registered with the Bureau of Alcohol,

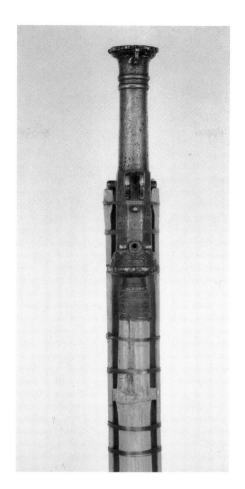

Replica of the first gun cane, a Chinese cannon held under the arm by a bamboo shaft, 38 3/4" high. It was fired by placing a burning punk to the touch hole.

Upper third of shaft pulls away to reveal a pistol. The handle operates as the firing pin, 36" high.

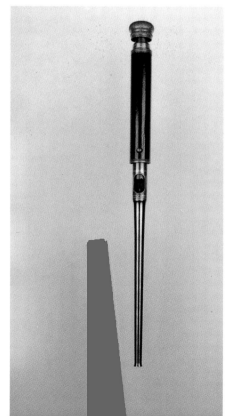

Tobacco and Firearms. In compliance with the law, I have registered all my gun canes. I understand that the British have just recently enacted a similar law.

Gun canes first appeared shortly after the invention of gun powder. They were initially used by the Chinese as hand cannons, then by others in flint-lock, air, cap and ball and, finally, cartridge varieties. In addition to the varying types of firing mechanisms, there were several styles of guns incorporated into sticks; rifles, pistols, revolvers, machine guns and combinations of these with concealed daggers and bayonets.

As expected, gun cane design originally emulated the prevalent gun design and style(s). Consequently the barrel of some earlier types curve upward from the mid-section when held horizontally so that one could place the handle of the cane under the arm pit and sight forward toward the end of the barrel. As this was a dead giveaway (no pun intended), in later examples the entire shaft was straightened and topped with a typical crutch handle.

One of the earliest and most desirable gun canes is a flint-lock pistol concealed in a wooden cane shaft. A particular specimen in my collection is a small, perfect gem manufactured by Henry William Vander Kleft, who obtained an English patent dated 1814 for its prototype. It is one of my oldest gun canes and is perfectly disguised. Its bec de corbin (semi-crook) handle doubles as the handle of the pistol which is withdrawn from the shaft by pressing a side button release. The flint-lock is at half cock when inserted in the cane and, of course, the pistol would have been loaded with powder and ball before insertion. When the pistol is drawn, a folding trigger immediately springs out. Then, when the flint mechanism is pulled to full cock, it is ready to be fired. This gun cane is beautifully made and bears the signature "W. H. Kleft, Inventor" on one side of the barrel and the inscription "London" on the other amid scrolled engravings.

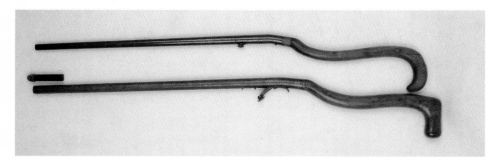

Two Day percussion cap gun canes.
Right: 38 1/4" high.

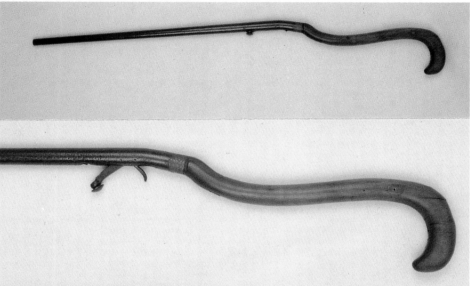

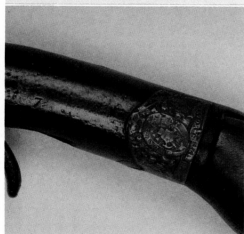

Day's patented percussion cap and ball
gun cane, 36 1/2" high.

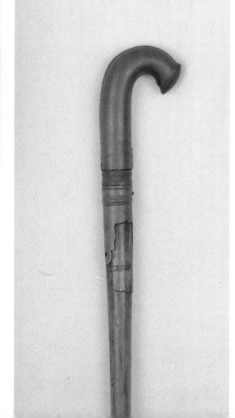

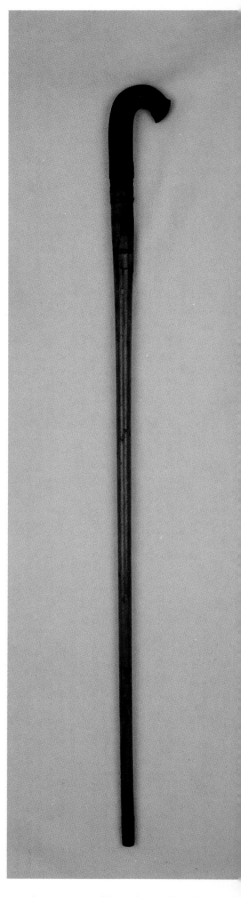

Early air gun cane with entire shaft as the
barrel and a bec de corbin handle. 43"
high.

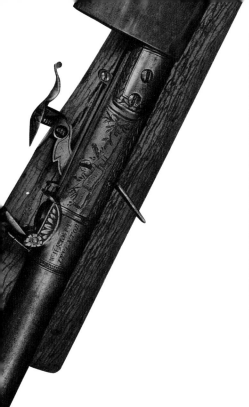

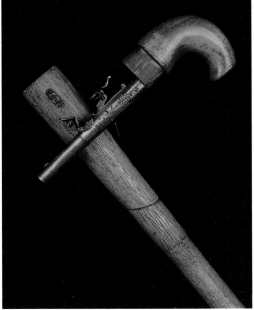

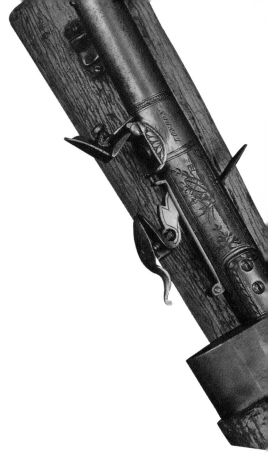

Flintlock pistol pulls from within the shaft. The barrel is engraved on the left "W.H. KLEFT INVENTOR" and on the right "LONDON," 35 1/4" high, pistol measures 8 1/4" in length.

Interestingly, while American Revolutionaries were still making and using flint-lock guns, the Austrians were perfecting powerful air guns. These were considered so lethal that Napoleon hanged every Austrian soldier he captured who carried one. Bonaparte claimed their use was immoral and an affront to decency as the air gun made no sound and did not emit a pall of black smoke indicating from where the shot came, as did the black powder flint-locks of that day. Even the Pope issued a bull prohibiting their use in humane, Christian warfare.

George Washington is said to have sent Benjamin Franklin to Europe to buy such guns for his Revolutionary Army, but the project had to be abandoned when it became clear that there were insufficient American smiths familiar with the repair and use of the touchy air valves employed in these guns. Furthermore, our government was poor, and the guns were costly. Early colonists made their own flint-lock guns from native materials. Later, Lewis and Clark carried an air gun on their exploration trip West. Its lack of noise and powder pall so astounded the Indians that they knelt in awe of the explorers.

It was inevitable that the air gun should be incorporated into a cane. Many of these were manufactured in England after 1848. They became very popular and were even cased with fine accouterments. Some of these air gun canes had interchangeable barrel which could shoot either ball or shot. The barrel for the ball was even rifled. Both barrels are in the cane, the rifled barrel inside the shotgun barrel. If one wishes to use the rifle, the gun is all set. If one chooses to use shot, one just unscrews and takes out the rifled barrel. All air gun canes could be inflated with the pumps that came with them, then fired 15 to 20 times without repumping. As Napoleon had discovered, they were noiseless, lethal and left no lingering smoke to indicate from which direction the shot came. They became the perfect poacher's weapon and were often used in England to deplete the game on noble estates by, apparently, innocent cane-toting peasants.

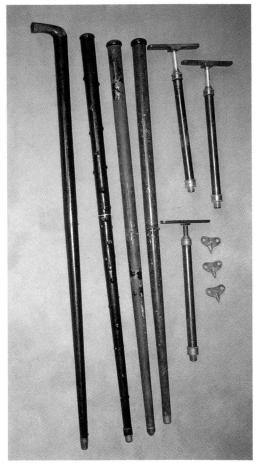

A grouping of British air gun canes with the pumps and keys necessary for firing.

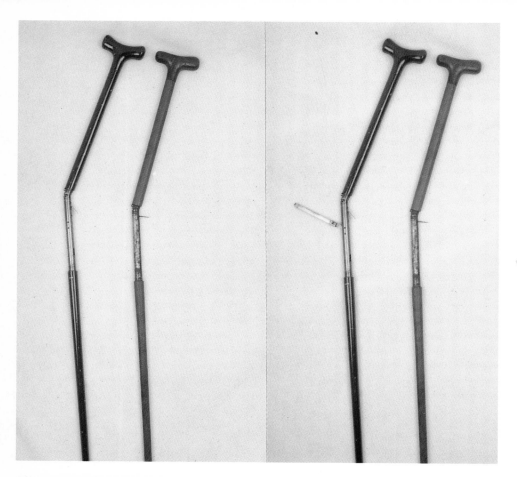

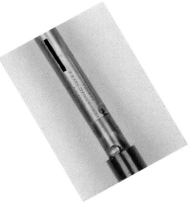

Lang's air gun canes cocked and ready, inscribed above: "Patent J. Lang 22 Cockspur Street, London, No. 222"; below: "7 Market Steet, London, No. 100."

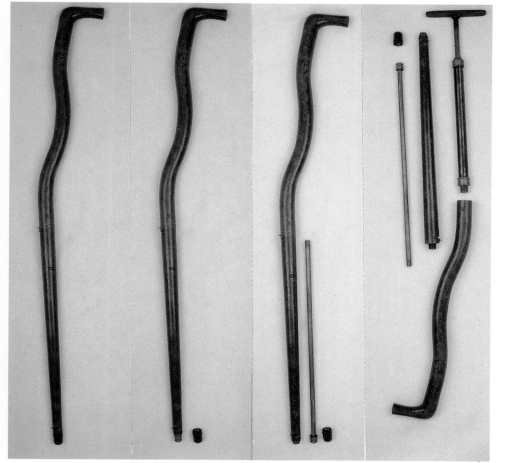

Air gun cane with pump, brass rifled insert. When the brass rifled insert is removed, it's a smooth bore shotgun. 37 1/2" high.

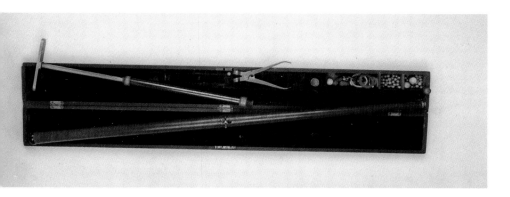

Complete air gun cane kit with pump, 36"
high.

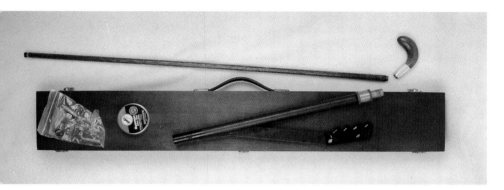

Modern American air gun cane kit by
Beeman Precision Arms.

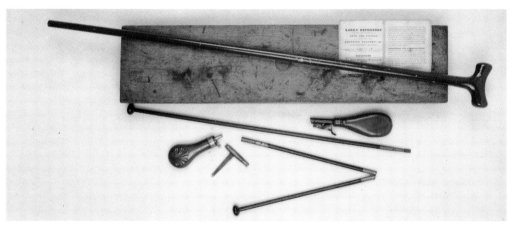

Concurrent with the appearance of
the air gun came the cap and ball canes.
One which is particularly sought after, by
stick *and* gun collectors, is the cased cap
and ball set by Joseph Lang, an early 19th
century London manufacturer. This
prized item contains many accessories:
cocking and capping tools, powder flask,
bullet mold, nipple wrench, vent prick,
oil can, caps, ramrod, replacement parts,
etc.

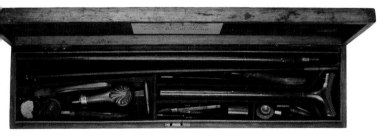

Rare complete percussion cap and ball
gun cane kit by Joseph Lang, 36" high

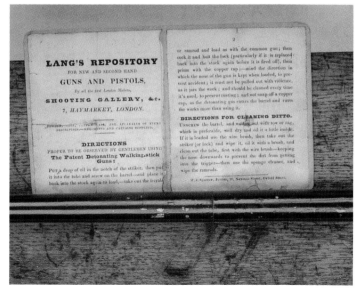

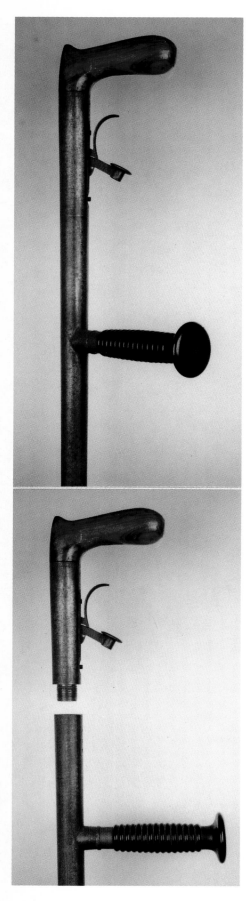

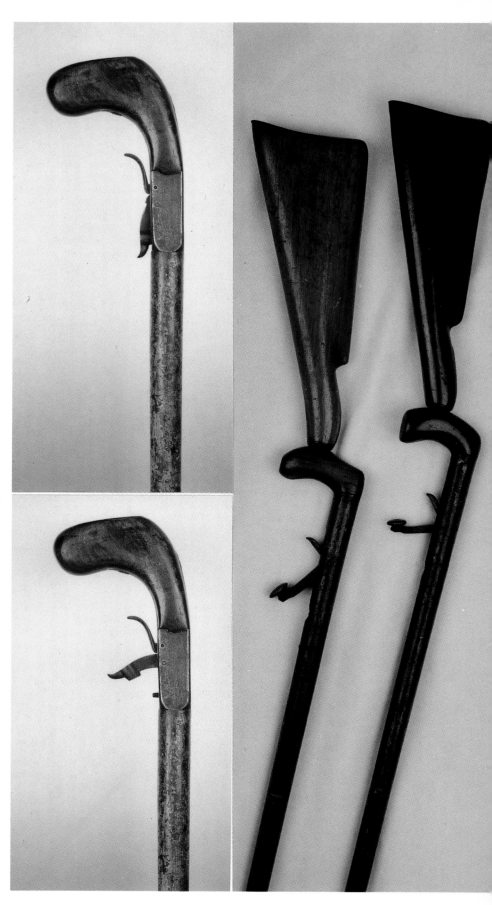

Large percussion cap and ball Chartelsworth (?) gun with underhammer mount and elevator handle, 35" high.

Underhammer percussion cap and ball model with fitting for a rifle stock at end of handle, 35 1/4" high.

Two underhammer percussion cap and ball gun canes with removable stocks.

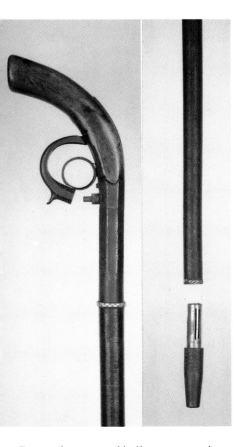

Percussion cap and ball gun cane, trigger guard is the hammer and trigger holds it in cock, 35 3/4" high.

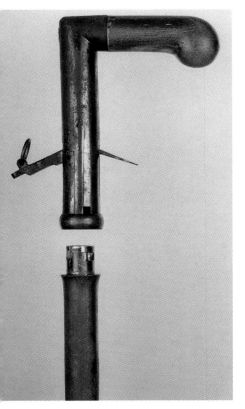

Cap and ball gun cane. Lift the ring to cock the hammer and set the trigger. Horn handle, 32" high.

In the U.S., the most widely acclaimed cap and ball canes were made by the Remington Arms Company from 1858. These were designed by J.F. Thomas who obtained a patent February 9, 1858. Remington also produced a cartridge gun cane through 1889. The latter are prized items and were made of gutta-percha over steel. Gutta-percha is the sap of a tree and served as a forerunner of hard rubber and plastics. The most desirable of the Remington gun canes is the dog head model in both cap and ball and cartridge types. These were made for .22-caliber short or .32-caliber short rimfire cartridges. Remington discontinued making these gun canes about 1910. Nevertheless, the Remington gun cane has always been the most beautiful and most well-balanced of all gun canes to date. Hence its great desirability.

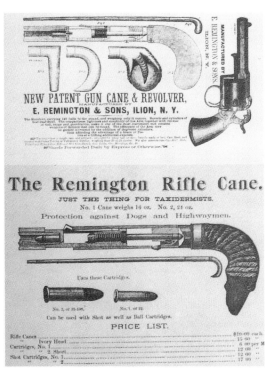

Remington Arms Company gun cane advertising.

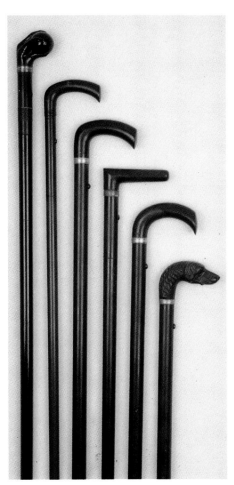

Six Remington Gun canes. Among the finest and best known of the American gun canes. The model with the bird's claw handle contains a percussion-cap firing mechanism of the type first patented in 1858. The remainder are cartridge models.

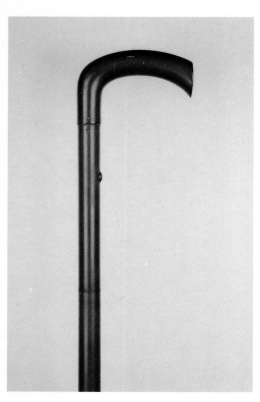

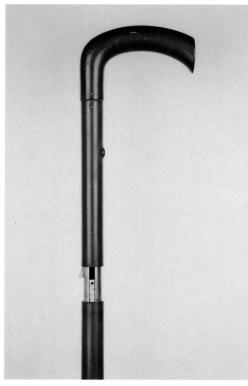

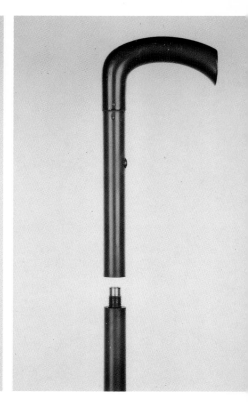

Lady Remington gun cane, 22 caliber, gutta percha shaft, 35 3/4" high.

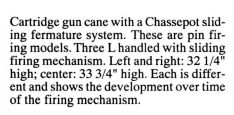

Cartridge gun cane with a Chassepot sliding fermature system. These are pin firing models. Three L handled with sliding firing mechanism. Left and right: 32 1/4" high; center: 33 3/4" high. Each is different and shows the development over time of the firing mechanism.

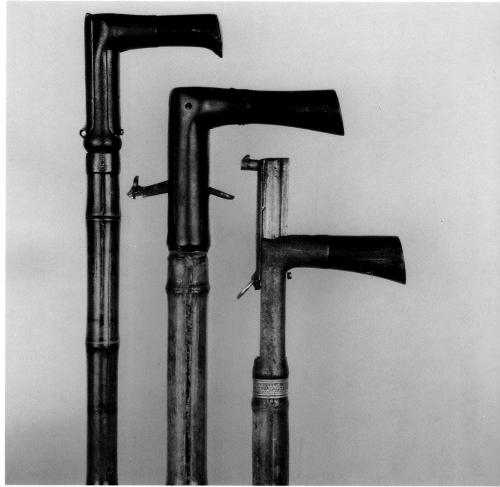

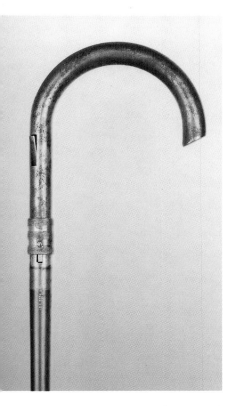
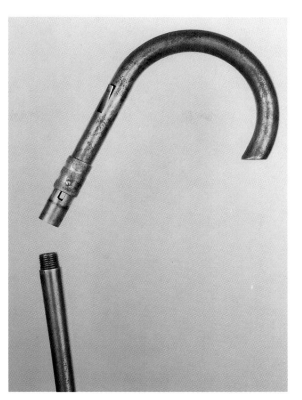
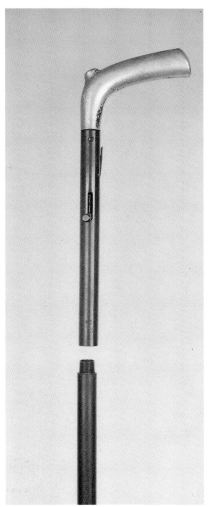

Pull back collar to expose trigger on this cartridge gun cane. The collar snaps back into place when fired. Silver shaft and crook handle, 33 1/2" high.

Pull bolt forward and back to set trigger for firing, silver handle, 34 3/4" high. A fine cartridge gun cane I purchased from the commander of the dirigible Macon.

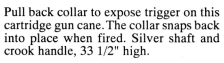
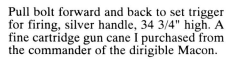
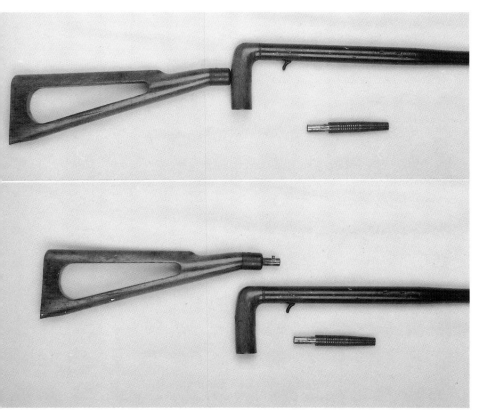

Breech loader with a hollow stock and tampion.

In 1877 Marcelin Daigle patented a repeating rifle gun cane which is very rarely found today. It had a metal shaft with a spherical or knob handle. A few inches below the handle, the shaft slid open to reveal a breech. From there to the bottom, the shaft contained two parallel tubes: one the rifle barrel, the other a cartridge magazine. A push button release on the side of the shaft near the handle would spring open, cock the breech and eject the previously spent cartridge. When the handle is pushed forward, the breech closes and the gun fires. This "push-pull action" causes the gun to eject a spent shell, chamber a new cartridge, cock the mechanism, close the breech and fire the gun. The procedure is repeated as often as the handle is pushed and pulled. The magazine holds about 20 cartridges of .22-caliber.

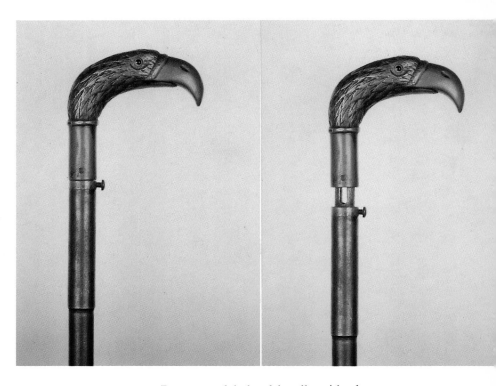

Bronze eagle's head handle with glass eyes, pull up and down to cock, then push the button to fire, 37" high.

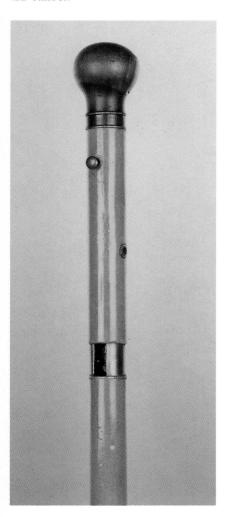

Rare Daigle repeating gun cane featuring a horn knob handle with eyelet. Push the handle back and forth to automatically load and discharge, cock and fire by pushing the button each time, 33" high.

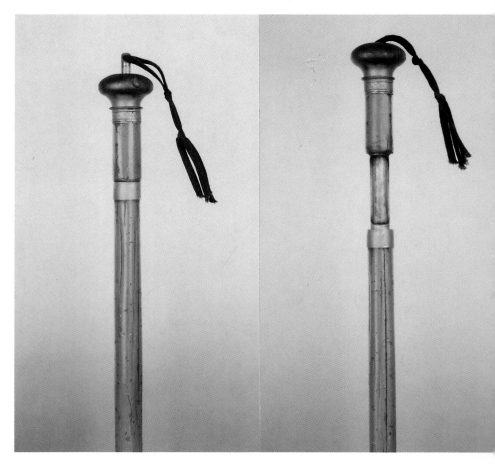

Breech loader with vertical firing pin, released by push button on handle, step malacca shaft, 33 1/2" high.

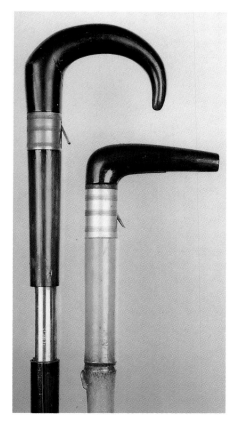

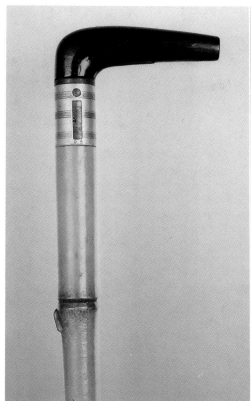

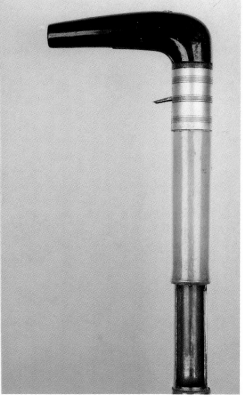

Two breech loaders, horn crutch and L-shaped handles, turn collars to reveal triggers, 35 3/8" high.

Black horn handle, malacca colored iron shaft, sight, breech loading, 35 1/4" high.

Pull back firing pin at end of gold handle, breech loading, 35 1/2" high.

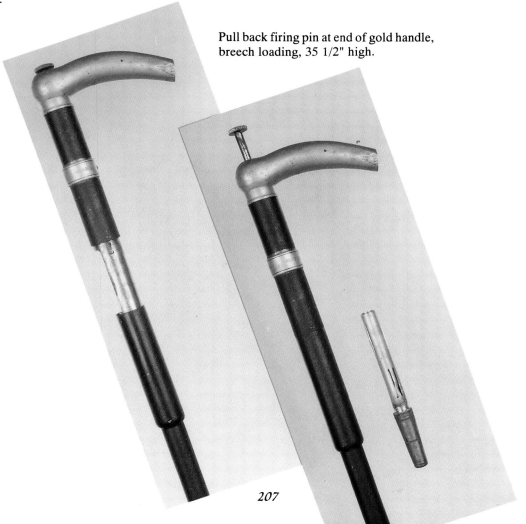

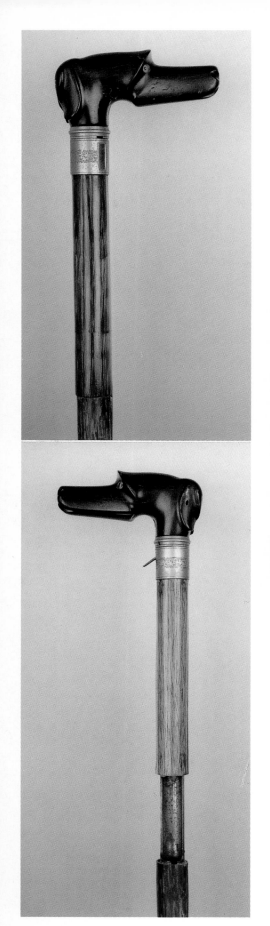

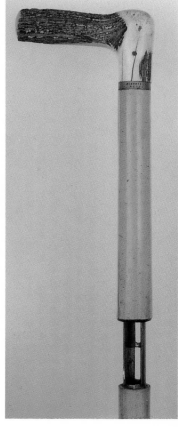

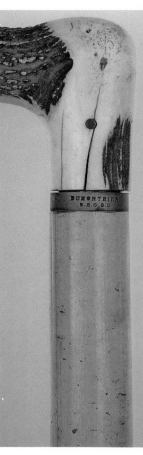

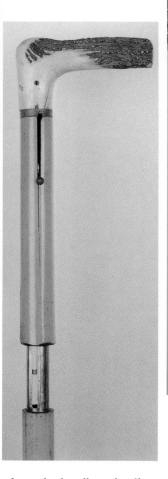

Turn the antler handle and pull to expose the breech of this breech loader by Dumonthier, 34 1/2" high.

Horn dog's head breech loader, turn the collar to expose the trigger, 36" high.

While many other types of gun canes were manufactured, most were of single shot design. In Europe, the most popular were the rifle and shotgun types made by Dumonthier in the mid-19th century. When their crutch handle is twisted to the left and pulled back while the shaft is held stationary, a breech opens. Into this, one can load a rifle or shotgun shell, depending upon the type of gun. The handle is then pushed forward to close the breech and turned to the right. The weapon is now loaded, cocked and set. Still, it appears just an ordinary cane to the casual observer. By turning a slotted band under the handle, it will pass over a concealed cavity from which a trigger will drop. The gun can then be activated and fired, providing the tampion/ferrule closing the end of the cane barrel is first removed.

The aforementioned gunsmith who fired my gun cane had neglected to do this, and blew the tampion so far he never found it. He had to make a new one in addition to hammering down the ballooned barrel resulting from the compressed gas explosion. Had the tampion not been blown out, he most certainly would have mutilated his hand, as the barrel would have burst in the resulting discharge.

These accidents must have occurred many times in the early development of the gun cane, as later models are cocked by an entirely different mechanism. The tampion in the bottom of the barrel, which also serves as the cane's ferrule, was altered so that it had to be removed in order to cock the gun as it was designed as a tool for this purpose. The tampion has a small hook extending outward from the inside of the removed ferrule. This hook fits into a hole in the back of the cane handle. The hole is an upward extension of the gun barrel which holds the firing pin device. At its top end, the firing pin is designed to be hooked by the tampion and pulled back. In this way, it is locked in a cocked position to be activated by the trigger. The tampion hooks were safety devices preventing explosions caused by the failure to remove them from the barrel.

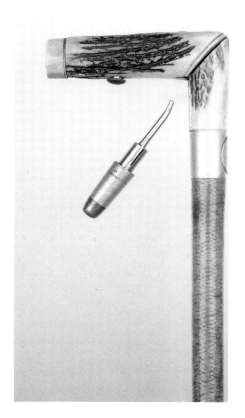

The ferrule operates under the handle to cock the gun. Antler handled German gun cane, c. 1875, with a metal shaft covered with cloth weave and varnished. 35 1/2" high.

Use the clip on the ferrule to pull back and cock the firing pin. Crook horn handle, wood covered metal barrel, 36 1/4" high.

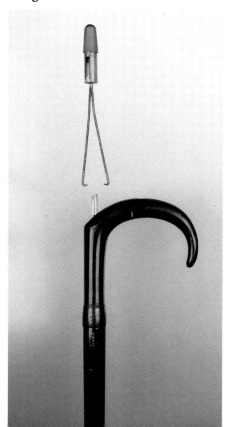

Even in the U.S. these tampion safety features were patented before 1840, although one cannot obtain the patent papers through the usual sources. While I have accumulated all the available patent papers ever issued on canes in the U.S., England and Germany, I do not have this one. One example of these gun canes in my collection has a hinged ferrule on the bottom with no tampion inserted in the barrel at all. The metal cane is covered by a wood sheath in which the barrel floats — i.e., it can be moved backward very slightly manually, then lurches forward by spring action. Dr. Roger Lambert filed this patent in 1832, the first for a gun cane in the U.S. When the bulbous ivory knob handle is pulled back after first being unlocked by twisting a brass band, the cane's intricate firing mechanisms are activated. Simultaneously, the hinged ferrule drops and hangs out of the way.

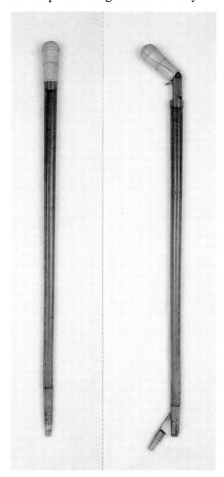

First American patented gun cane by Dr. Roger N. Lambert. The ferrule is spring loaded and pops down, freeing the barrel when the ivory handle is pulled back to reveal the trigger mechanism, c. 1840. 33" high.

Other gun activating mechanisms of German design prior to 1900 are completely hidden in the handle, and the gun is cocked by pulling a lever down from under the grip. This movement cocks the firing pin and ejects the trigger.

Some canes enclose complete 6-shot revolvers, often with attached daggers, and their shock value is enhanced tremendously when they are pulled from an innocuous stick. Such sticks are often referred to as "pepper boxes."

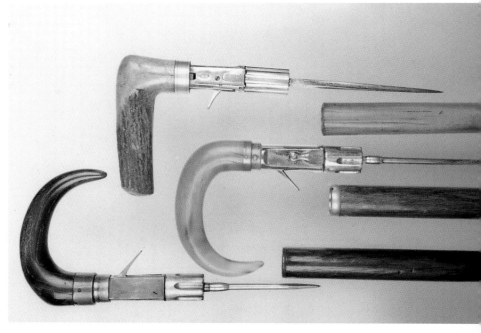

Three rare pepper box gun canes with stilettos of Belgium make. The ferrule on these pull out and reveal long plunger rods used to push the spent cartridges out of their chambers. This is a feature frequently overlooked.

Two German models, pull out lever to expose trigger, c. 1890. Left: 36 3/4" high; right: 34 3/4" high. These are the finest single shot German gun canes, c. 1880. One is rifled and the other is a shot gun.

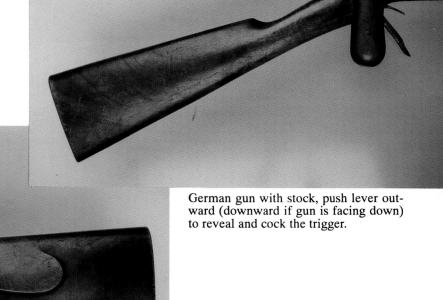

German gun with stock, push lever outward (downward if gun is facing down) to reveal and cock the trigger.

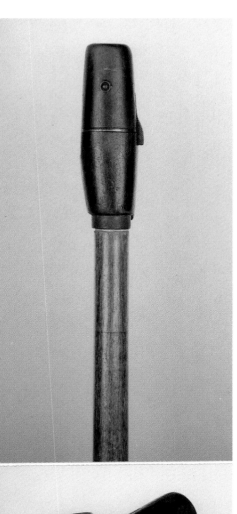

What is not generally known and therefore overlooked is that most of these canes have a removable ferrule which has a long inner extension that is used as a probe to eject spent shells from the cartridge holder.

Most gun canes require the use of two hands to cock and activate the firing mechanism. Seeing his opportunity, in 1921 an enterprising Frenchman named C. Joriot invented a gun cane which could be operated with only one hand. In addition, it shoots two cartridges. This is a pistol cane that has an indiscernible activator on the inside of its soft, black leather handle. When the handle is pressed by the right thumb on its left side, it releases a spring which blows the entire shaft from the breech, leaving only the pistol in the hand. Then, using the same pressure activator, one can fire up to two cartridges. All this is easily accomplished with one hand.

Another of my canes is a combination gun and sword which is quite heavy, but has a fine staghorn handle mounted on a beautiful dark wooden shaft. It is said to have been made in France, but the only inscription is "M. DEPOSSE" on the silver band connecting the handle to the gun mechanism. The wood veneer covers a thin, iron barrel which, in turn, conceals a round 19" tube with a 3" stiletto or bayonet affixed to its far end. This gun barrel fires a .38 center fire cartridge. It has a long, thin, steel rod ejector. At its distal, end, it contains a hollow brass tube for storing three reserve cartridges. This particular stick is so heavy it could easily be used as a bludgeon in a pinch.

It is rare for a gun cane to contain a pistol rather than just a rifle or shotgun, and rarer still to house a rifle-pistol-sword-dagger combination. Some splendid examples of the latter were made for Indian maharajahs and are constructed of steel inlaid with gold, silver or brass in ornate scrolled and floral patterns which cover the entire cane. One in my collection was made about 1850 and conceals a percussion pistol, rifle, sword, dagger and elephant prod. It even contains its own firing balls and other accouterments in the handle's compartments. Again, as would be expected, this is an extremely heavy cane which provides a clue that it is more than it initially seems to be.

In addition to the typical types, there are the odd-ball gun canes such as cartridge canes activated by blowing a floating firing pin with one's mouth at the end of the rounded cane handle. The original version has a covering cap which is removed to reveal a mouth piece into which one forcibly blows. This propels the floating firing pin against and discharges the single cartridge which is centered in the shaft half-way down the stick. Evidently the recoil from this discharge could be sufficiently violent to knock out the front teeth of the user. Later examples have rubber-cushioned mouth pieces.

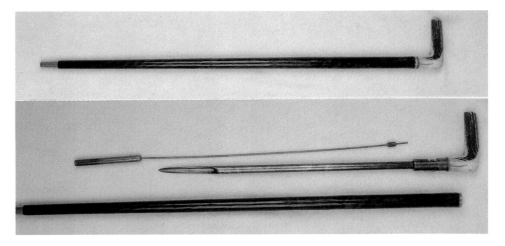

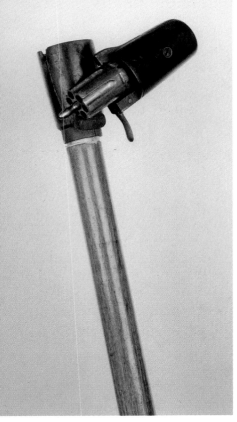

Bicycle handle pepper box pistol converted into the handle of a gun cane, 35 3/4" high.

Unusual antler handled cane with a gun that has a bayonet for a barrel end, all inside the outer shaft, 36 3/4" high.

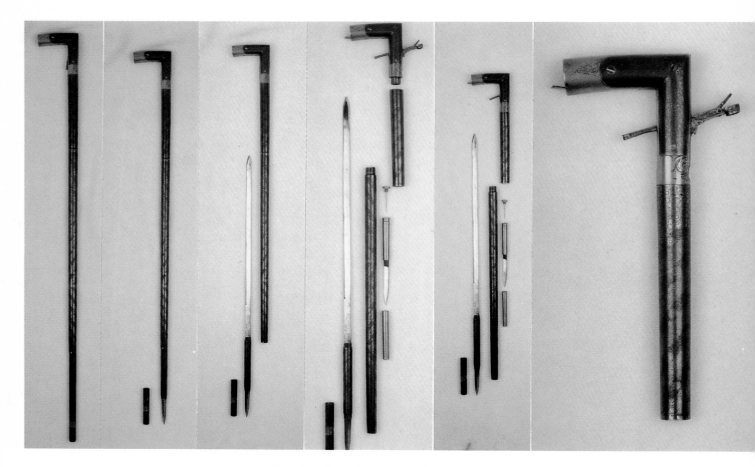

Nineteenth century percussion cap gun cane of East Indian Maharajah royalty in six parts.

Arabian gun cane with silver inlay on a Dumonthier gun cane.

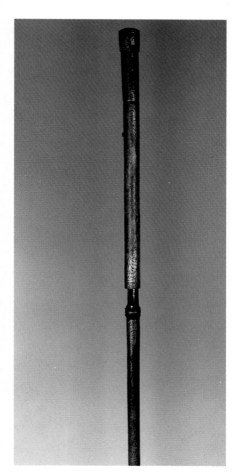

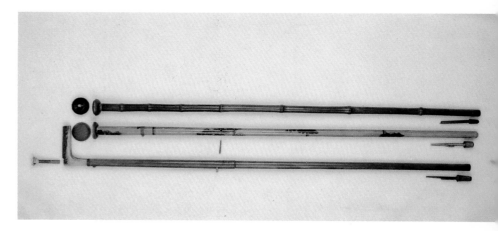

Three blow pipe canes. Left: with antler L handle, blow hole revealed with removal of piece of handle, 37" high; center: 34 1/2" high; right: 34 3/4" high.

The English passion for darts encouraged the development of a system stick made up of a blow gun with which one might shoot darts or, more lethally, arrows. In 1867, the British advertised these "Walking Stick Blow Tubes" for shooting vermin, birds and rabbits — a pleasing outdoor amusement. Some years back, however, we all read about the Bulgarian secret police using a somewhat updated version of these canes in London to mortally wound one of its defecting agents. The pellet used was filled with spider poison and was presumed to have been ejected from a tube by compressed air. It was so small that the victim did not know for days, even as he lay dying in a hospital, that he had been shot. All he remembered was that a suspiciously-looking man had pointed an umbrella at him and, a few hours later, he became ill.

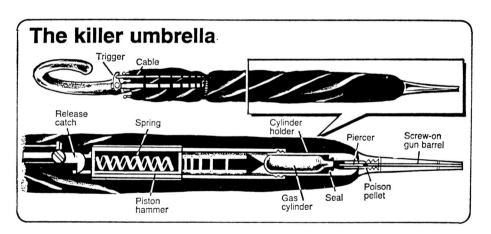

English blow gun cane, malacca shaft, c. 1900, 35" high.

Mississippi River boat gamblers used a simple gun stick similar to the Chinese cannon cane. A small, tilting 'cannon' is mounted horizontally at the top of the cane's shaft. It has a touch hole at the top rear of the handle. When a lighted faggot was placed to the touch hole, it activated the cannon. Our gentleman gambler merely pointed his pre-loaded cane handle toward his victim and, while keeping up his "Who, me?" gambit, nonchalantly passed his cigar over the touch hole thereby detonating the cannon. As the cannon barrel was tilted upward, it invariably caused a wound in a vital abdominal area. Because these sticks were cigar activated, they are known as "cheroot" canes.

Many of my canes are real Rube Goldberg contraptions. Others are so mysterious that, though I know what they are, I cannot discover how to work them. I hope that any readers who recognize these pictures and can tell me how they work will be kind enough to write me.

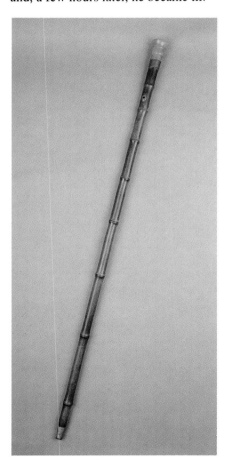

Blow dart cane with false eyelets, handle is mouthpiece, c. 1885, 38 1/2" high.

The killer umbrella

Trigger Cable

Release catch   Spring   Cylinder holder   Piercer   Screw-on gun barrel

Piston hammer   Gas cylinder   Seal   Poison pellet

The Killer Cane.

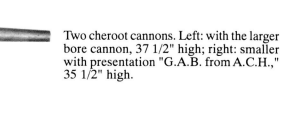

Two cheroot cannons. Left: with the larger bore cannon, 37 1/2" high; right: smaller with presentation "G.A.B. from A.C.H.," 35 1/2" high.

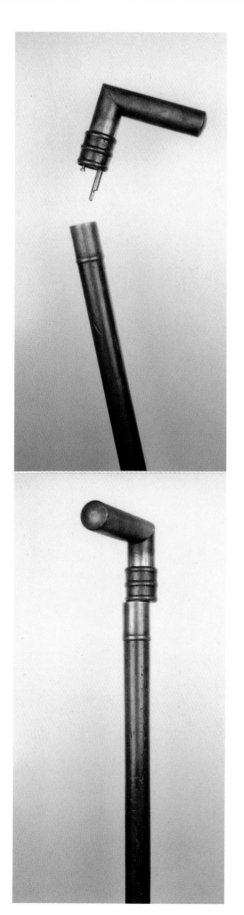

Sword Canes

Every beginning cane collector prides himself on his first sword cane. This category is so varied that this in itself would make a fine sub-specialty to collect. There are canes with long swords inside the shaft ; with daggers inside the shaft ; with short blades in the handle itself that flick out by a sudden downward thrust of the head when the shaft is held at the middle and there are walking sticks having blades that shake and flick out of the bottom. Others contain a sword and a dagger so one can use the dagger in the left hand for close combat while paring and thrusting with the longer blade in the right hand.

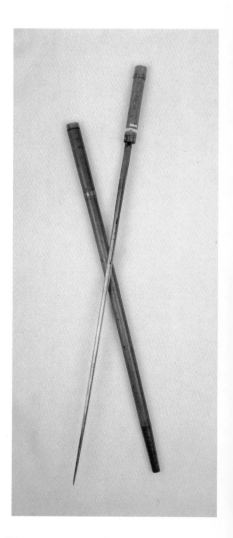

Handle pulls back and down to reveal the firing pin, 35 3/4" high. This is a complicated mechanism — a real "Rube Goldberg."

A very mysterious gun cane mechanism. Pull back the collar and the handle turns and comes loose, 32 1/2" high.

There are canes with long swords inside the shafts. Old English sword cane engraved with the date "Sep 22 1786, Hennery Peak," on silver handle, triangular blade, 35 3/8" high with a 4" high ferrule.

214

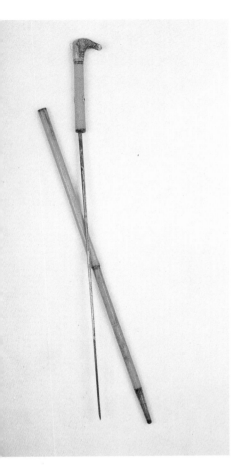

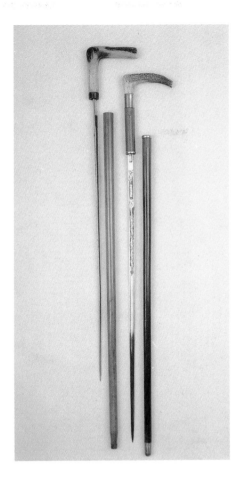

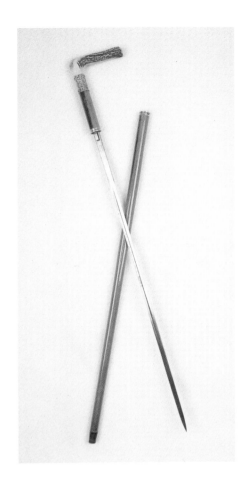

Bec de Corbin antler handled sword cane, c. 1730, malacca shaft, very old, etched blade, eyelets, 35 1/4" high, ferrule 3 1/4" high.

Silver knob handle marked "Paris 10 Dec 1888." Twist the handle to unlock the double edged blade. This cane has a malacca shaft, 35 3/4" high.

Two antler handled sword canes. Left: three sided Toledo blade, black collar, malacca shaft, 35 1/2" high; right: silver collar, triangular Toledo blade, 36 1/2" high, twist malacca shaft to release blade.

Antler handle Toledo blade, twist the malacca shaft to release the blade, the shaft separates at silver collar, 36" high.

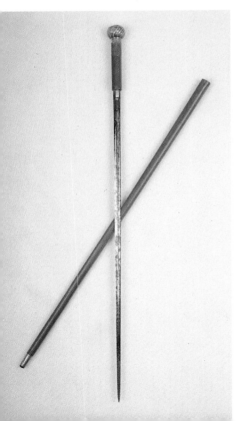

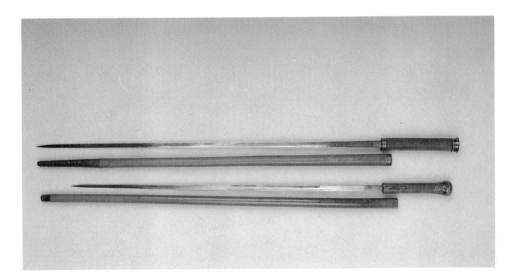

Two malacca shafted straight handled sword canes with Toledo blades. Left: silver end cap, three sides blade, 36" high, 5" ferrule; right: silver knob handle with triangular blade, 35 1/2" high, 1" high ferrule.

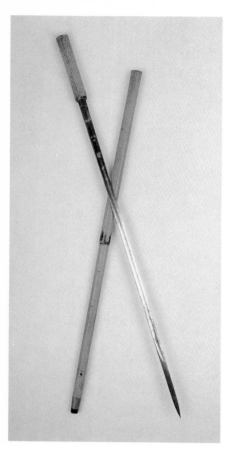

Straight handle with small ivory cap, etched single edged blade, c. 1860, 35 3/4" high.

Other canes hide daggers within their shafts. Ivory hand handle with dagger, four sided marked "IN SOLIGEN" on blade, 33 1/2" high.

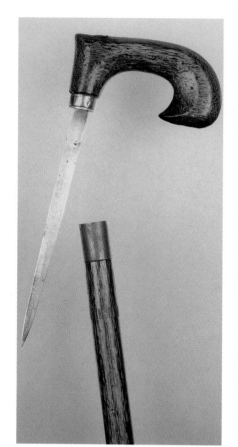

South American dagger.

Some canes house short blades in the handles themselves that flick out with a sudden downward thrust of the cane head when the shaft is held at the middle. Three flick sticks, all with knob handles. Left: black knob, bamboo shaft, 34 1/2" high; center: wood handle on a malacca shaft, 36" high; right: all wood, remains in natural — almost folk art — condition, 35 1/

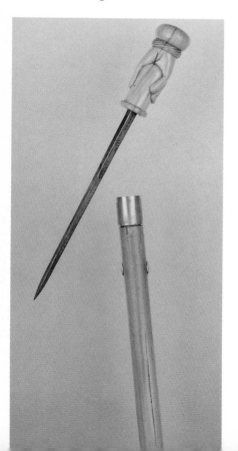

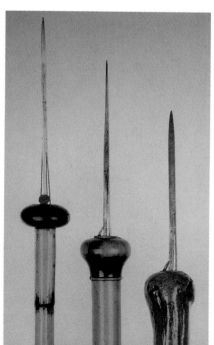

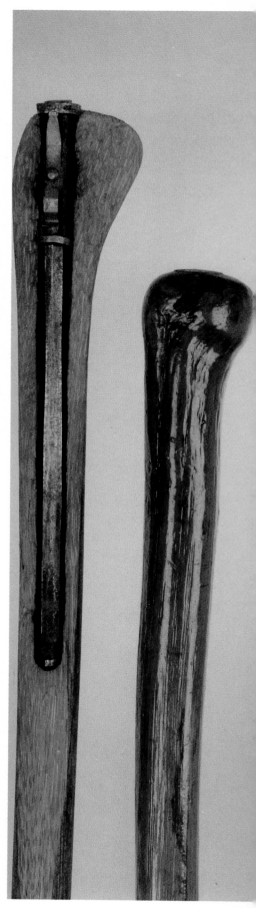

The inner workings of a flick stick.

Some canes have beautifully etched blades and finely carved handles and all are cleverly concealed in innocent appearing shafts. The second gadget cane patented in the U.S. was a sword cane. Many of the blades are locked into the shaft and it takes a knowledgeable collector to find how to open them. Some handles are turned half clockwise on the shaft and then pulled to withdraw the blade; others have a push button somewhere on the handle. It may be so ingeniously hidden that it may be merely one of several protrusions such as a branch knob that appears to be part of the handle, or one of many decorative precious or lesser stones.

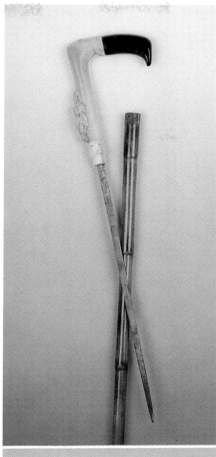

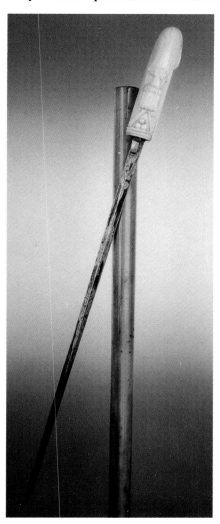

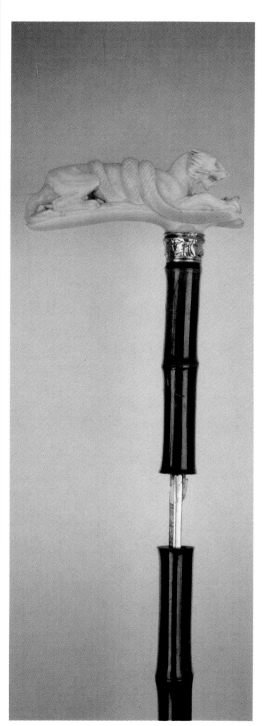

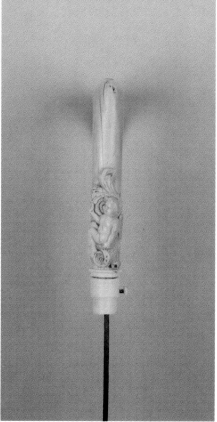

Some blades have beautifully etched blades and finely carved handles. Ivory handle engraved with Southern Civil War military equipment including a back pack, cannon balls and a Southern cap, concealed dagger cane with a beautifully decorated blade. Malacca shaft. The cane opens by pressing the right cannon ball. This cane dates from c. 1860. 34 3/4" high.

Old French ivory and horn L handle sword cane with cherub on handle, partridge wood shaft, c. 1600. 35 3/4" high.

Bone tiger and snake in battle, silver collar, decorated sword blade, 36" high.

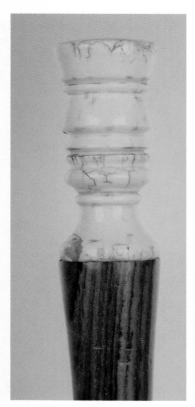

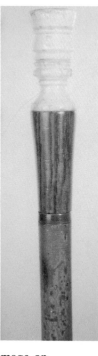

Napoleon shadow cane, casts image on wall, ivory handle, sword blade within, 35 1/4" high.

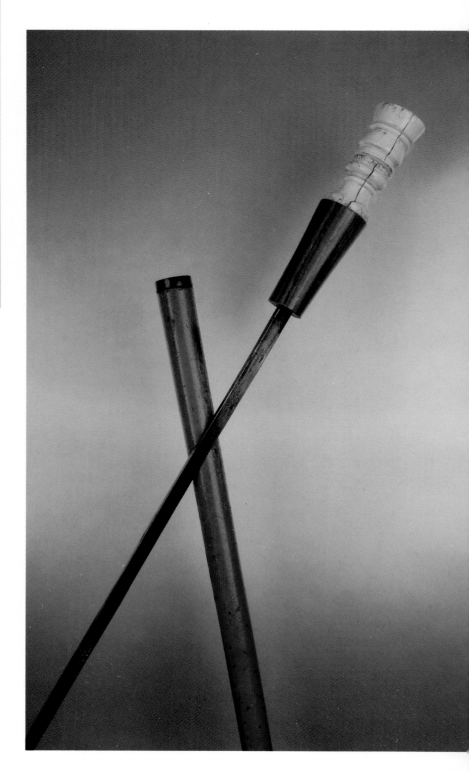

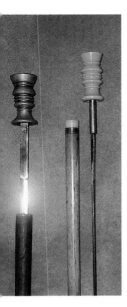

Two Napoleon shadow handle sword canes.

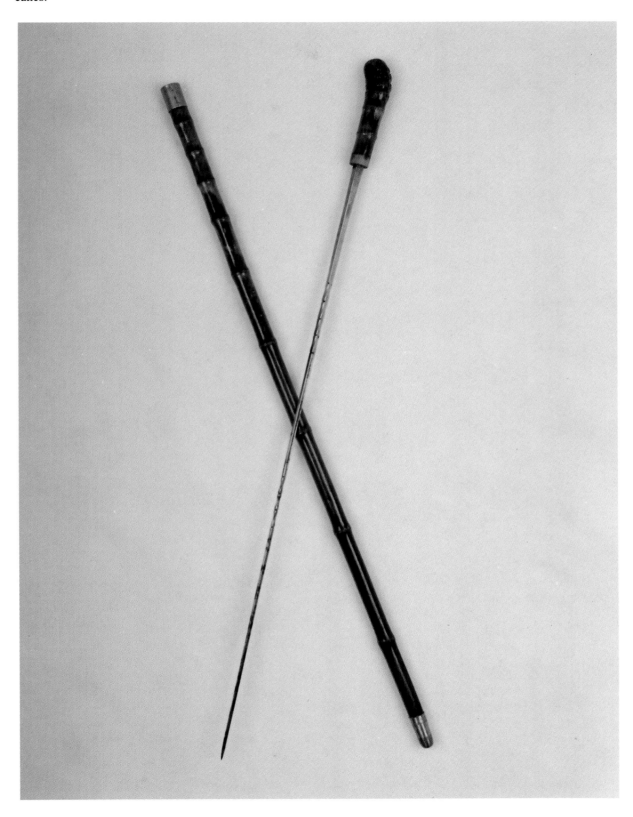

Some swords are very well hidden in the canes. Bamboo shaft and root handle, four sided blade within, serrated at intervals, 36 3/4" high.

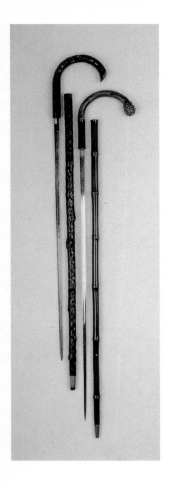

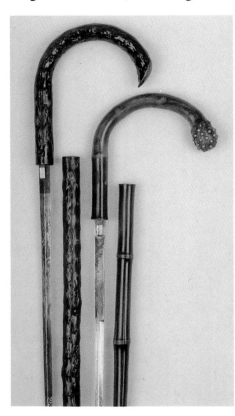

Two crook handles with swords, very well hidden. Left: push button releases double edged blade from within vine shaft, c. 1900, 35 3/4" high; right: crook handle with silver beads in the end of the handle, triangular sword blade, 37 1/2" high.

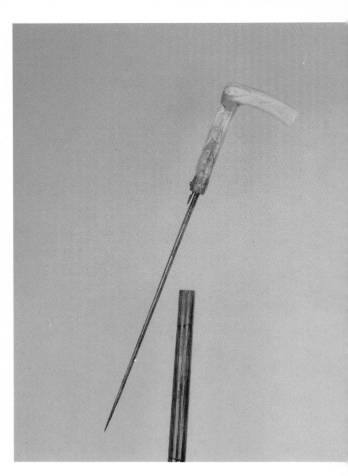

Bone L handle carved with leaves and acorns, brass collar with push button, small knife blade within, c. 1850, 35 1/2" high.

Originally all upper class citizens in England and Europe carried swords as defense weapons, a step above in a society where the lower classes were limited to their staffs and cudgels. Because of the constant warfare amongst the nations, people were already accustomed to the swords carried by men in the army, and now these soldiers upon discharge from the kings service kept the swords as mementos and emblems of their patriotic service.

As seen from old pictures and prints, all officers when in civil society carried the fashion-demanded cane in addition to their military swords. This made a most encumbering picture indeed, and now all the discharged soldiers were carrying their swords into their civil lives.

As every man was now armed, when disputes arose in taverns amongst the ale and wine drinking citizens, bloody clashes would arise because of some imagined slight or slur. As a result, the various nations and countries forbade the

carrying of a sword in civil life except by the authorities or the upper classes. Almost naturally now the swords were concealed in hollowed-out canes.

Stickmakers did not limit themselves to the usual soldier's sword for the blade but designed various others. Thus we find hidden in or by a stick, long swords, shorter swords and daggers. These blades were rapier-like in some instances so that only a pointed blade was employed; others were flat blades sharpened on one or both sides. Then there were four-sided, pointed blades not intended for defensive usage but mostly designed for the customs and taxing officials who would stick them in bedding on horse-drawn carts, bales of wood or cotton to see if any contraband was being smuggled over the border.

Still the eruptions between inebriated or insulted individuals did not abate. You could always assume your assailant had a sword in his cane. A soldier with a regular military sword had a hand guard

to protect himself against his opponents sword, but a civilian with a sword cane containing a long sword had no such protection against a sword blade sharpened on one or both sides. The thug need merely slide his sharp blade down the raised sword blade of his victim and cut his hand so badly that the accosted one had to let go of his sword. Once his hand was slashed in the clash, the outcome was determined. As a defense against such an event, some sword canes were soon constructed so that as one pulled out his sword from his cane, a pair of folding cross bars sprung out and locked into place to form a hand guard. These hand guards were called quillions. For the sword cane collector, these are an advanced and more desirable type of sword cane.

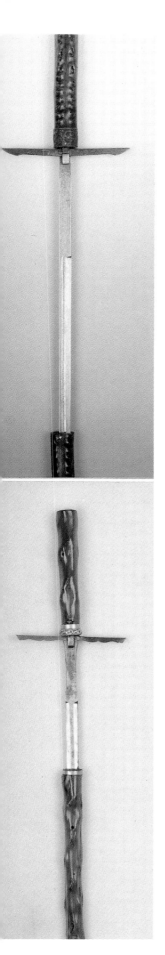

Some sword canes were constructed with a pair of folding cross bars that sprung out and locked into place to form a hand guard. Toledo blade with hand guards springing to action when the blade is released, 35 1/2" high.

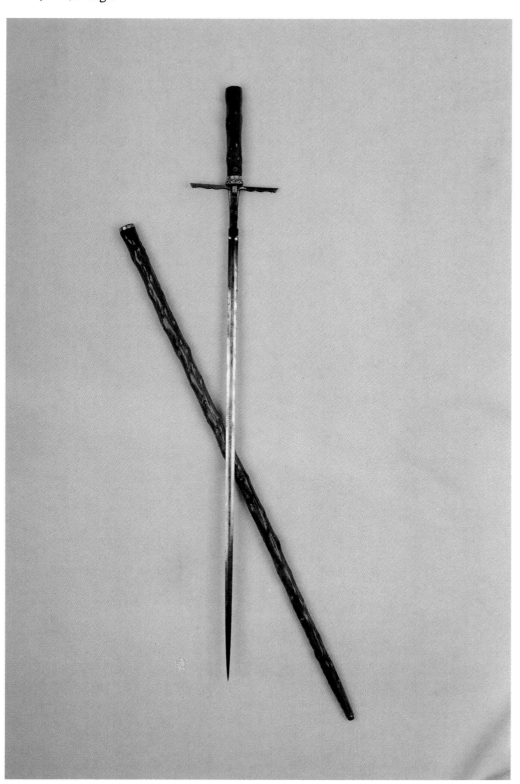

Old sword cane c. 1780, silver on vine, push knob and pull, blade is released and hand guards spring out, 35 1/2" high.

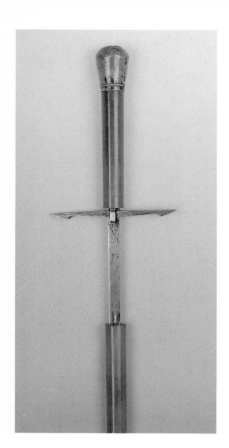

Toledo blade, silver knob handle, malacca
shaft, hand protectors spring forth when
blade is removed from shaft, 37 1/2" high.

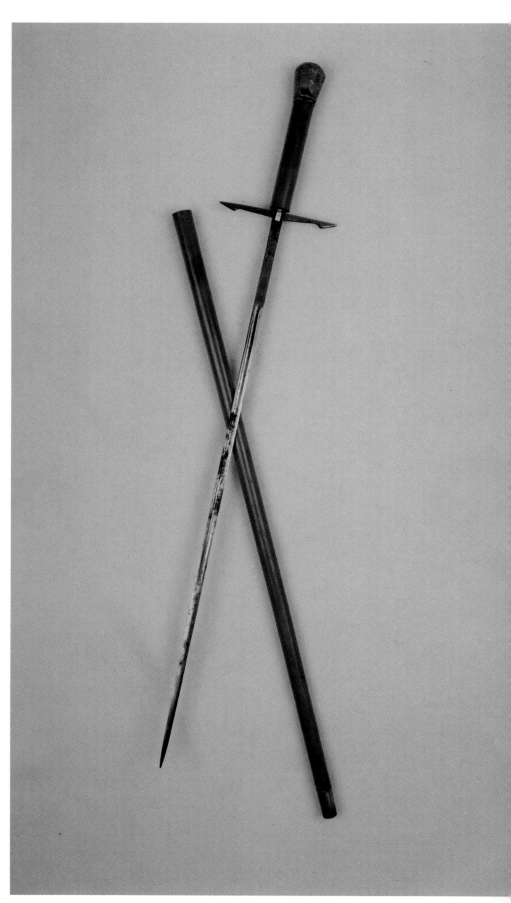

As in all warfare, each new weapon brings out a new defense. Sword canes were made that had a concealed gun barrel in the handles in addition to the hand guard.

Most antique western sword canes have blades that could be called "stickers" because of their sharpened point as distinguished from the Japanese sword canes which have straight blades that are very sharp on one side—the lower side—only and could be called "slashers." This is in conformity with their Samurai swords which in fighting were held by two hands and used to behead or dismember an opponent.

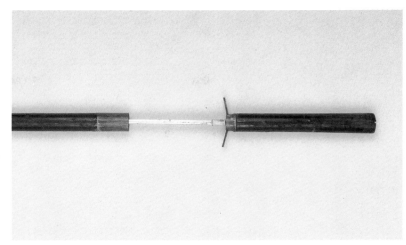

A Japanese sword cane, this one has small spring out hand protectors, single edged blade, 35 1/2" high.

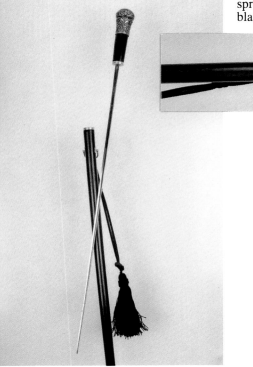

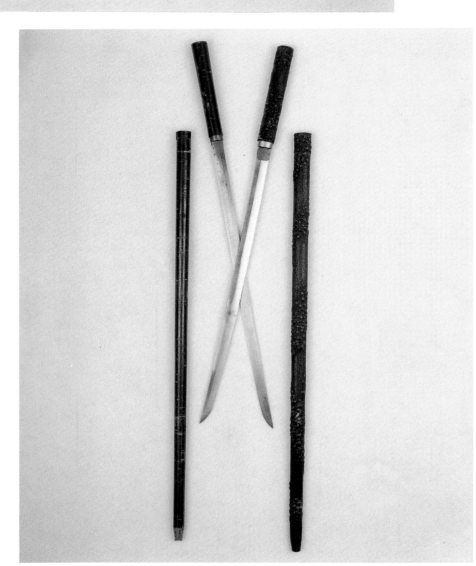

Most antique western sword canes have sharpened points for stabbing. Silver handled sword cane, ebony shaft, eyelets and thog ring, c. 1880, three edged decorated blade, 35 1/2" high.

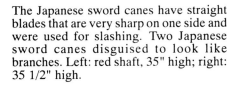

The Japanese sword canes have straight blades that are very sharp on one side and were used for slashing. Two Japanese sword canes disguised to look like branches. Left: red shaft, 35" high; right: 35 1/2" high.

Then there are sword canes that are double whammies. They contain both a spear-like sword and a knife side by side in a cane to be used in the clinches where the opponent has only a simple sword. This cane parts at the usual place but the top or handle is pulled out with the left hand and a regular dagger slides out from where it lay alongside the spear blade of the shaft which is now held at its ferrule end by the right hand and has the advantage of length. While both the combatants are in a clinch with their weapons locked at the wrist, the one with the knife has the advantage as he can just slide it under the guard of his assailant and dispatch him.

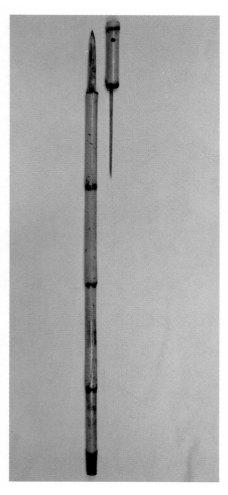

There are sword canes that are double whammies. They contain both a spear-like sword and a knife, side by side.

A less effective type of this sword cane, but nevertheless a desirable collectible, has two blades which lie alongside each other in a common shaft - one having its handle at the ferrule end and the other at the regular upper end. For some reason this is called a dueling sword cane - with a blade for each combatant - as though the owner would not take out and use for himself the better of the two. But then perhaps this dueling sword cane may have been the property of the referee alone.

Andrew Jackson, seventh president of the United States, was known for his hot temper and the sword cane he constantly carried. Once he was attacked by a would-be assassin, Robert Lawrence, and there is a print in the New York Historical Society of Andrew Jackson on the steps of the Capitol in Washington brandishing his unsheathed sword and exclaiming to his restraining friends, "Let me at him, gentlemen, I am not afraid." With his sword cane available, Jackson was not afraid. Earlier he had killed his own cousin, Samuel Jackson, with it. Pleading self defense, Andrew Jackson was acquitted of the crime by a petit jury.

In July 1907, Francis Bannerman published a Catalogue of Military Goods in which he advertised a physician's sword cane, and stated it was the same as carried by priests in the Philippines under Spanish rule. He also advised that it would be sold only to incorporated museums under seal, physicians or collectors who could furnish them with a letter from the chief of police or magistrates of their town under official letter showing right to own such a weapon. Other mail order houses made similar restrictions.

Of course, blades come in all sizes and so do their concealing shaft. Some canes are thinner than a pencil. These are presumed to be ladies' sword canes. Just look at the sinister blade on this Spanish model. When the wicked lady would withdraw it from her victim half his insides would come out with it. Isn't this proof that the female is the more bloodthirsty of the species?

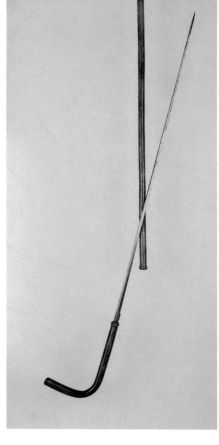

A ladie's sword cane. Very pretty with a narrow L handle cane and double silver collars above a four sided blade, c. 1880. 36" high.

Blades come in all sizes and so do their concealing shafts. Some canes are thinner than a pencil and presumed to the ladies' sword canes. Silver and abalone shell inlay handle with ivory top, shaft unscrews and a long stabbing blade removes, wrist cord, 32 1/4" high.

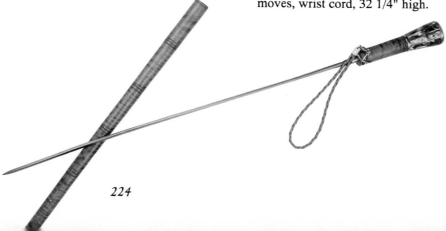

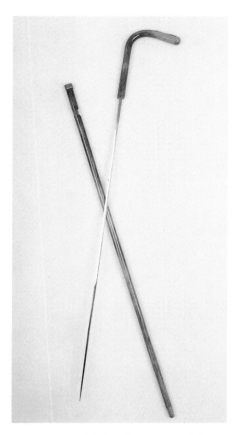

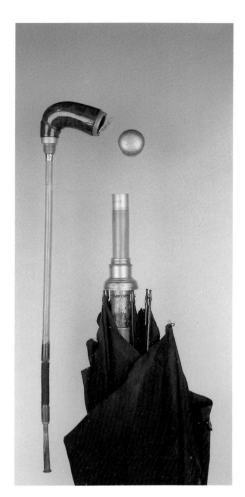

Modern sword canes were being made for the African planters during the Mau-Mau uprising and could be purchased in London. These have Wilkinson sword blades that for quick action, in case the shaft were grasped by an opponent, merely pulled out without any latching device. I purchased one of these at the Wilkinson sword shop on my first trip to London and I carried it all through Europe - but then that was before the metal detectors were installed in all airports.

In this category we must include the sword umbrellas and the gun umbrellas, because umbrellas, like canes, conceal many other objects.

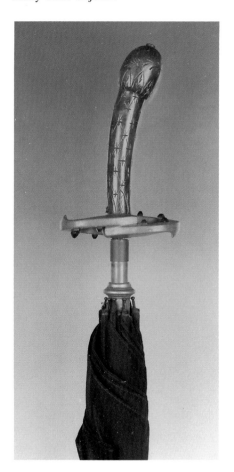

Partridge wood L handle cane, push button to release blade, 35 1/2" high.

A sinister blade is found in this Spanish model. Beautiful bone handled ladie's dagger, push button release, notched cruciform blade, bone ferrule, 33 3/4" high.

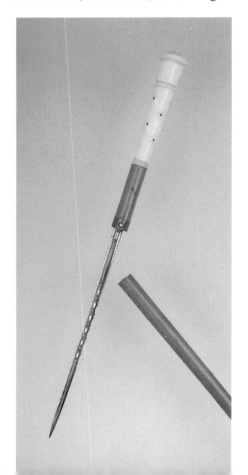

Sword umbrella cane with hand guards, c. 1885, 34 1/2" high.

One particularly interesting old item is an umbrella, the top rain shedder of which can itself be shed on a fine day to use solely as a walking stick. The handle in turn can be unscrewed to furnish a convenient smoking pipe.

Smoking cane and umbrella, German patent, 35 1/2" high. On sunny days the umbrella slides off the shaft and one has a fine walking stick. Should the stroller want to smoke, the handle screws off and a long stemmed pipe emerges. The pipe has a wind and rain cover. The bowl is meershaum lined.

About sword canes, it should be mentioned again that there was a sword cane made and used in Great Britain which was not either an offensive or defensive weapon. It was made for and used by custom officers on the border in the 18th and 19th Century to plunge into bales of wool, etc., to test for concealed contraband. As such, these were usually four sided, heavy blades with a wooden crook handle that fit into a heavy wooden sheath and could be carried like a regular walking stick.

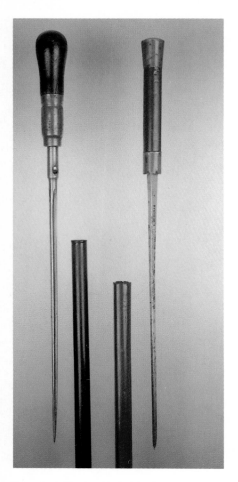

Two short blades. Left: black knob handle with cruciform blade, silver collar marked "LUTZ FILE AND TOOL CO. CINCI/O," 35 3/4" high; right: metal handle and collar, four sided short blade, 35 1/4" high.

Mention of the British custom agent reminds me of a story I heard in Ireland. A very haughty lady was returning from a trip to the sacred shrine at Lourdes, France. The English custom agent at her home port went through her luggage and found a bottle. Taxation on importing spirits was high and he asked what was in this large bottle. She said "honest, it's holy water from Lourdes and I'm bringing it to a sick friend." The custom agent eyed her suspiciously and on a whim he unscrewed the cap and smelled the contents. "It smells like gin, he said." "It can't be," she said, "It's holy water for the sick." The custom agent took a swig and said, "It not only smells of gin, it tastes like gin!" The Irish lady rolled her eyes to heaven and exclaimed, "Glory be to God, a miracle already!" Had she known of and carried a topers stick, she might have gotten away with her ruse.

Another most unusual and sought for sword cane is the so called "flick out"

bladed cane. This is a cane that, when held in about the middle of the shaft with the handle end upward and forward and is rapidly slashed downward, a small blade of about 6-8" ejects out of the handle and locks into place to be used as a jabbing weapon. When the adventure is over, one need merely press a catch at the top - or handle end — of the cane at the base of the extended blade, and tap the bottom of the cane on the floor and the blade will disappear inside the handle by gravity. To top it all, a little spring activated trap door now automatically closes over the opening where the blade disappeared and the top looks as normal and innocuous as the top of any stick. There are even variations of this "flick out" cane where the blade shoots out of the bottom by wrist action alone but these are very rare. I have many of these "flick out" sword canes and some have blades over 24" long. All are of great shock value that in itself can immobilize an opponent.

Among the more unusual and most sought out of the sword canes are the "flick out" bladed canes. Silver knob handled flick sticks. Left: silver handle, malacca shaft, extra-long blade, c. 1870; right: small handle, no collar, malacca shaft, 35 1/4" high.

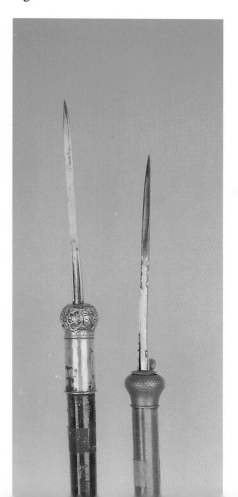

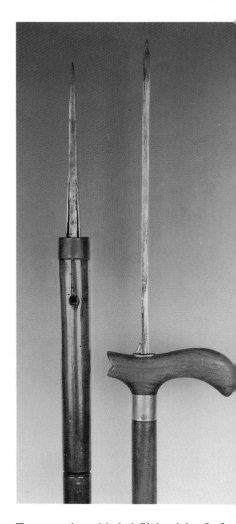

Two very long bladed flick sticks. Left: large wood shaft with single hole, 37" high; right: large blade springs from a regular wood handle, 37 1/4" high.

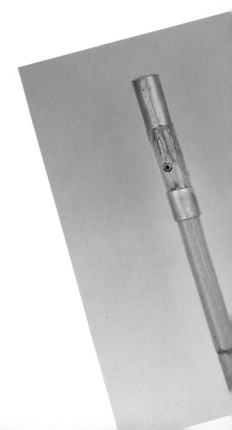

The most unusual of all sword canes is the spring activated sword cane known by the French as Cannes a. Dard. With this cane, one need merely press a button at or near the handle and a long blade shoots out the bottom of the stick and locks in place all by spring action giving that stick wearer a sword almost twice the length of his cane. How ingenious some of our ancestors were in hiding such shocking weapons in a mere but sometimes beautiful stick.

I hunted for a long time before finding such a sword cane, finally finding one at a flea market in Cannes, France, but I am always looking for a finer and better one.

Once while in an antique shop in Cleveland, Ohio I inquired of the dealer if he had or knew where I could get a spring activated sword cane. He rolled his eyes upward and told me he had had an experience that really terrified him. Having recently obtained a cane collection from a widow whose cane collecting husband had died, he was sorting out the sticks and thought one deserved greater interest because of its weight. As he held it up closer to a light hanging over his desk, he pushed several protrusions of a design and suddenly a blade shot out of the cane bottom and pierced and embedded itself in his desk with such force that he had great difficulty extracting it. He was so frightened that he became sick at the recollection and handled every cane thereafter very gingerly making sure he touched no protrusions. He subsequently sold the cane to a person unknown; much as I tried to jog his memory of the name and address of the buyer so I could track him down, I was unsuccessful. He had one bit of advice for me - he said unless you know what you are doing, never push any button on any cane unless you have both the bottom and top pointing away from any person or object dear to you. He still shook, he said, when he recalled the incident.

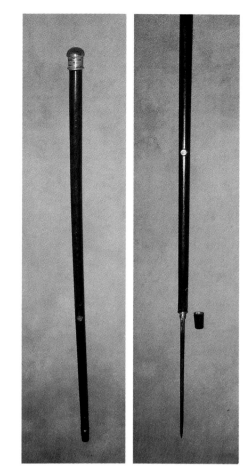

Press a button low on the shaft and the blade flies out and locks in place.

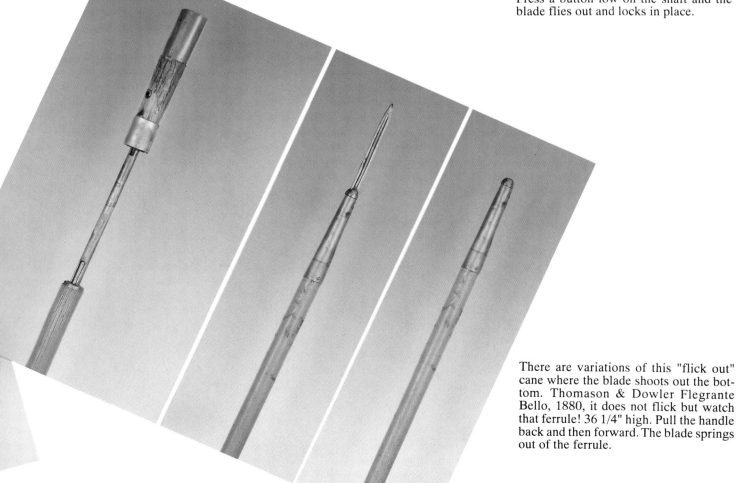

There are variations of this "flick out" cane where the blade shoots out the bottom. Thomason & Dowler Flegrante Bello, 1880, it does not flick but watch that ferrule! 36 1/4" high. Pull the handle back and then forward. The blade springs out of the ferrule.

Sword canes are almost as interesting in their various mechanisms as gun canes. The average sword cane is a pull out affair. One merely pulls on the handle while holding the shaft and the blade slides out. Others have a locking device requiring one to push a button called a thumb spring that presses down on a catch and releases the blade when it is pulled outward. The finest of the sword canes, however, have a cam device holding it locked. One must twist the handle 1/2 turn to the right and a cam rolls over a spring catch and releases the blade when it is pulled. Upon replacing the blade, one must turn the handle a half turn counterclockwise and the blade is perfectly and securely locked. I have found and bought these from owners who never knew they were selling a sword cane.

I have variations of this cane where one merely turns the ring or band between the handle and shaft of the stick to unlock the device.

Needless to say, not only are these latter canes rare and hard to find, but unfortunately if you are so lucky as to find one, you shortly discover that the locking device is broken. This presents a great problem as they are most difficult and sometimes impossible to fix. If you can find a repairman, invariably his charges are far greater than you ever paid for the cane as you are paying his time for learning how the cane works before he can figure out how to repair it.

Another very rare and, therefore, desirable sword cane is what I call the assassin's stick where the blade comes out of the bottom as one pushes on the handle of the cane with the lower end of the cane pressed against the victim. The entire blade is stationery but the lower shaft of the stick slides over the stationery blade into its upper overriding shaft and compresses a spring holding it over the blade. The blade pierces the victim and upon releasing the pressure on the handle and pulling the stick away, the blade is completely covered by the spring-activated, lower section of the shaft and the assailant walks innocently away. Incidentally, one of the first cane patents in the United States was such a stick. I have one and its ferrule states, "Hudson Patent, September 9, 1851."

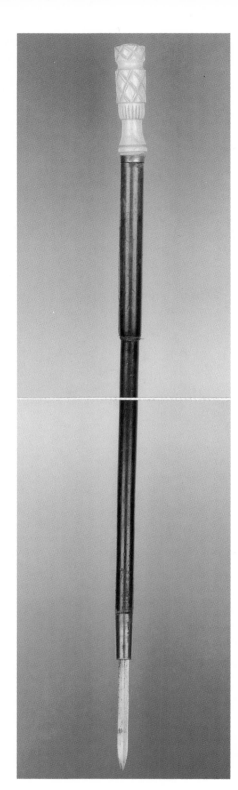

Bone handled assassin's stick with retracting lower shaft to reveal the blade, 35" high. Push the bottom of the cane against a person and the blade pierces him as the lower shaft retracts from the stationary blade. When the deed is done and the blade removed, the lower shaft glides back over the incriminating blade.

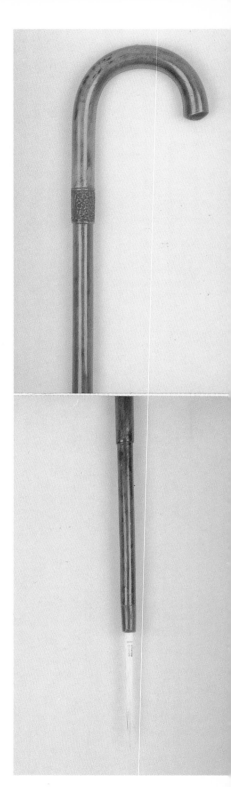

Another sinister assassin's stick. The lower half of the shaft pushes up into the handle as the stationary blade beneath plunges into its target, marked Louper Solingen on the blade, 36 1/2" high.

Clients of my law practice were frequent sources of interesting canes. To break the ice at times I would discuss my hobby with them and ask if they knew of any unusual cane. One such young man had just come back from the island of Okinawa where he had been stationed during the war. He said that he and his fellow marines had a hobby too - collecting strange Oriental weapons amongst other things. As a consequence, the officers would frequently raid their barracks and search all lockers in the presence of the marines. As this young mans locker was opened, the sergeant found a small package wrapped with an old sweat shirt. My marine seeing the officer handle this was terrified and hollered out, "Don't touch that and I mean (he amplified) be very, very careful or that may kill you."

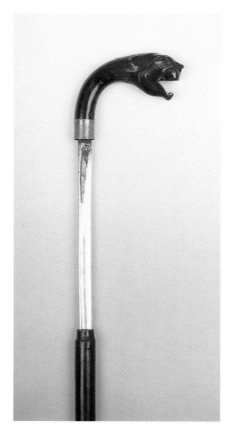

Oriental sword cane, tiger's head of horn, 37 1/4" high.

He then explained that it was a native shooting knife - if you pressed the button on a small thick baton, a knife blade would shoot out the bottom by spring action. It would not, however, stop and lock into place, but keep going for about 30 feet, embedding itself in any-

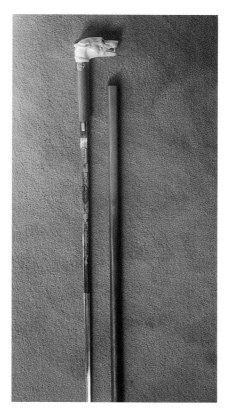

Sword blade marked "TOLEDO" on a very fine sword cane with an ivory dog's head handle.

thing in its way. It was a spring device and had a separate mechanism that was needed to insert and lock the blade against the strong spring in the baton. His superiors confiscated the device but he was not punished. I asked and he said he had seen canes with such devices. I wrote every place he suggested in Okinawa where he thought I could purchase one, but I never received any reply so I am still looking for such a sword cane.

Four sided blade marked "IN SOLIGEN." Hand shaped ivory handle with dagger. 33 1/2" high.

Many of the old sword canes have etched on the blade the names "Toledo" or "Birmingham" or "Solingen." This does not necessarily indicate that the sword cane was manufactured there. These famous geographic names of Spain, England, and Germany were noted steel centers long famous for the quality of their fighting blades. Many companies in these centers made only the blades and stamped thereon these well-known names and shipped them all over the world where they were ultimately purchased and used by local cane makers who inserted them into sticks of their own manufacture.

One manufacturer in London told me that before World War II his company sent all their sticks to Germany to be drilled for the insertion of blades because, he said, only the Germans could drill a hole straight through the shaft and not come out the side.

While with this world-famous London dealer, I managed to inveigle myself into their work room. Imagine my surprise when I found that they had purchased a number of antique canes and sawed them asunder from the top to bottom. Both sides were now partially gauged out on their inner side which was then filled with glue. A greased blade - one carrying their world-famous brand name was laid on top of one glued side. The other glued side was then placed on top and the two taped tightly together.

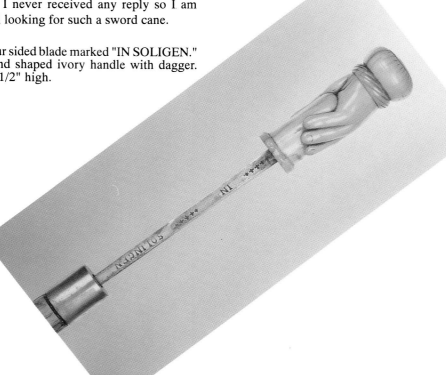

When the glue hardened, the blade was pulled out leaving a perfectly bored receptacle as a container for the blade. The cane was so well put together I could not see the line of demarcation where the two sides met. Fortunately, I was able to purchase one of their last German-bored malacca sword canes which I still have.

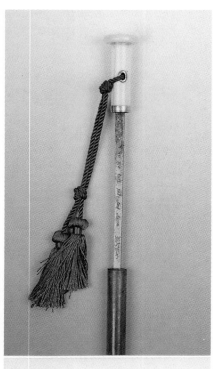

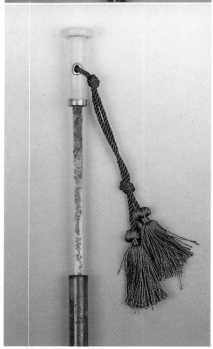

Ivory handled French blade with eyelets and malacca shaft, French phrase on blade the gist of which is "Do not remove me without reason, do not replace me without honor," c. 1780, 34 1/8" high.

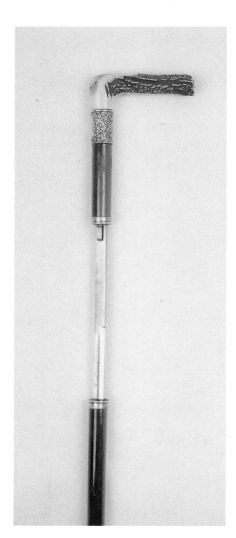

Antler handle Toledo blade, twist the malacca shaft to release the blade, the shaft separates at silver collar, 36" high.

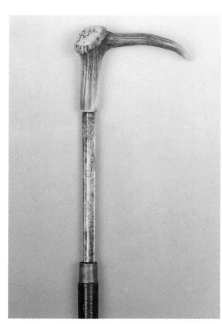

Antler handle marked "R.M.," sword cane, double edged blade with small decorations on the upper third, 34" high.

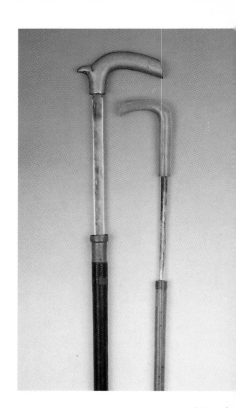

Two L handled sword canes. The left hand sword cane has a brass handle and a single edged blade; the right hand sword canes has a horn handle with a double edged blade, c. 1890. Left: 34 1/4" high; right: 34 3/4" high.

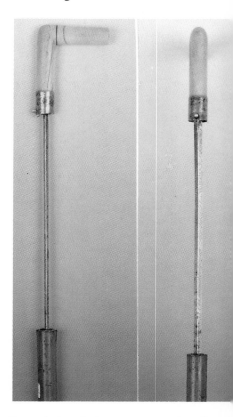

Ivory L handled sword cane with silver collar dedicated to "E.S. McNeal from his friend Alfred Jacould," ornate blade, c. 1810, 31 1/2" high.

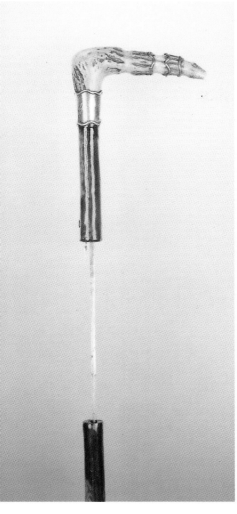

Antler and silver handled Toledo blade, silver collar marked "W.P. Coffin," 35 3/4" high.

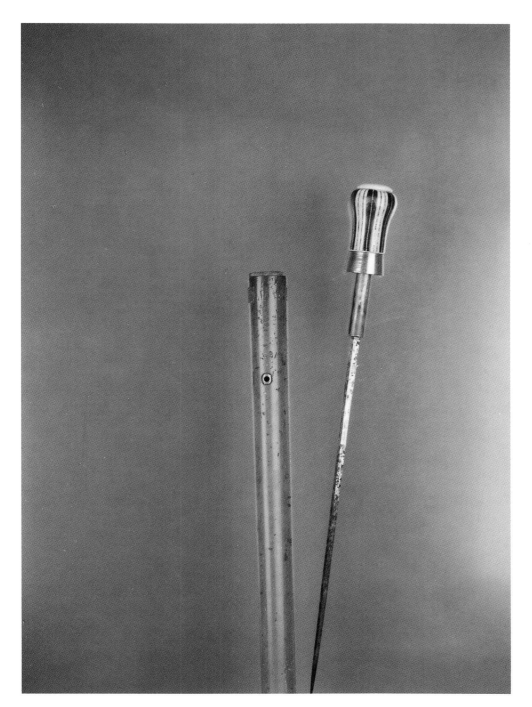

Old striped ivory knob handle with dagger, four sided blade marked "NETTER," malacca shaft, eyelets, c. 1780, 36" high with a 4" high ferrule.

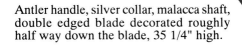

Antler handle, silver collar, malacca shaft, double edged blade decorated roughly half way down the blade, 35 1/4" high.

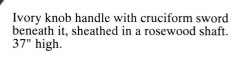

Ivory knob handle with cruciform sword beneath it, sheathed in a rosewood shaft. 37" high.

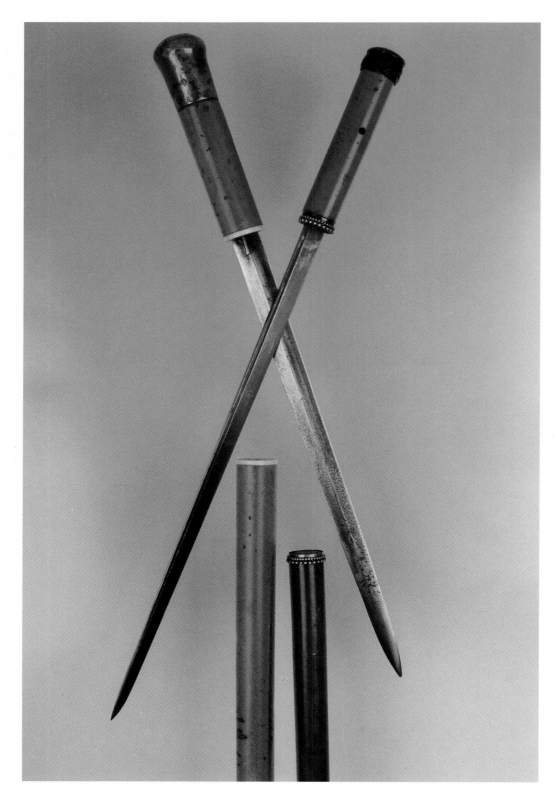

Two broad but short bladed sword canes.
Left: silver knob handle with "EAG"
monogram on top, double-edged blade,
white collar, malacca shaft, 34 1/2" high;
right: black handle with rope design,
small black eyelets in handle, silver
beaded collar, triangular blade, c. 1800,
37" high.

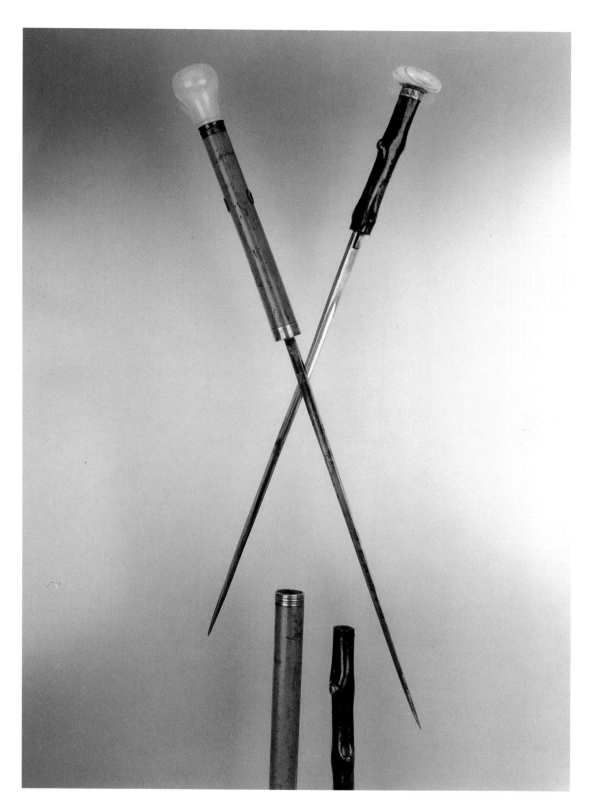

Two ivory handled sword canes. Left: very old, c. 1790, ivory knob handle with signature in top, silver eyelets, step malacca and short blade, 34 3/4" high; right: small ivory handle, copper collar, button to release four sided blade, 33" high.

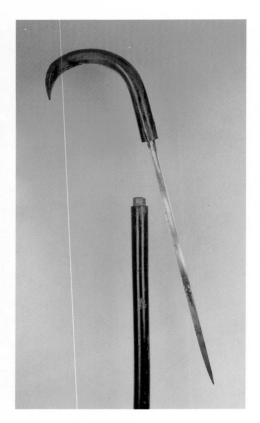

Black crook handled sword, short triangular blade, c. 1820, 36 3/8" high.

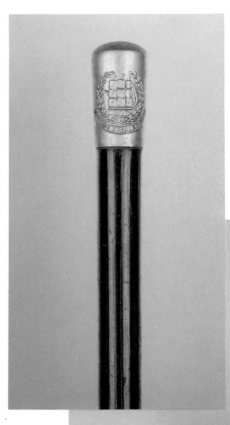

British Guiana Police sword cane with silver handle and stamped ship and laurel insignia, 35 1/2" high.

German long antler horn handled sword cane with "HK" monogram at the crest of the antler, 36 3/4" high.

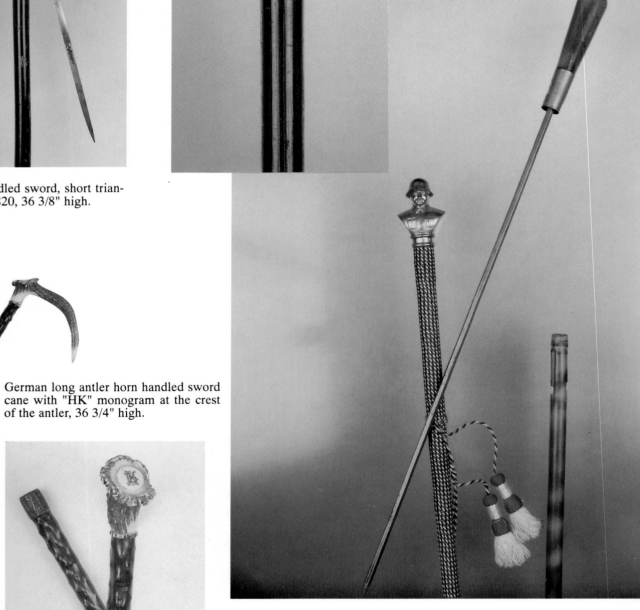

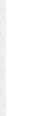

Two Nazi canes — left: soldier's bust with the word "RESERVE" marked on the handle in front and "HAT RUHI" in back, 36 7/8" high, shaft covered in weave; right: Nazi sword cane, enameled swastika on top, 35" high.

234

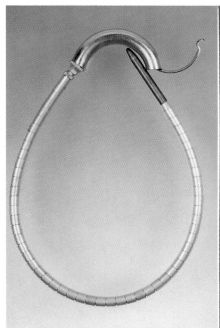

Steel traveling cane, International Patent, "SCHUKRA," c. 1935, 35 1/2" high. Pull off the ferrule to uncover a spear blade.

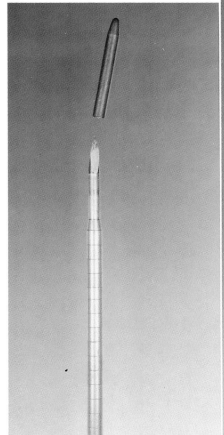

The blade beneath the ferrule of the steel traveling cane.

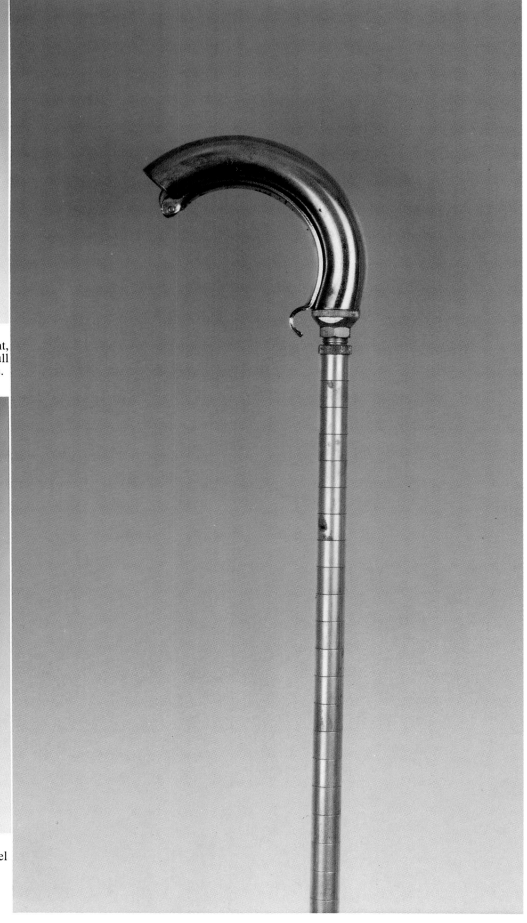

Other Weapon Canes

There are black jack canes, that have an inner pull-out striking rod, made of rubber, or steel cable, or steel spring making a quick-draw concealed cudgel; other innocuous appearing canes have just weighted heads , or rod reinforced shafts; all having the sole purpose of striking a would be opponent.

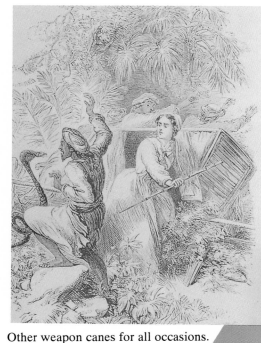

Other weapon canes for all occasions.

German cane with a spring black jack an a crook handle, c. 1930. 35 1/2" high.

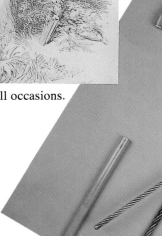

Three bludgeon canes. Left: thinnest with spring striker; right: with horn handle has cable striker. All have crook handles and malacca shafts. Left: 36 1/2" high; center: 35 3/4" high; right: 36 1/4" high.

British Military & Police Fighting Stick of Hickory with hand guard, 35" high.

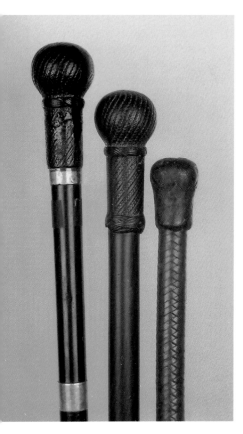

Three knob kerrie canes with weighted handles. Left and center canes are gutta percha, right is leather wrapped. Left: 35 3/4" high; center 33 3/4" high with silver collar, dating c. 1870; right: 35 1/4" high.

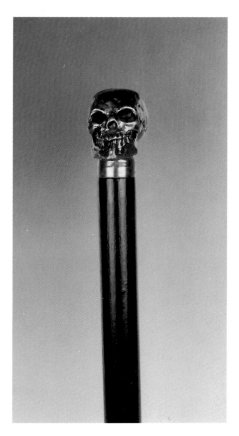

Brass skull knob kerrie cane of modern Oriental make, 36" high.

One intricate cane has a screw off top so designed that when the cane is held at mid shaft and swung toward the victim, a leaden ball attached to a spring flies out and hits him and then springs back inside its shaft.

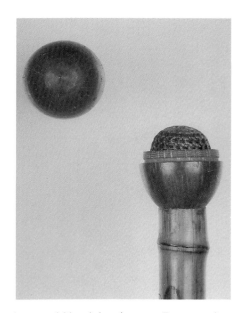

A very old knob kerrie cane. Remove the top and a lead ball on a spring can be whipped out and back, 34 1/4" high.

Some effective clobbering canes have hatchet-shaped handles. Two Polish shepherd's canes with rattles and axe heads, both 35 3/8" high. Both have a guard on the sharp wolf-repelling axe heads and have mountain spikes for ferrules.

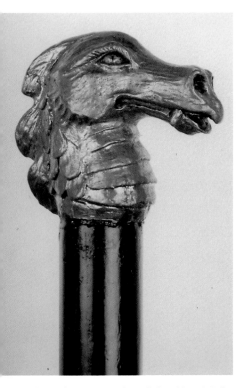

Modern silver coated, weighted lead Oriental dragon handle on a black shaft, 36" high. This is a heavy clobbering cane.

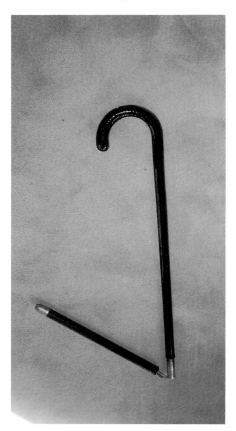

Nunchaku cane, a most vicious weapon.

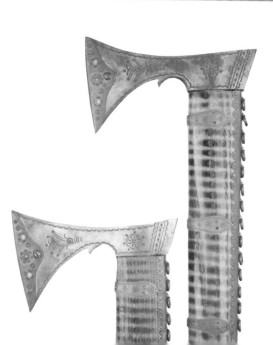

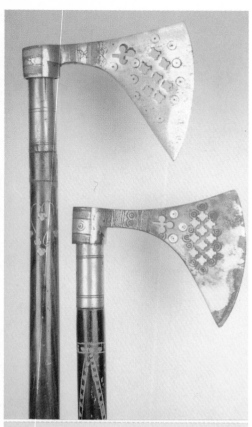

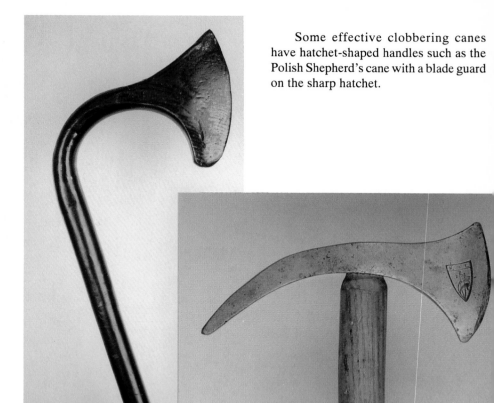

Some effective clobbering canes have hatchet-shaped handles such as the Polish Shepherd's cane with a blade guard on the sharp hatchet.

Black painted light wood cane with handle shaped as a hatchet, 37 1/2" high. Very light in weight but effective in defense.

Small hatched handled cane with a shield with the initials "K.L." impressed into the blade, 33 1/2" high.

Small hatched shaped handle, painted and carved haft with a foliate motif, gold painted pointed metal ferrule. This cane come from Eastern Europe. 35 3/8" high.

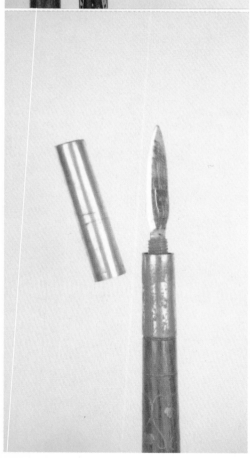

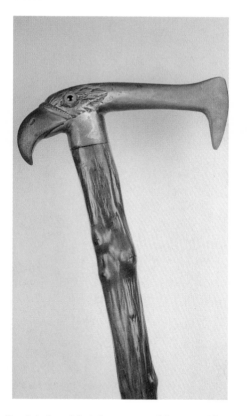

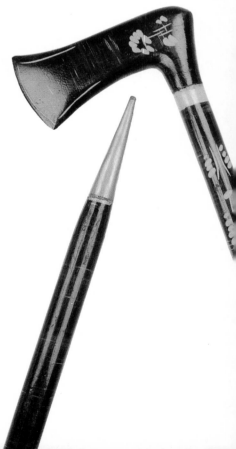

Two East Indian hatchet handled canes with spear points beneath the ferrules. Left: brown shaft, 34 1/2" high; right: black shaft, 31" high.

Eagle's head hatchet cane of brass with glass eyes, gnarled wooden shaft, 36" high.

Canes carrying deterring noxious liquids far antedate the modern chemical mace container. They usually operate by pressing a button on the side of the shaft near the head whereupon a spray, usually of ammonia, would squirt out of the mouth of a human or horse's head that is part of the handle. Other handles are in the form of Chinese faces and are operated by lifting and depressing the queue of his head dress.

Canes carrying deterring noxious liquids operate by pressing a button on the side of the shaft near the handle whereupon a spray, usually ammonia, would squirt out of the mouth of the figure designed into the handle. Grinning man squirting cane. A push button model measuring 35 1/4" high.

Squirting horse with saddle and dog, push button, 36" high.

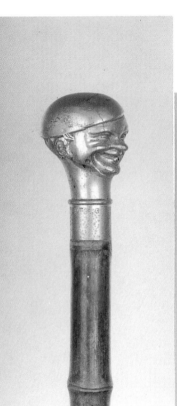

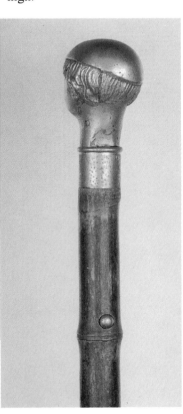

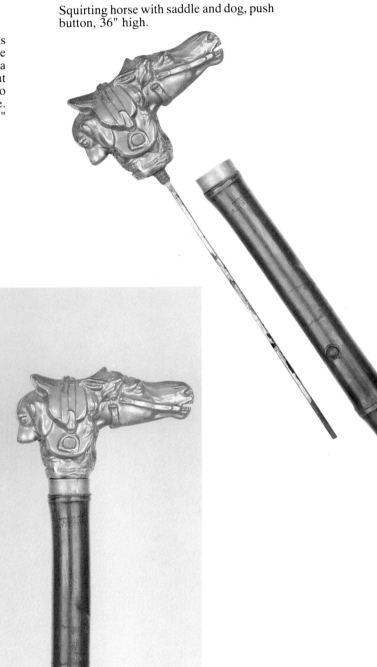

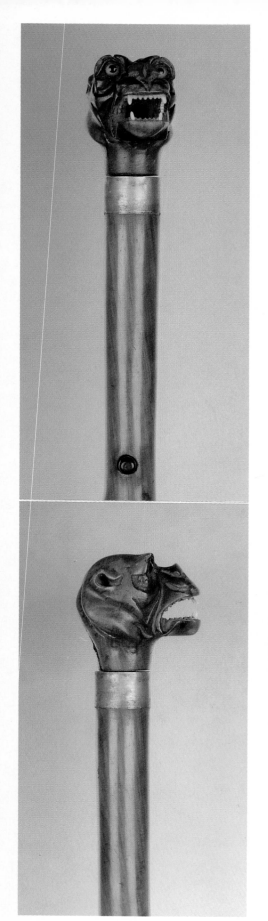

Spear canes are also to be found. An old European version used in the mountains between Spain and France has a heavy steel ferrule, apparently for traction on slippery slopes. In reality this heavy ferrule is meant to give heft and balance to a spear that appears when the long leather covered handle is screwed off. These are called Makhila and are throwing spears or hand thrown weighted arrows.

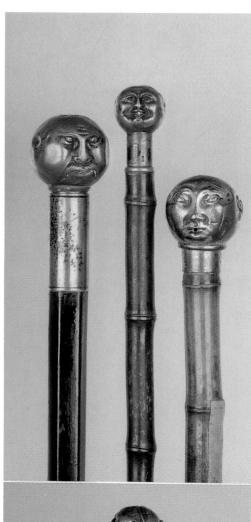

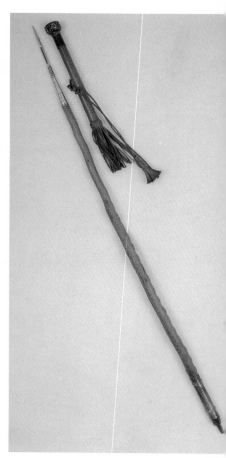

Mountain cane with spear beneath handle called Makhila Cane. This cane sports a purple and white stone handle, leather wrap on upper third of shaft, blade marked Keller Laria, 35 1/2" high.

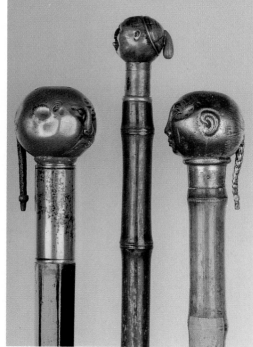

Squirting cane with mastiff's head, ivory teeth, and glass eyes, 37 1/2" high.

Three squirting China men, raise the queues, press them back down and the handles squirt. These were used with water for fun or ammonia for defense. The original (liquid) mace cane. Left: 35 1/2" high; center: 36 1/2" high; right: 35" high.

240

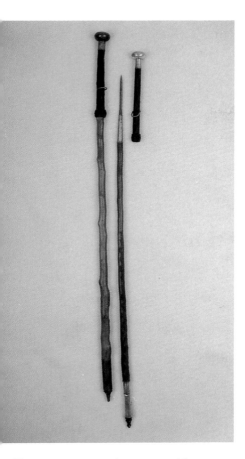

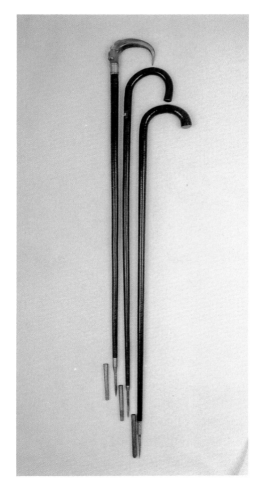

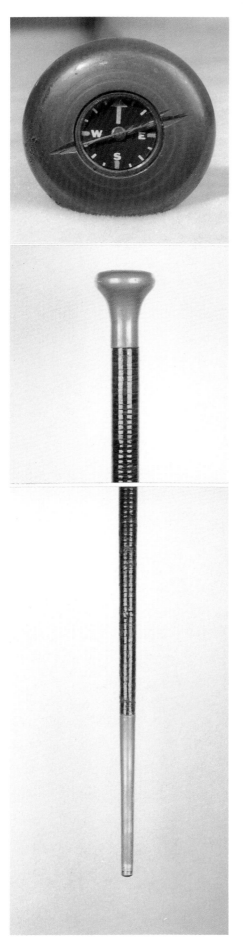

Two more mountain canes with spears called Makhila, from the mountains between France and Spain. Left: bone knob handle, leather wrap on upper third, 35 1/2" high; right: silver knob handle, 35 3/4" high.

A different example is one containing a compass in the heavy brass handle of a walking stick made of leather washers or discs, threaded on a steel rod, the bottom ferrule of which pulls off to reveal a wicked barb. This cane can be used as a whipping club, a black jack, a spear, and a direction finder. I use it when searching for mushrooms, which reminds me of a collector I met in Rome, Italy who's pride was a truffle cane with a small silver spade as a ferrule. This man was head of a large insurance company and a mutual friend took me to his home. He bragged of his cane collection and as he showed me his prized sticks one by one, I said I too had such a one; in desperation, he showed me a rare violin cane. I almost didn't tell him I had one of those too. But when he showed me his truffle cane, he had me stumped and I looked far and wide for a duplicate, eventually finding it in my own small town of Lake Forest. You can never tell where you will find a treasure!

Three heavy metal canes, wrapped in leather, with blades beneath the ferrules. Left: horn handle, silver collar, 35 1/4" high; center: tightly crooked handle, 34 1/2" high; right: more open crook, 35" high. The ferrules quickly slip off in an emergency.

Leather wrapped metal cane with a compass in the top of the handle, long ferrule, 35 1/4" high; ferrule, 4 3/4" high. A spear blade is hidden beneath a pull off ferrule.

Musical Canes

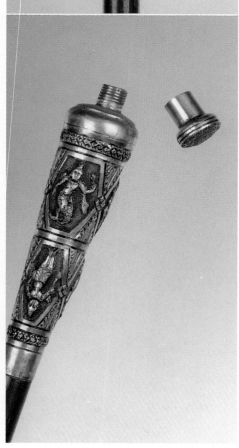

Ladies poisoning cane in East Indian motifs, c. 1880s, 38 3/4" high.

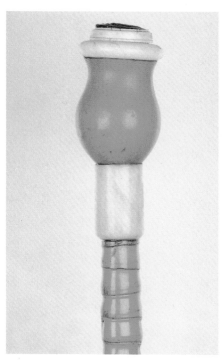

Chinese pet cricket cane. Carrying the cricket along gave the owner of this cane natural music wherever he or she went. Ivory and bamboo cane, c. 1900. 38" high.

In the late 1700s and early 1800s, the Jewish people were harrassed in middle Europe. They were not allowed to practice the professions, were limited to what trades they could engage in, and were relegated to living in ghettos. Anti-semetic uprisings would occur frequently. Many Jewish people, being dedicated to music, were able to eek out a living teaching violin lessons. When, however, they left the ghetto with their violin cases, ruffians would pounce on them, yank their side locks, open the cases and crash the violins on their heads. Thus in 1815 in Bohemia a need for a new gadget cane arose and the violin was disguised as a common walking cane.

Many gadget canes contain <u>whistles</u>, which were utilized to hail horse-drawn cabs or otherwise attract the attention. What is not generally known is that very professional instruments such as the aforementioned violins, flutes and banjos were also made into walking sticks.

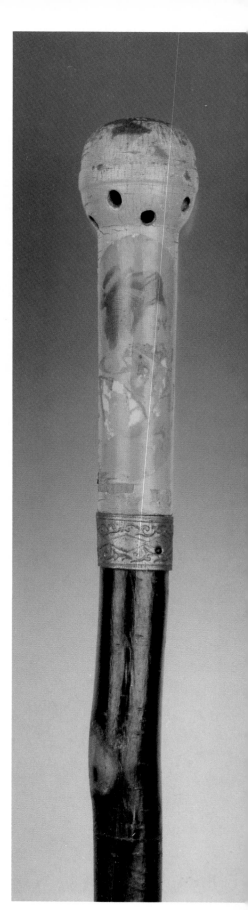

Japanese wolf siren whistle with Asian woman on the handle, a thin collar and a bark covered shaft, c. 1910. 36" high.

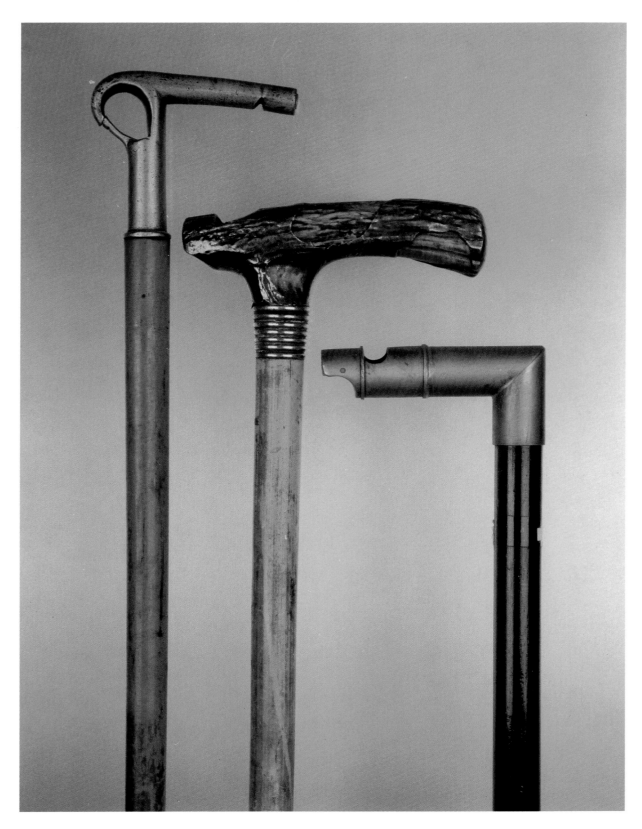

Three whistle canes — left is a dog lead
or leash with a key ring to attach to dog
collar. The other end is a whistle to call
the dog. Malacca shaft, 31 1/2" high. Center is an elaborate antler and silver shaped
as antler whistle handle on a malacca
shaft, 34 1/4" high. Right is a simple brass
whistle L handle on a black shaft, 36 1/4"
high.

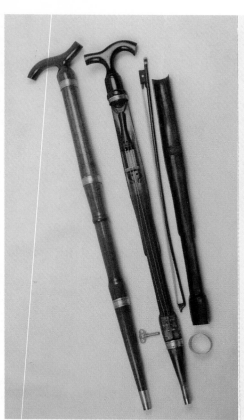
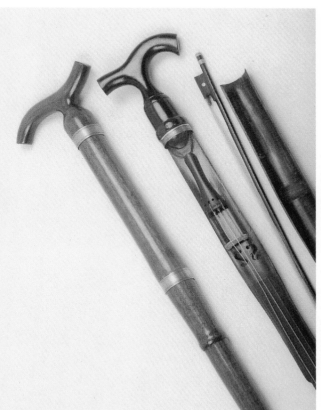
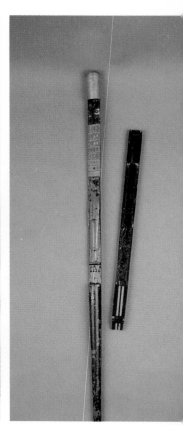

Two violin canes, top: 35 1/2" high; bottom: 34" high.

Metal guitar cane, U.S. patent, 36 1/4" high.

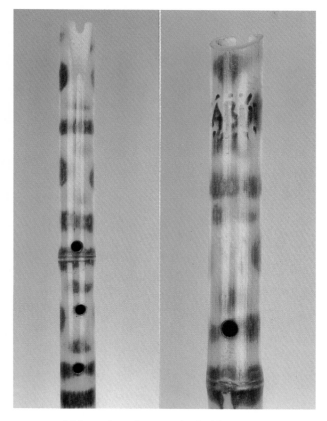

African-American reed wind instrument made by Abu of Baltimore, Maryland and marked "ABU" on back, 31 1/2" high.

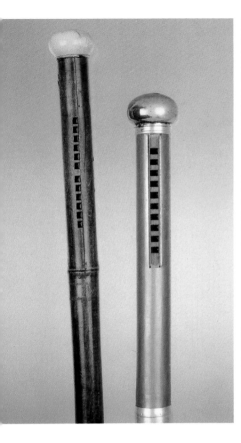

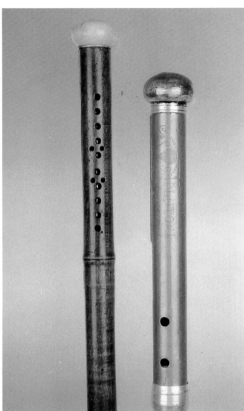

Two harmonica canes. Left: wood with ivory knob and fingering holes, 35" high; right: metal harmonica "Meinel's Flutonica", malacca shaft, 38 1/2" high. German make.

Music stand cane, 34 3/4" high. The entire top folds into the handle.

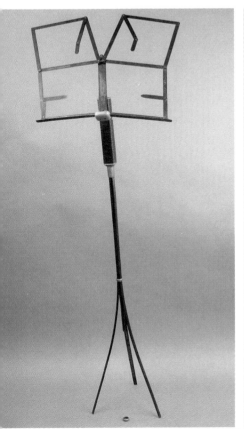

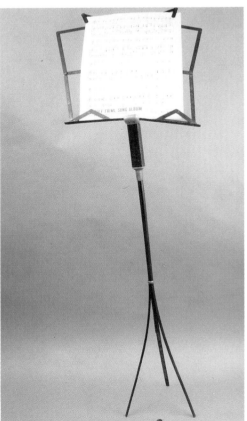

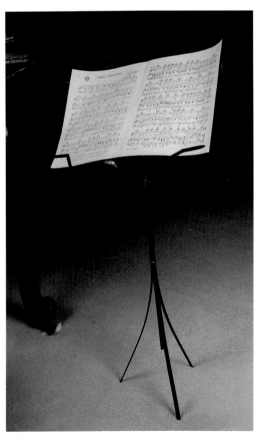

So we read about the Czakn [Hung. csakany], (Fr. canneflute a bec; Ger:. Stockflote.) as being a recorded Hungarian instrument probably of Bohemian origin which was much in vogue in the 1820s. It was first mentioned in the Wiener Zeitung of October 1, 1808 and is said to have been invented by a musician named Anton Heberle. "—-Two small holes were bored in the knob to serve as a blowhole. The tube was of inverted conical form, fitted with six front fingerholes and a rear thumbhole.—-" (Musical Instruments. A Comprehensive Dictionary by Sibyl Marcuse. Doubleday & Co. Inc. Garden City, NY, 1964).

In the same source we find a definition for an *Umbrella flute,* as a walking stick flute adapted to the British climatic conditions by flutist, J. Clinton.

Walking-stick flute (Fr. canne-flute. Ger. Stockflote) is defined as a 19th Century flute made in the form of a walking stick and it defines walking stick oboes, and a walking stick trumpet invented by T. Harper of London in the 1840s. A walking stick violin (Fr. canne-pochette; Ger. Stockgeige) is described as a kit in walking stick form invented in the mid-18th Century by Johann Wilde of St. Petersburg, and resuscitated in the 1880s by A. Lutz & Co. of Vienna.

I have four fine flute canes, but through the courtesy of the curator of the music department of the Library of Congress, I have been permitted to photograph, and here for the first time, picture the flute canes of the extensive flute collection of Dayton C. Miller.

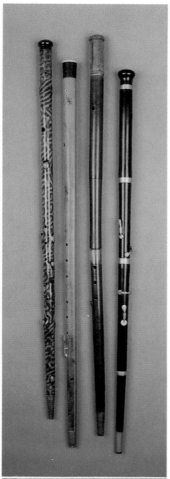

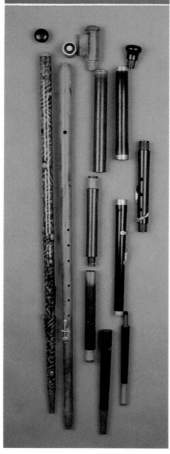

Four flute canes ranging from 34 3/4" to 36" high. These four date from c. 1830 - 1900. From left to right: the first flute (with four keys) is beautifully disguised by means of smoke brands, the second is a fine malacca flute with a single key, the third is a very old flute that separates in the center and has a snuff box or ditty kit as a handle, and the fourth is a fine ebony three key flute that disassembles into four parts and is said to be a concert flute.

The Dayton C. Miller Flute Collection

Dayton C. Miller was born in Strangville, Ohio, in 1866 and became a scientist devoting much of his life to collecting source material for the history and development of the flute from prehistoric times to the present date. His collection of flutes was reputed to be the world's largest. He became a professor of astronomy and physics and wrote several books on sound: *The Science of Musical Sounds* (1906-revised 1922), *Sound Waves, Shape and Speed* (1937), *Sparks, Lightening & Cosmic Rays* (1937). He translated Theobald Boehm's *The Flute and Flute Playing* (1908-revised 1922, reprinted 1960). He died in 1941 and bequeathed his entire collection to our Library of Congress which published *The Dayton C. Miller Flute Collection,* a checklist of the instruments, compiled by Laura E. Gilliam and William Lichtenwanger (Music Division. Reference Department. Library of Congress, Washington, 1961). There are over 1600 flutes in this collection, but only 21 are in the shape and design of a cane or walking stick which indicates the rarity of these walking sticks. The checklist is now out of print. Here are the flute canes in the collection, giving the number, type, maker, description and date of purchase for each. Two were not photographed due to their deteriorated condition.

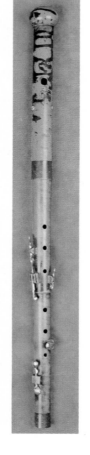

228. <u>Walking Stick Flute in C</u>, Scalvini, Brescia, Italy, early 19th Century. 1 key, boxwood (cut to look like bamboo) with brass key and black ebony knob; 936 mm bought from G. Meriggioli, Milan, February 1, 1922.

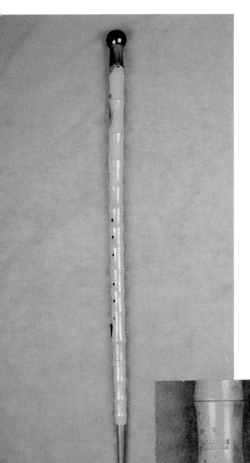

390. Walking Stick Flute in C. - Anon., early 19th Century. 1 key; mahogany (?) with brass key, ivory ring, silver ferrule, and iron tip; 870 mm. Bought from C.W. Unger, Pottsville, Pennsylvania, February 14, 1924.

271. Walking Stick Flute in C with other instruments by Anthony.

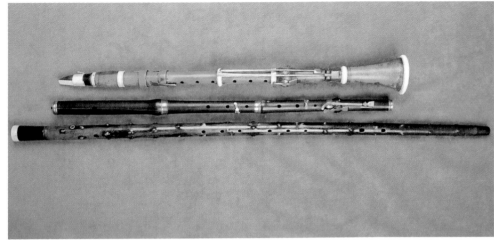

228. Walking Stick Flute in C by Scalvini, Brescia, Italy.

390. Walking Stick Flute in C — Anon. Early 19th century, 1 key.

271. Walking Stick Flute in C. - Anthony, Philadelphia, 1794-1830. 4 keys; wood stained brown & black and covered with "thorns"; ivory cap: 957 mm. Gift of W.P. Harrell, Portsmouth, Virginia, August 24, 1922.

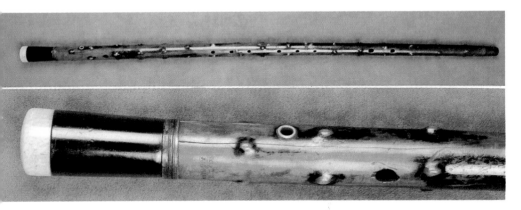

271. Walking Stick Flute in C by Anthony, Philadelphia.

420. <u>Walking Stick Flute in C</u>. - Anon., early 19th Century.
6/1, 5 keys, grenadilla with silver fittings and horn knob, 903 mm. Bought from Sumner Healey, New York, June 7, 1924.

613. <u>Walking Stick English Flageolet</u> - Anon., early 19th Century. 7/1, 1 key, yellow wood with brass key and ivory and brass rings; 753 mm. Bought from Andre Rossignol, Pores, July 28, 1926.

684. <u>Walking Stick Czakan</u> - J. Merkleim, Vienna, C. 1825-47. 7/1, 4 keys; boxwood with brass keys, ivory rings, and brass ferrule; 84 mm. Gift of Allen Loomes, Elkhart, Indiana, November   18, 1926.

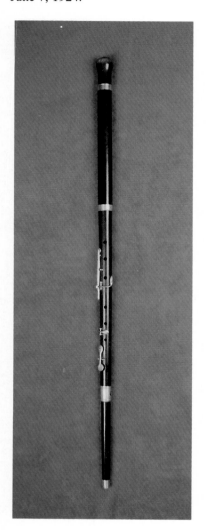

420. Walking Stick Flute in C — Anon. Early 19th century, 5 keys.

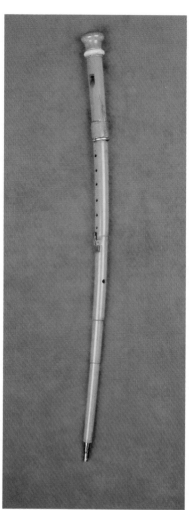

613. Walking Stick English Flagolet — Anon. Early 19th century, 1 key.

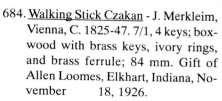

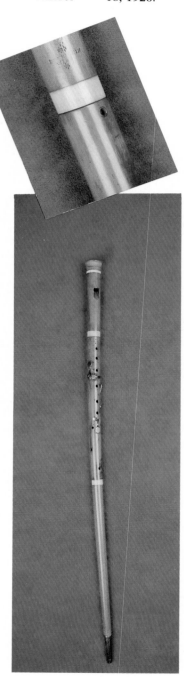

684. Walking Stick Czakan — J. Merkleim, Vienna, c. 1825-47, 4 keys.

612. Walking Stick Flute in C — Anon. Early 19th century, 1 key.

612. <u>Walking Stick Flute in C</u>. - Anon. early 19th Century. 1 key; brown wood with imitation knots, wood key, and brass and iron tip; 860 mm. Bought from Andre Rossignol, Paris, July 28, 1926.

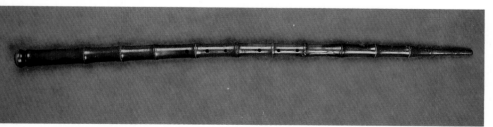

726. <u>Walking Stick Flute in C</u>. - Stoudinger (?), Dresden (?), C. 1820. 1 key; wood varnished black with brass key, ivory ring, 2 black horn rings, and brass tip; 862 mm. Exhibited at the Music Loan Exhibition, London 1904 (p.187). Formerly in the T.W. Taphouse Collection. Bought at Brownsea Castle Sale, No. 1864 (C. Van Roalte Collection), Bournemouth, England, August 6, 1927.

727. <u>Walking Stick Czakan</u> - Anon., early 19th Century.

7/1, 2 keys; wood with silver keys, horn ferrule and brass ferrule; cane has hammer-shaped head; 811 mm. Exhibited at the Music Loan Exhibition, London 1904 (p.184). Formerly in the T.W. Taphouse Collection. Brought at Brownsea Castle Sale, No. 1866 (G. Van Roalte Collection). Bournemouth, England, August 6, 1927.

805. <u>Walking Stick Flute</u> - Anon., early 19th Century. 1 key, plum wood (?) with brass key, ivory rings, and iron tip covered with brass, 940 mm. Bought from Henning Oppermann, Basel, August 7, 1928.

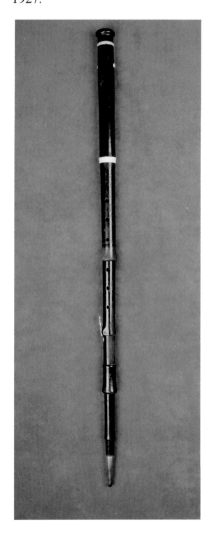

726. Walking Stick Flute in C — Stoudinger (?), Dresden (?), c. 1820, 1 key.

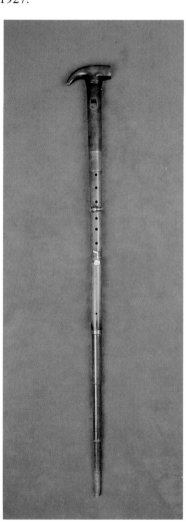

727. Walking Stick Czakan — Anon. Early 19th century, 2 keys.

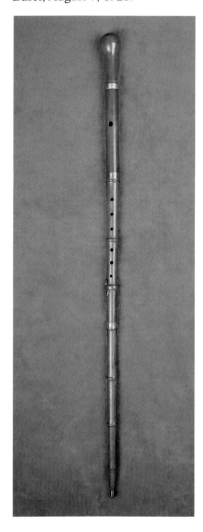

805. Walking Stick Flute — Anon. Early 19th century, 1 key.

824. <u>Walking Stick Flageolet</u> - Anon., early 19th Century. 7/1, 4 keys; decorated with wavy burned-in streaks; brass ferrule with iron tip; 875 mm. (without handle). Bequest of Carolyn A. Alchin, Los Angeles, December 15, 1928.

841. <u>Walking Stick Flute</u> - Anon., 1851. 4 keys (7 key for right thumb); light colored wood with mottled stain or burn, keys of same wood; ivory knob; 895 mm. Bought from G.L. Tilden, Northboro, Massachusetts, April 5, 1929.

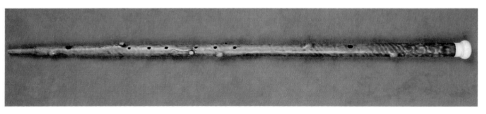

841. Walking Stick Flute —Anon. 1851, 4 keys.

904. <u>Walking Stick Flute in C</u>. - Anon., early 19th Century. 6 keys, rosewood with silver fittings and ivory knob; 877 mm. Gift of John T. Shiel, Walkdew, England, December 5, 1929.

908. <u>Walking Stick Flute in C</u>. - Lambert, Paris, 18th Century. 1 key; light colored wood with key of the same wood and brass ferrule; 890 mm. Bought from Sumner Healy, New York, January 10, 1930.

982. <u>Walking Stick Flute</u> - Anon., early 19th Century. 1 key, light wood with brass fittings; 817 mm. Bought from Sigmund Koch, Munich, August 27, 1930.

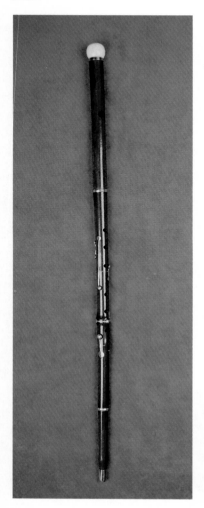

904. Walking Stick Flute in C — Anon. Early 19th century, 6 keys.

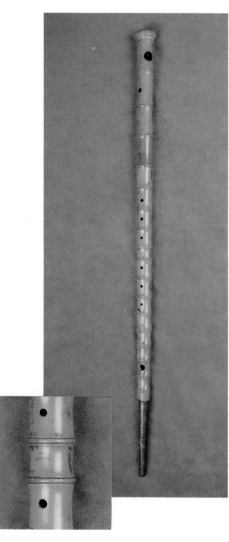

908. Walking Stick Flute in C — Lambert, Paris, 18th century, 1 key.

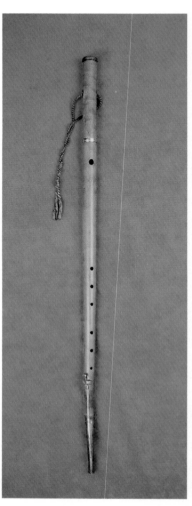

982. Walking Stick Flute — Anon. Early 19th century, 1 key.

1040. <u>Walking Stick Flute in C</u>. - Anon., early 19th Century. 1 key; reddish brown wood tube and key with brass rings and ferrule and black horn cap; 870 mm. Gift of estate of John T. Fagan, Portland, Maine, April 8, 1931.

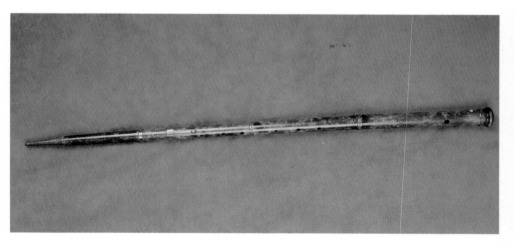

1040. Walking Stick Flute in C — Anon. Early 19th century, 1 key.

1090. <u>Walking Stick Flute in C</u>. - Anon., early 19th Century. 1 key; curly and knotted wood with silver fittings; 833 mm. Bought from J. L. Hessey, Wallasey, Cheshire, England, September 21, 1931.

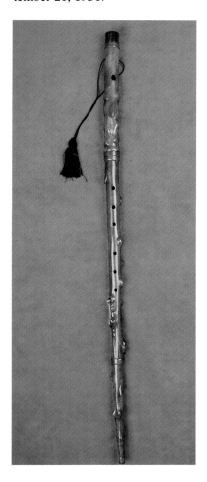

1090. Walking Stick Flute in C — Anon.

1218. <u>Walking Stick Flute in C</u>. - Anon., early 19th Century. 4 keys; light colored wood body and keys with ivory cap and brass tip; 925 mm. Bought from Boston Antique Shop, Boston, June 17, 1934.

1232. <u>Walking Stick Flageolet</u> - Anon., mid 19th Century. 7/1, 1 key; wood stained black with brass key and tip, 827 mm. Bought from James D. Price, West Hartford, Connecticut, December 6, 1934.

1391. <u>Walking Stick Flute in C</u>. - Paul Walch, Berchtesgaden, 1850-73. 1 key; wood with brass key and ferrule; 904 mm. Bought from Sadie I. Huntington, Pittsfield, Massachusetts, November 2, 1939.

Other Gadget Canes

For the woods stroller there are nut cracker canes ; for the city walker there are coin receptacle canes that carried a number of nickels in the handle to pay for a street car should one tire of the journey and wish to ride back.

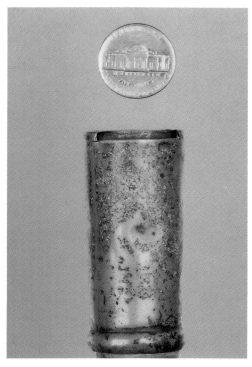

Simple nickel dispenser, 35 3/4" high.

Two nut cracker canes. Left: with hinged head and beard, 36 1/2" high; right: screw driven model, put a nut in the mouth and screw down until the nut cracks, 38 1/4" high. Made at Oberamagau, Germany.

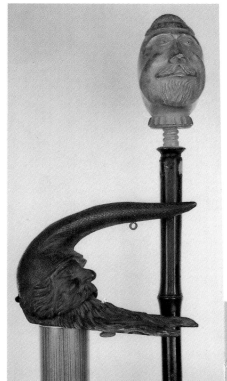

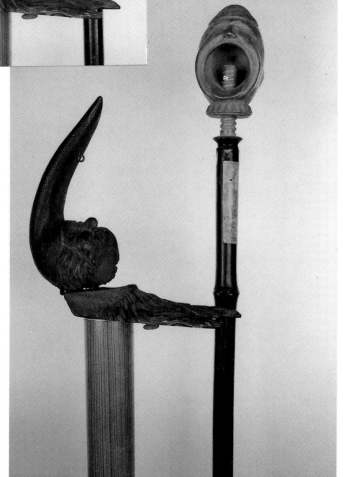

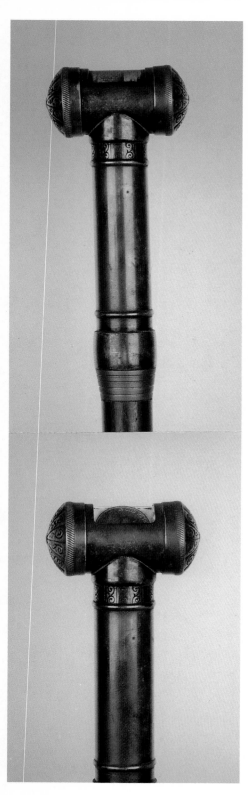

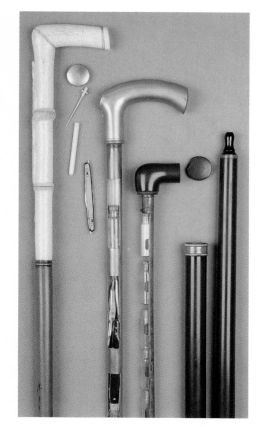

Three physicians canes: left bone handle with snake entwined on shaft, 34 1/2" high; center: brass handle opens, hollow handle holds instruments, shaft holds medical instruments and medicines, 36 1/2" high; right: gutta-percha cane, part of cane reassembles to form stethoscope, rest holds medicines, 35 1/2" high. American patent.

Physicians' Canes

Silver handled nickel and pill dispenser, Pat. Dec. 11, 1888, 37 1/4" high. The open chamber on the left held the pills while the center opening dispensed nickels.

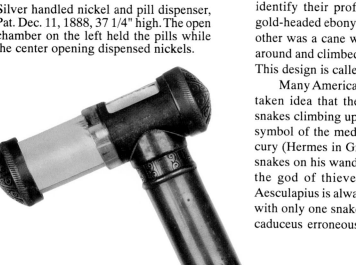

Silver handled nickel and pill dispenser, Pat. Dec. 11, 1888, 37 1/4" high.

Medicinal canes covered physician and patient; the doctor had his with medical vials, stethoscope and other instruments and canes with disinfecting handles used when entering a sick room , and the patient dutifully carried one with all the pills the doctor prescribed.

Originally every physician's cane had a perforated hollow knob of gold, silver or ivory, the inside of which concealed a sponge soaked in an aromatic concoction that could be inhaled by the physician to ward off contagion from the sick room. It is said that a favorite preparation was Marseilles Vinegar, also called "vinegar of the four thieves," who confessed they had successfully evaded contracting disease during the plague of Marseilles while in their ghoulish trade of plundering dead bodies of victims fearfully avoided by relatives and friends alike.

In a rare 1865 book, "Family Walking Sticks" by George Mogridge, this practice is still mentioned though it indicated the practice had died out saying:

> "It was formerly the practice among physicians to use a cane with a hollow head, the top of which was gold, pierced with small holes like a pepper box. This box contained a small quantity of aromatic powder or snuff; and, on entering a house or room where a deceased, supposed to be infectious prevailed, the doctor struck his cane on the floor to agitate the powder and then applied it to his nose. Thence all the old prints represent physicians with cane to their noses. In my youthful days, I used to think that the act of the physician, in holding his cane to his nose or mouth was a mere affectation of deep thought and profound meditation; but I did not then know that he had a reason for his conduct."

In very early days medical doctors adopted two types of walking sticks to identify their profession. One was the gold-headed ebony or malacca stick. The other was a cane with a snake entwined around and climbed upward on the shaft. This design is called a Caduceus.

Many American doctors have a mistaken idea that the caduceus with two snakes climbing up a wand is the proper symbol of the medical profession. Mercury (Hermes in Greek) always had two snakes on his wand or baton, but he was the god of thieves. The healing god Aesculapius is always shown with a stick with only one snake on it, not two as the caduceus erroneously portrays. This error is confined solely to the United States as the two snakes are on the emblem of hospital stewards of the U.S. Army, and on the seal of the U.S. Public Health Service, and in 1902, on the uniforms of the U.S. Army medical officers. The true Aesculapian symbol, as now employed by the American Medical Association, has only one snake climbing up a staff or cane. Collectors of medical canes should be aware of this.

I have a very old malacca cane with a fine ivory handle carved with the figure of a robed seated man I thought was an early disciple or apostle, but though it may be such, I now notice he is holding a long thin staff with a caduceus emblem carved on it so I believe it is an early doctor's cane. Most of the early European doctor's canes have merely one snake on it and no wings, which is proper historically.

Other doctor's canes that I have, mentioned above, contain medicine vials and instruments. Look in my detailed index of patents appended to this book and you will find many canes patented for a doctor's use.

The soldier not only had his cane to conceal his baton or dress blade when traveling as a civilian, but his sergeant had a cane that would calibrate the necessary stride when marching in formation. Smokers had humidors, snuff boxes, pipes, cigars, cigarettes, lighters, matches, flints, and cigar crimpers all in a walking stick and our lady had not only her perfume in a cane, but a siren to call for aid should she be the object of unwelcome attention. Surveyors, carpenters and lumber buyers all carried their measuring devices in their sticks. Even fans were concealed in a staff for when needed. The gadget wonders are unlimited and once you have bought one you are like the addict who took his first dose thinking it would not be habit forming. Soon he will recognize he is mercilessly hooked, and so will you.

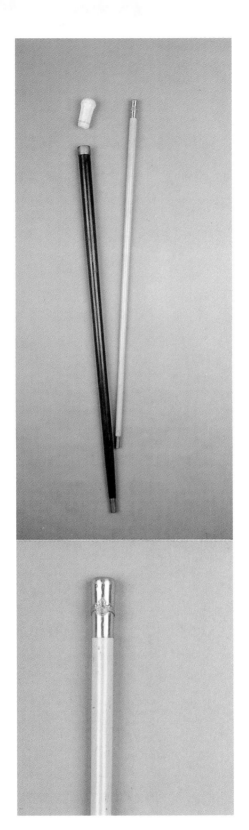

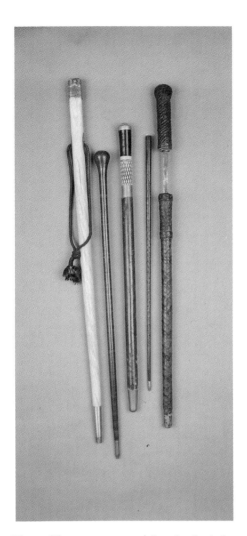

Five military swagger sticks, the far left is a narwhal tusk shaft, the far right is a leather wrapped dagger with a four sided blade marked "FRANCE," ranging in height from 20" to 28".

Walrus ivory handle with a hollow metal shaft containing an RAF swagger stick inside, 33 1/4" high.

Two tourist swagger sticks, left with eyelets is marked "KOREA," the right has a sticker "MADE IN THE PHILIPPINES." Left: 16 5/8"; right 19 1/2" high.

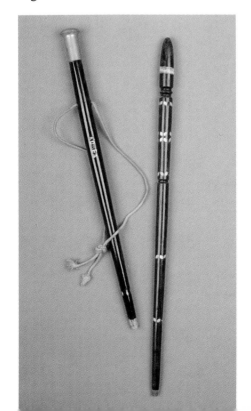

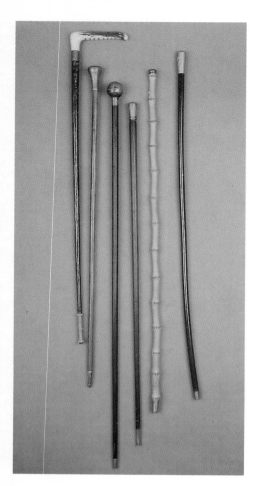

Six military swagger sticks, the second and third from the left have photos of the tops of their handles, ranging in height from 24 1/4" to 30 1/4".

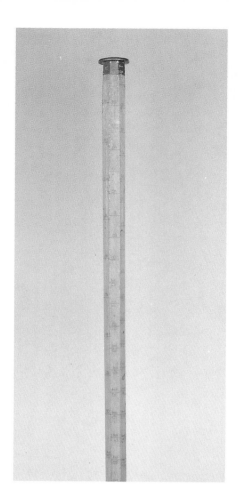

Lumber measuring cane in various scales, 36 1/4" high.

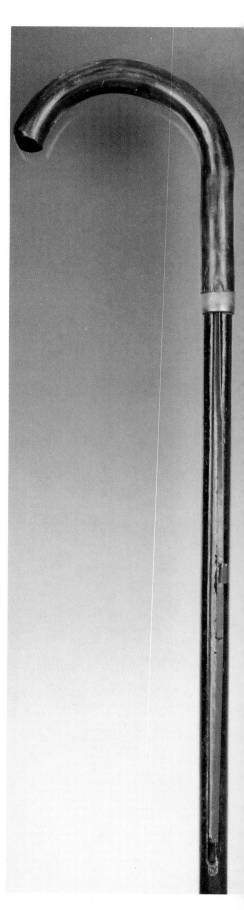

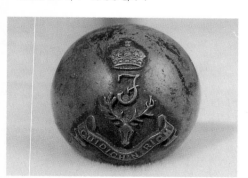

Swagger stick with regimental insignia on top featuring an "F" and the phrase "GUIDICH'N RIGH," 30 1/2" high.

Silver knob swagger stick with American eagle and shield on top, 25" high.

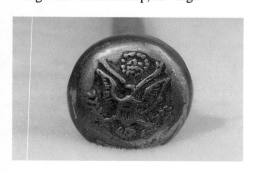

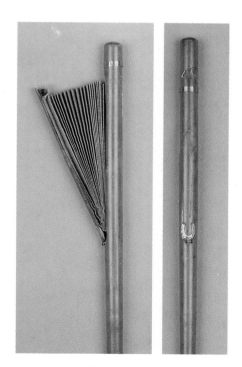

Ladies cane with a fan, hinged at horse-shoe, 35" high, gold collar holds fan in place.

Crook handled map cane of Boston, closed, c. 1939, 35" high.

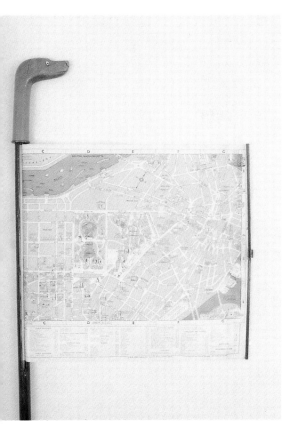

Old map (map of Boston) cane with a dog's head wood handle with glass inset eyes, 33 1/2" high.

Map canes are still to be found that had been sold to conventioneers and tourists at American Legion Conventions, Worlds Fairs, etc. These usually have a crook handle and the shaft is constructed like a window shade roller. An almost indiscernible tab midway down the shaft is pulled at right angles and a cloth map unrolls from inside to depict all the cities' streets and other points of interest. Upon pulling the map further and releasing it, it snap-rolls back into the shaft.

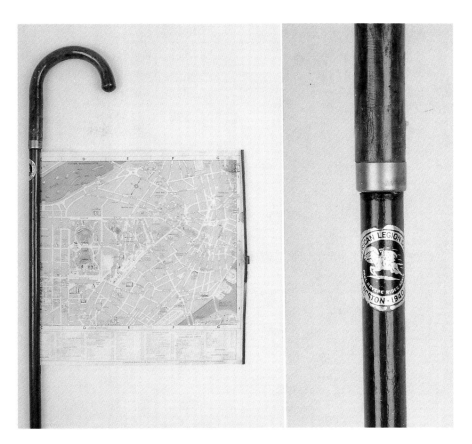

American Legion map cane of Boston, 1940, 35" high.

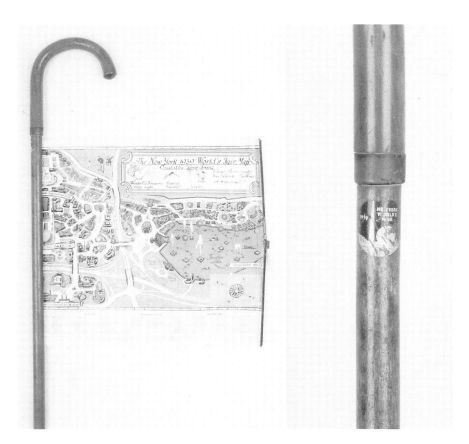

New York World's Fair, 1939, map cane with crook handle, 34 3/4" high.

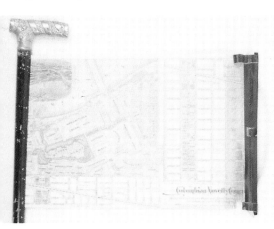

Silver handled cane with a map by the Columbian Novelty Company, 35" high.

Spectators at British parades, golf matches, and such customarily carried box type periscopes to see the activity over the heads of crowds. Until then they sat in the crowd on what the English called "shooting sticks," named so because initially the country gentlemen sat on these while shooting skeet, grouse, etc. It was but a matter of time before someone would patent a combination cane seat and periscope. Surprisingly this came just a few years ago in what is known as the Peristick.

English school masters ingeniously hid their disciplining switch in a walking stick. When we remember that in days gone by a gentleman, or one who thought himself so, was never without or far from his cane, we can see the teacher in his class with his stout cane. As necessity arose he could extract from it a slender bamboo lash that he could alternately use as a pointer or a pliable disciplining rod for which the British school system was famous.

So close were men to their canes that they became a problem at restaurants, operas, lectures and such. The checking of canes caused so many losses that some establishments refused altogether to check sticks. The problem must have been tremendous when several hundred men gathered at one social function, each with his most prized stick of the moment. As a consequence, an ingenious inventor patented a device for quick identification of canes, etc. Another patented an accessory for attaching the cane to the body on a suspender like the early toters who first "wore" their canes so that checking was unnecessary.

Watch canes at about the turn of the century were very popular, but in primitive and early settler days watches were scarce and far too costly and fragile to be placed on or in a walking stick. Yet the time was always an essential inquiry. In early days, up to almost 1900, sun dials were used and many are the various types of portable sun dials, all worthy of collection in their own right. The shepherds of the environs of Lourdes, France were noted for the pillar dial on their sticks as also were the early pilgrims to Benares, India.

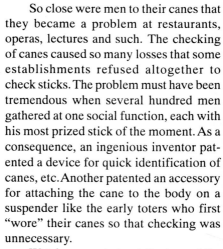

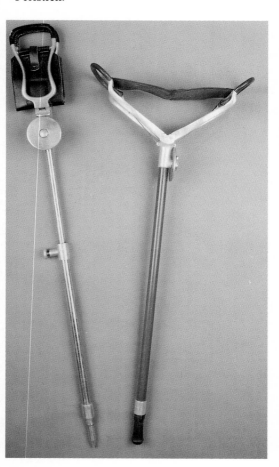

Two shooter's seat canes. Black leather seat, 36" high; brown leather seat, 34" high.

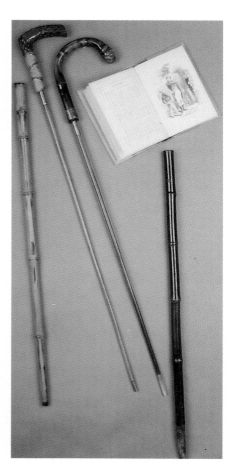

Two school teachers' pointer and discipline canes. Left: L handle measuring 36" high; right: crook handle measuring 36 1/2" high.

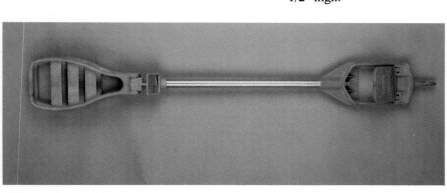

British seat cane with periscope for looking at parades over the heads of the crowd. Blue plastic and aluminum cane measuring 33 1/2" high.

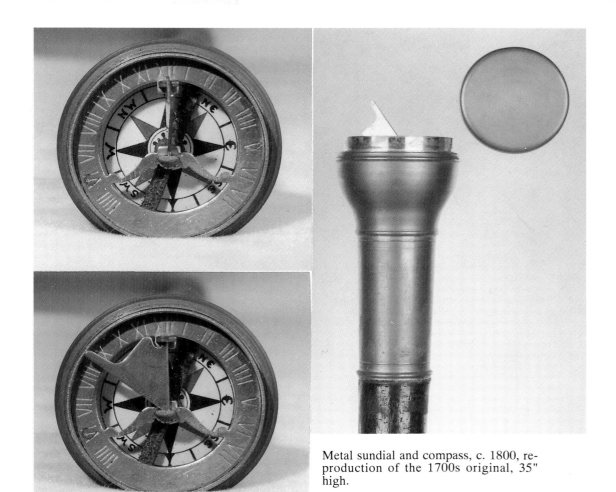

Metal sundial and compass, c. 1800, reproduction of the 1700s original, 35" high.

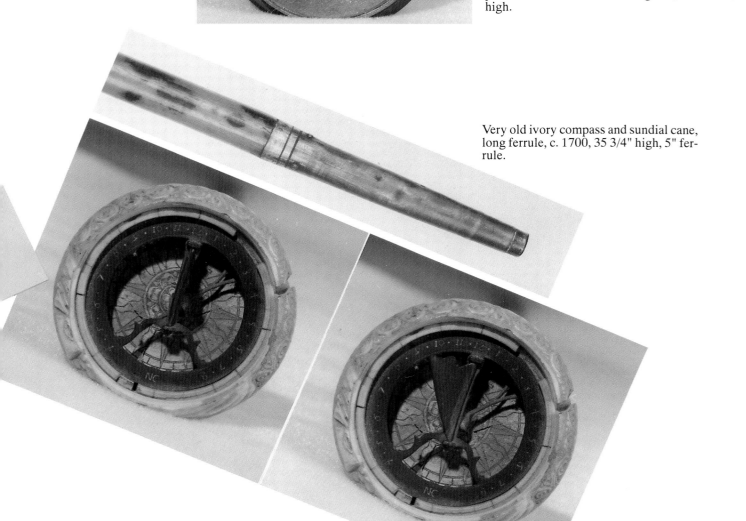

Very old ivory compass and sundial cane, long ferrule, c. 1700, 35 3/4" high, 5" ferrule.

In France near Lourdes shepherds used the "pillar dial" atop a cane or shepherd's staff. The religious pilgrims to Benares, the site of the most famous shrine in all of India, would carry a cylinder dial on their staves. These were 4 1/2 to 5 1/2 feet long, eight sided and the sun dial was the upper portion that contained the half hours from sunrise to sunset. It was merely necessary to point the retractable gnomon or style, also called an indicator, toward the sun and its shadow on the shaft would designate the hour of the day.

In later years very fine gold watches and time pieces of other precious metals, often jewel encrusted, became integral parts of canes and are to be found to this day.

Even the theater usher had his cane with a light at the bottom to conduct patrons to their seats.

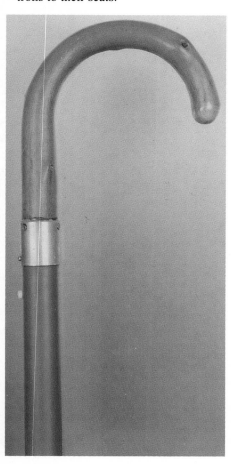

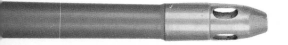

Theater usher's cane with push button, the light is in the ferrule to seat theater-goers, 36 1/2" high.

The military had their canes, aside from those previously mentioned, i.e., the sergeants marching step calibrator, the traveling officers cane (carrying his sword blade, while his suitcase carried its handle.) The Second World War brought out a cane with an involved range finding calculator that would quickly determine the distance an artillery shell should be set to detonate.

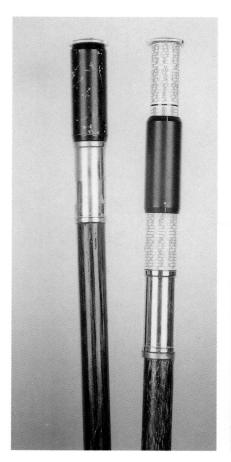

Two artillery canes for calculating the ballistic arc and angle for firing the guns, c. 1918. Left: 37 3/4" high and stamped Made In England; right: 39" high.

The older gun and weapon canes now have a sinister modern development. Within the past 10 years, we have read of pellets carrying lethal and undetectable diseases being propelled from canes and umbrellas by foreign enemy agents. Even our own intelligence departments have specialists designing such weapons according to testimony given at a recent Senate inquiry.

World War II also brought out several black-out canes that could be used to shine a most infinitesimal beam of light to light one's way in the darkness. One

such has a further development for use by the military in sending out coded signals by merely pressing a button on the top of the handle. Right after that war, a Japanese company manufactured a cane containing a transistor radio. All this production went to New York in the amount of many hundreds, yet to date I have been unable to find one though a crystal wireless cane was patented in England as early as 1924. I did, however, find an Italian radio in the handle of an umbrella.

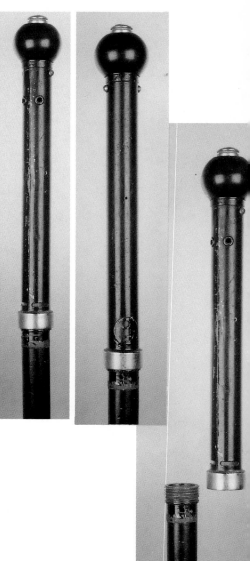

Military signal light cane, push button knob handle, five lights, two up top and three just above the screw joint for the battery, c. 1914, 35 1/8" high.

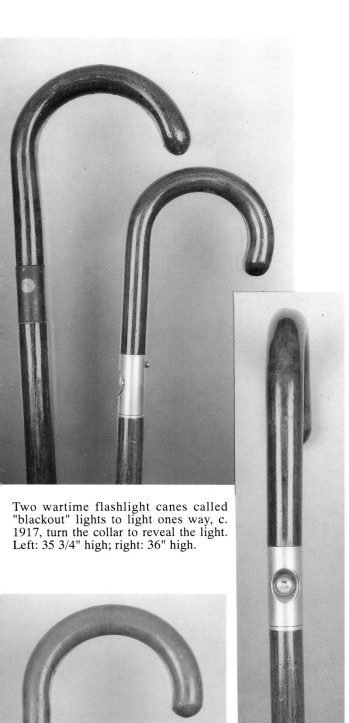

With so many millions of canes available at one time and with prominent stores carrying them in the hundreds, it was but natural that a cane-seller's cane should be patented and in general use by such establishments. This cane looks like an ordinary walking stick, but the bottom ferrule pulls out telescope-wise and this portion has calibrations so that the buyer of a cane need merely grasp the cane handle, hold the stick in the usual fashion and press down until a comfortable height is reached. The seller, by looking at the measure at the bottom, can now immediately tell the length of cane this buyer requires.

Many a GI who had the dangerous job of finding and defusing land mines with a general-issue long probe, consisting of a tubular aluminum shaft with a long spike on the bottom, used this instrument as a cane or walking staff as the spike probe could be pulled out, reversed and reinserted to become the ferrule for his walking staff. To lengthen it to his cane or staff requirements he merely extended the top by using a readily available sporting item in GI camps - a handle from a baseball bat.

Two wartime flashlight canes called "blackout" lights to light ones way, c. 1917, turn the collar to reveal the light. Left: 35 3/4" high; right: 36" high.

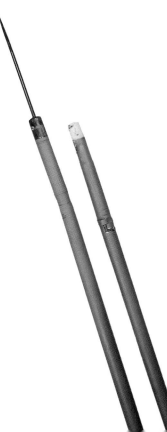

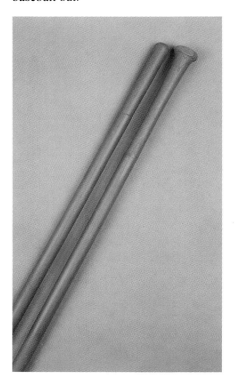

Another wartime model, the flashlight is revealed by pulling the collar upwards, 35" high.

Two American military mine seeking canes with reversible spike probes — left: with rounded top, 50" high; right: a baseball bat was used to extend the handle to a more comfortable marching position, 53" high.

259

The horse racing addict had his pencil cane to handicap his selection. On the press of a button or pull of a tab, a silver pencil would eject from the top of the stick. Surveyors had their tripods in their canes or their marking sticks. Patients had various canes to carry not only pills, but with compartments to carry a whole set of pills. Of course, anyone of any vintage recalls the rash of walking sticks for toting spirits by the toper during prohibition - affectionately called tipplers or decanter canes.

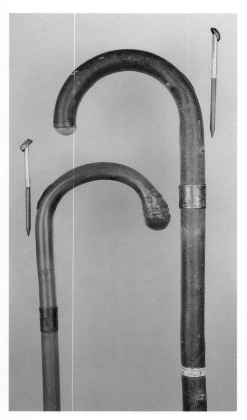

Two pencils in canes for the race track. Left: 37" high; right: 37 1/2" high.

Pencil cane, the handle unscrews to reveal the pencil, 36 1/2" high.

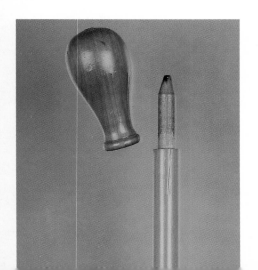

Golfers who could not play golf on Sunday because of "blue laws" could carry a cane whose handle was a golf head and could surreptitiously practice his shots.

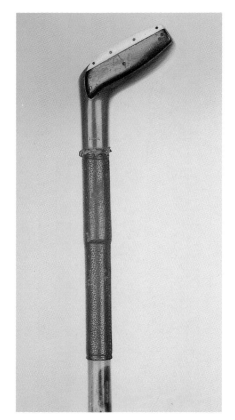

Old golf cane for puttering around. 36" high.

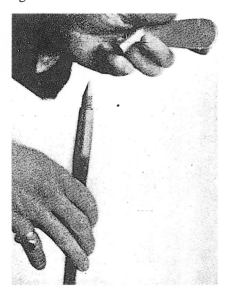

A golfer's gadget cane advertised as "Making the golf stick and the walking stick one."

The golfer who liked to walk over the course, but not the necessity of carrying a heavy bag with a multitude of clubs, had a cane whose handle could be reset as needed to the right pitch with a key to form a perfectly functionary golf club. Another golfer's cane consisted of a metal skeletal frame attached to a walking stick for the purpose of holding the clubs and the pointed end of the stick was stuck into the ground to stand this "bag" upright. The drinker had his cork screw concealed in his stick. Whatever could be combined in a walking stick has been thought of, tried and/or patented. The 1700 or so patent descriptions I have covering all applications in England, Germany and the United States are filled with bizarre and ludicrous ideas that make most interesting reading on rainy afternoons.

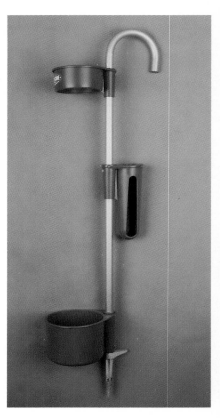

Caddie-Cane — a cane golf bag that holds clubs, balls and tees. This cane stands up when the bottom spike is shoved into the ground. 35 1/2" high.

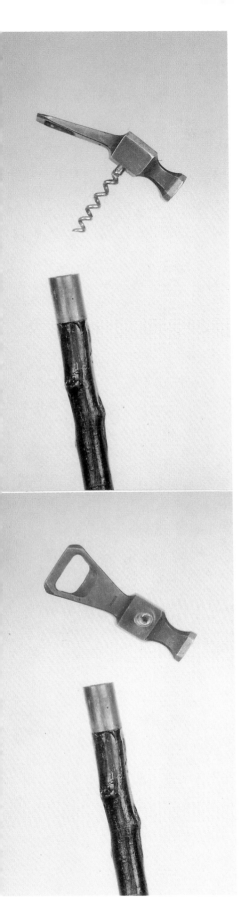

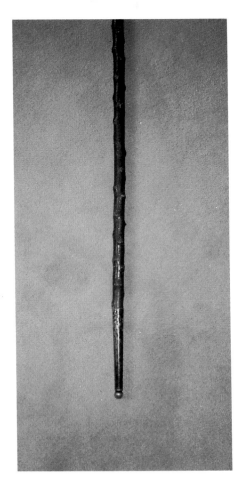

Note the long ferrule on the toper's cane with the bottle opener and cork screw.

English rent collector's cane, c. 1890, shown with a book illustration, 35" high. A protective ferrule is mounted at the end of the L-shaped handle which is used to knock on the doors of renters.

The English renter, rapping with his cane, out to collect the rent.

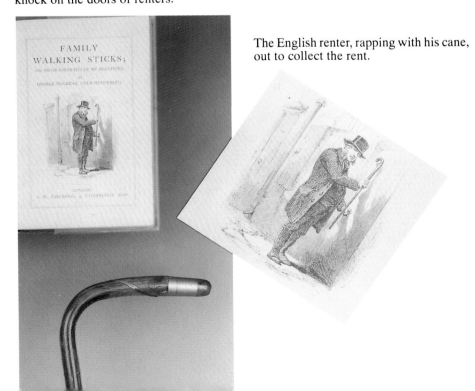

Toper's cane with a bottle opener and cork screw on Irish blackthorn shaft, 34 3/8" high.

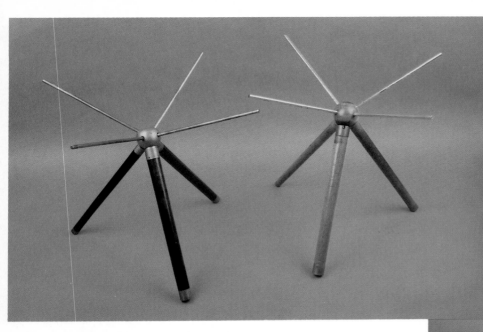

Fold away camp stool slides into shaft, steel L handle. This was made in Chicago, Illinois in 1905.

Two camp stool canes, everything sockets into the handles. Left: with steel handle, 36 1/4" high; right: with wooden handle, 37" high, U.S. Patent 194175, Aug. 14, 1877. The canvas seat covers are missing.

Luggage carrying cane with wheels, 39" high.

Old mountain pick handled cane, 33 1/4" high.

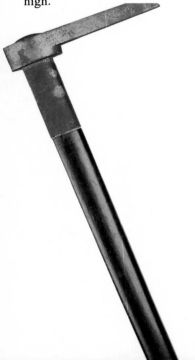

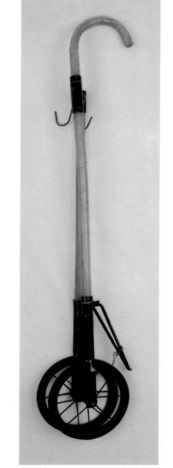

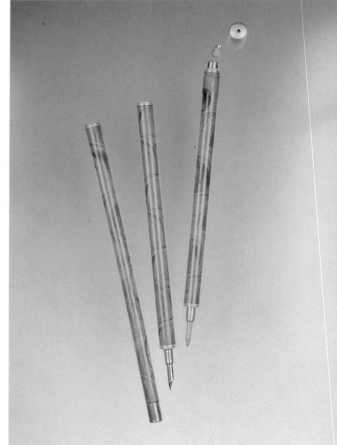

Pen, inkwell, and pencil in a cane, c. 1900, 34 1/4" high.

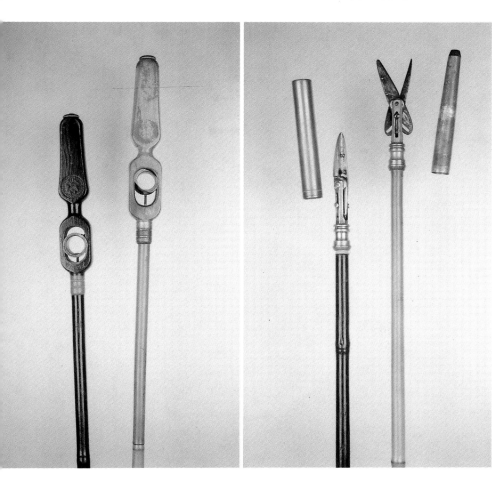

Two French rose and/or grape picking canes. Left: black, 39 1/2" high; right: 44 3/8" high.

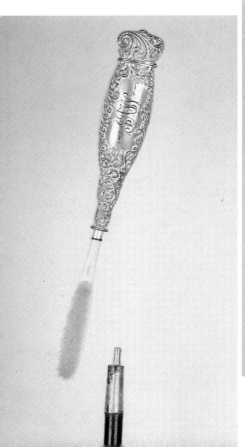

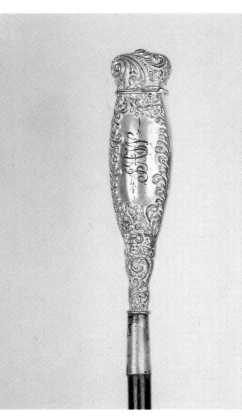

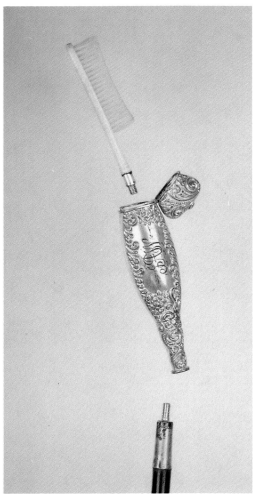

French ladies tooth brush handle cane, 36 3/4" high.

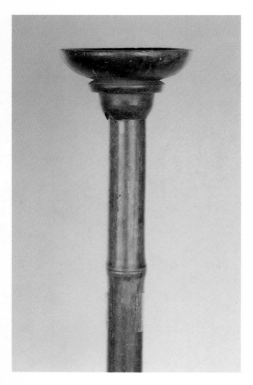

English water inspectors cane. He would place his ear to the top of the dish-like handle and ferrule on the ground to listen for broken water mains. 34 3/4" high.

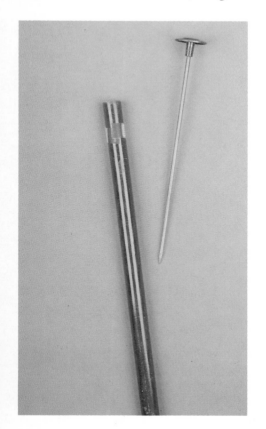

Veterinarian's "stomach sticker" cane to relieve gas from horses and cows, c. 1920. 36 3/4" high. The flat top can be slapped in through the tough hide by the palm of the hand without injury to the vet.

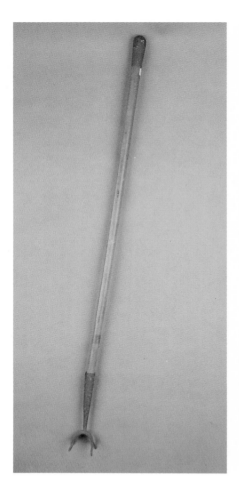

Snake catching cane, c. 1900, 38 3/4" high.

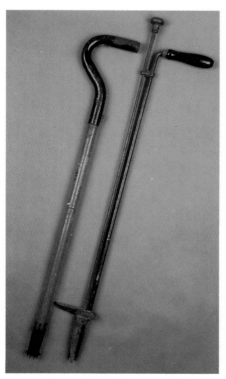

Two cane-shaped garden tools. Left: Rifle Weeder, 33 1/2" high; right: green with black handle and a plunger, 35 1/2" high.

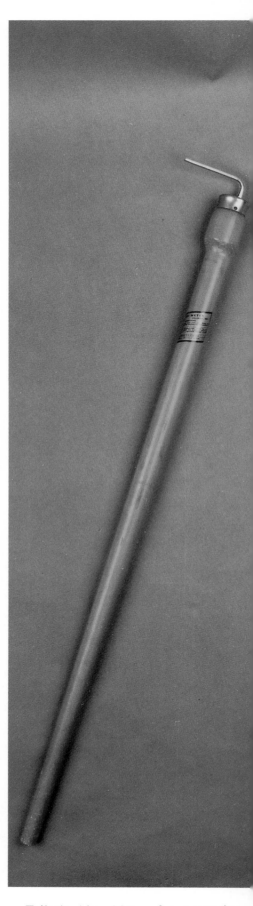

Tailor's Alter-Meter, for measuring outseams, c. 1930, 38 1/8" high.

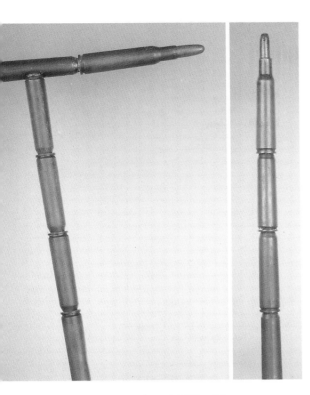

Patented gun shell cane from WWI with gun shell ferrule, 33" high. (See U.S. Patent Index)

I have an early cane of a much traveled tourist with 23 such shields. Each is an embossed picture of a city or place, some in enamel, some brass, some silver, one is gold plated:

Bod Reichenhall
Hohensalzburg mit Gaisberg
Munchen-hofbrauhaus
Lucerne
Starnberger See
Rigi-Kulm 1800M
Gegenstanserhorn U Bergenstock
Vitznau
Jungfrau Joch 3457 M U N
Interlochen - Jungfrau 4766M
Kleine Scheidego m Eiger u Monch
A shield with no name, merely a red
  background with a gold cross
  in the center.
Bern Gegen Berner Oberland
Zurich Utogai
Nurnberg am Henkersteg
Praha Steromestsk Rodnice
Praha Hradeany
Wien Panorama Mit Burctheater
Rothenburg O.T. Partie Markus
Turm Brandenburger Tor. Berlin.
Kochel am See
Volkerschlacht-Denkmal. Leipzig
Innsbruck mit Nordkette
Lanchid Budapest

Once while in Washington, D.C., I stopped in an electronic eavesdropping laboratory to inquire if they had or had heard of any canes embodying their items. I was surprised to learn that they were not uncommon in that field and was told that they had manufactured an innocuous looking walking stick for an elderly and wealthy gentleman who feared kidnapping. Upon such an eventuality, his activated cane would emit a constant and silent electronic beep to allow his guards with their surveillance equipment to readily locate him wherever he might be. These specialty canes that are made to order are most scarce and would be highly prized in a collection.

Early in this century while the custom still persisted for all — especially tourists sightseeing in Europe — to carry a cane, it was the practice to obtain a shield from each city, shrine, or famous spa visited and affix it to one's cane. This was much like what travelers do today in posting city stickers on the back window of cars, or wearing location souvenir pins on their caps and hats, or sleeve shields on jackets.

As I have stated before, thirty years ago I had purchased through the mail a dog head Remington gun cane, but one most rare in that the dog head handle was made of fine elephant ivory. I had sent my money and awaited the cane breathlessly. It was slow in coming and in the meantime I had a massive heart attack and was in intensive hospital care. Every day that my wife visited me I asked if my cane had arrived yet. This went on for many weeks, but I every day looked forward eagerly to receive my ivory Remington. This kept me alive said my doctor even though I never received the cane. I eventually found that the seller - way out west - was a fraud and I helped the U.S. government prepare its prosecution against the man. This dragged on for months and finally when all he received was probation. I had come to my senses and did not complain as he had really saved my life.

Recently I found an old cane at a flea market that is most unusual. It is a society thief's stick with a very fine mahogany shaft, large silver straight cap deeply engraved, and a fine old German silver and steel ferrule. The real surprise is that it is a container cane. One unscrews the silver handle and there in the cavity of the cane is an 1890 glass cutter with a walnut or mahogany handle. It has a brass and steel head with a diamond cutter embedded in the steel head.

The elegance of this cane betrays that it was not a stick of an ordinary glass cutter carrying his work-a-day tool in his cane, but of a real gentleman - though also a professional - a house-thief or second-story man.

What a story this cane could tell - its gentleman owner strolling with his cane in wealthy neighborhoods sizing up suitable homes to break into. Or perhaps he was a gentleman party-guest with his cane which perhaps he did not surrender to the butler but kept close to himself so that when the guests had all drunk their fill, or the time was late and all had left, he would stroll in the yard, climb up a trellis and use his glass cutter to make an opening in an upstairs window through which he could insert his hand, unlatch the window, enter and rifle his sleeping hostesses' jewelry which she had carelessly strewn on her dresser.

Then, ever the gentleman, he would saunter down the street swinging his elegant stick and arousing no suspicion from any passers-by.

During my travels, I filled in the lonely hours visiting antique shops, other cane collectors, and patent offices. I would be content with my collection now if only I hadn't run down all those patents on canes in America and England. Now I know that there are many hundreds of gadget canes I do not yet have. This, however, is what makes tomorrow welcome as I may receive an offer of a trade for one I do not yet have. I can hardly wait for tomorrow's mail. Is not this what makes collecting so therapeutic and gives interest and zest to life? And now in closing this section, may I wish you all, "Happy Hunting!"

The Anemometer Cane

In the very early days of lighter than air balloons and dirigibles, one could visualize a gathering of aeronauts, each with his cane which — in reality — was an anemometer that calibrated the velocity of the wind. Each navigator would take a reading with the hand-held anemometer to determine the advisability of attempting to ascend.

I purchased the cane pictured herein in England from a shop that specializes in antique scientific instruments. Many aspects of its provenance remain a mystery, so any information readers might provide about it would be most welcome.

The stick consists of a long, black, metal shaft measuring 41.5 inches from the tip of the ferrule to the top of the handle. The handle of wood and brass is 3.6 inches in length, .75 inches in diameter at the base and flares in a tulip shape to 2.1 inches at the top.

At approximately seven inches from the handle's top is a knurled metal band on the cane shaft with a spring push-button above it. At the tip of the shaft is a brass ferrule which is removed when the wind meter is attached to the cane.

The anemometer stick comes with a leather case which has a carrying strap and two belt straps on the back that attach to the aeronaut's trouser belt. The case measures 6 inches wide, 4.75 inches deep and 3 inches high. On the left side of the lid is imprinted the name "DAVID" in black, and the word "BIRAM" is imprinted on the right. "DAVID" may be the name of the manufacturer. While I am not entirely certain what "BIRAM" refers to, Sterling P. Fergusson mentions Biram as

English burglar's cane used by a second story man masquerading as a gentleman. A glass cutter is hidden within the shaft. This cane dates from 1890 to 1905.

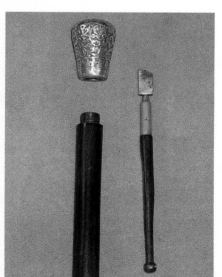

English military anemometer cane for military balloonists, c. 1850 - 1880, 40 1/2" high.

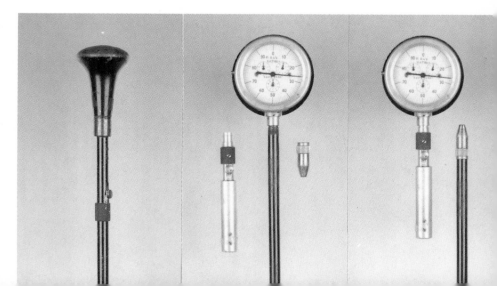

a designer of air meters in use during the latter half of the 19th century in his *Experimental Studies of Anemometers* published in Cambridge by Harvard University Press in 1939. The back side of the case is hand-lettered in white paint with the word "AREANDY".

Inside the case are two instruments: One is a shorter version of the black metal shaft, measuring only 5.1 inches long. The shorter shaft is made of white metal and contains the identical knurled band as on the longer shaft. The other instrument housed in the case is a round wind velocity meter measuring 3.1 inches in diameter and 2 inches deep. The face or dial of the meter is calibrated around the edges like the face of a clock with numbers running from zero to 100. In the center of the dial is a long hand which moves to point to the various calibrations. Around the meter's center are three smaller dials that give further refinements of measurement in the hundreds, thousands and ten thousands, much like a domestic gas meter.

"DAVIS DERBY" is printed in the center of the meter face. Near the top of the dial the words "B, 248, METERS" are handprinted in red ink. The base of the round meter has a cylindrical exposed tube threaded on the inside so that either the long or short shaft can be attached to it.

When I purchased this cane, I was informed that it was either a military or civilian anemometer that was used from the mid-1880s to the turn of the century by balloonists or zeppelin operators to measure the velocity of the wind before ascending, while in the air and before descending. The long shaft was employed to take readings aloft so that the meter could be held well away from the airship or balloon. The short shaft was used to take these measurements while on the ground.

To operate the anemometer, one attaches either the long or short shaft to the dial by screwing one into the other. This knurled band on the shaft is then pushed forward toward the dial. It moves about one-half inch and is locked in place by the threaded push-button. Next the windmill or propeller side of the meter is faced into the wind. After a designated time, the push-button is depressed and the knurled band springs back. This disengages an inner spindle in the shaft from a pinion

gear in the center and stops the instrument from recording. One then consults the meter to determine the mean wind speed for the interval measured.

When the anemometer is not in use, the dial and small shaft are stored in their leather case, and the long shaft and ferrule reattached to the handle so that the whole can be utilized as a walking stick. The case is of very fine craftsmanship and is imprinted with the legend "Hand Sewn". We might therefore assume that this particular cane was for civilian use and of English manufacture.

Although I've accumulated thousands of gadget canes of every conceivable sort, this is the only anemometer I've seen or heard about. If anyone has seen others or has any thoughts about the origin of this stick — particularly the inscriptions "DAVID", "DAVIS DERBY", OR "AREANDY", I would be delighted to hear from him or her.

Cane Umbrella

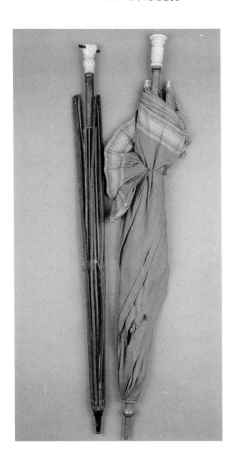

Two whale bone handled umbrella canes. Left: fist with baton, c. 1860, 36 1/2" high; right: marked J. White on top, has material of umbrella, c. 1880, 38" high.

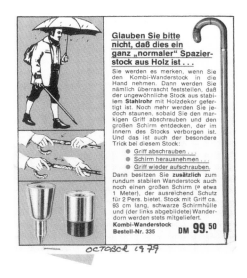

In Germany, a particularly useful stick was invented. It was a combination cane and umbrella, assuming that one needed a stick to walk for security and stability, and it suddenly rained. He could not carry both an umbrella and a stick. The umbrella could steady his progress when used as a cane, but when used as an umbrella, he was bereft of the security of the stick. This patented umbrella cane had an umbrella in the cane and it was taken out by unscrewing the handle and pulling out a separate umbrella from the inside of the stick. The handle was then screwed back on the empty (but steel cylindrical stick covered with wood veneer) and now the man could carry his open umbrella in his left hand and use his cane in his right hand for support or other security. This is a real boon for sportsmen as well as the disabled as it has an interchangeable ferrule with a choice of prong or rubberized bottom.

The Sergeant's Pace Stick

The pace stick was used by the British Regimental Sergeant Major. The standard infantry pace is 30" long and when training recruits, he checks that they are stepping the right distance. Different regiments, particularly the Light Infantry, have shorter steps.

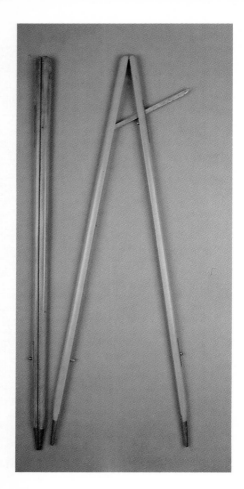

Two English military canes designed to measure marching gaits, both measure 36 2/8" high.

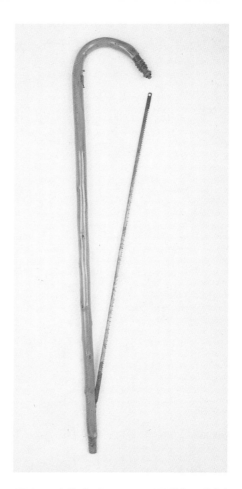

Holtzapfell & Company Walking Stick Pruning Saw of English manufacture. 37 3/4" high.

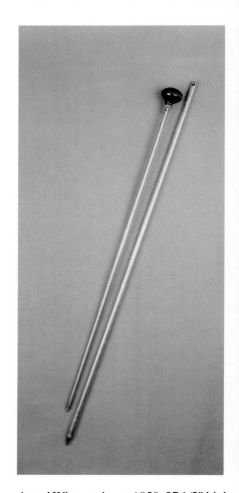

Angel Wing probe, c. 1950, 37 1/2" high.

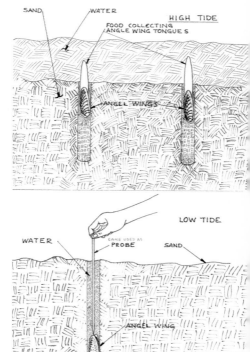

Holtzapffel & Co. Walking Stick Pruning Saw

This stick pruning saw was advertised in 1910 as being for gentlemen, sportsmen, fishermen, foresters and others. When used as a stick, the narrow saw blade was concealed, lying in the inner groove of the stick and retained in place by a sliding bolt on the inner side of the handle. To use it, one drew back the bolt which released the saw blade. The lower end of the saw is attached to the lower end of the cane. The end of the cane is then placed on the ground and the stick is bent slightly to allow the hole in the upper end of the saw blade to hook over a pin at the end of the handle. The milled ring then comes and covers the pin to prevent the accidental displacement of the saw. The necessary tension for the blade is obtained from the spring of the stick. This stick was made in two patterns. One as stated above where the blade simply falls back into its place in the stick groove and an improved pattern in which the saw blade after being released is pivoted at the bottom end and turned on itself before being put back in its place in the stick so that the back or safe edge is turned outwards and locked in place when not in use. I have the latter cane and it is displayed herein.

A Modern Gadget Cane

Although I collect many canes — numerous ivory figural sticks and other rarities — I particularly like gadget canes, i.e. those sticks that contain or do something.

Not only were gadget canes very popular during "the century of the stick" — 1820 to about 1920 — but some are still used today for convenience in carrying such items that are very useful in certain hobbies or pursuits, but are very cumbersome or dangerous if not protected in a cane-type sheath. I obtained such a cane about 10 years ago in trade with a friend from another state whom I met at a winter resort in Florida. We were on an island and met while collecting sea shells on the shore line. I found some long thin shells that had been tossed up by the waves and which he identified as "angel wings". These shells have very beautifully colored interior nacre, or skin, which shines with an iridescent hue similar to mother of pearl or black opal, and when spread open and apart, they look like a pair of wings of an angel.

When laying haphazardly on a beach, only one wing of the shell may be found. It may also be broken and it is not usually a shell in prime condition. When found alive they are very beautiful and there are some people who specialize in hunting for them as fine examples sell for 30 to 80 U.S. dollars. Hunting for them can be very profitable if one is knowledgeable in finding these mollusks, but getting them out of the sand is very difficult as they bury themselves 2 1/2 feet deep.

These mollusks are found in deep holes about 1 inch in diameter on salt water beaches and at low tide. The tops of these holes can be seen congregated in groups. Deep down in that hole there may or may not be an angel wing mollusk. They come up the hole to near the top at high tide when the holes are covered with water and they project out their long tongues above the top of the hole and feed, with their bodies still safely in the hole away from the mollusk's enemies. When low tide comes, they return to the bottom of the hole for greater protection. Only the hole is now visible. In it may be a prized undamaged angel wing mollusk.

To dig with a shovel 2 1/2 to 3 feet is very tiresome and time consuming, especially if all the holes are empty. Therefore came the invention of a new gadget cane. This man prepared a stainless steel probe that is about 31 inches long and pointed at the bottom end. Because of the point it is a dangerous tool unless enclosed. It has a cane handle on the top and when not in use, it is carried in a very close fitting stainless steel tube, like the sheath of a sword cane. As a cane, the tool is very easy, safe and unobtrusive to carry. It is 37 inches long and the outer tube is 1/2" in diameter. To use this probe, merely insert it down the hole 2 1/2 feet, wiggle the top, then raise and lower the probe until the sound of steel grating over the hard shell is heard. This grating indicates the desired angel wing is there. Needless to mention, this friend has a wonderful collection of paired angel wings.

Seemingly Endless Variety
Advertising Canes

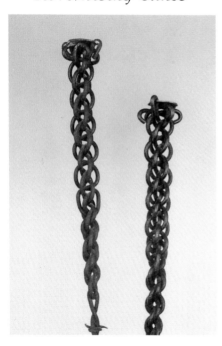

Two barbed wire advertising canes (one with and the other without barbs) with the advertisement "Compliments of J. Haish, "S" barb, Steel Fence Wire, Dekalb, ILL." on top, left 34 1/2" high; right 37 1/2" high. Haish owned one of the first large barbed wire factories in Illinois. One of his salesmen, "Bet a Million" Gates, became a competitor and founded the American Steel & Wire Co., U.S. Steel with J.P. Morgan and owned many railroads. He founded Texaco which became the third largest corporation in the world and he became known as "Bet a Million" Gates.

Advertisement from the top of the J. Haish barbed wire cane.

Seat Canes

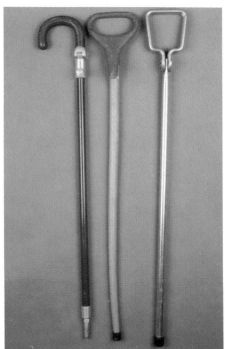

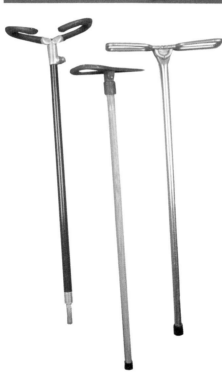

Three fold out seat cane, folded and unfolded. Left: 33 1/4" high; center: 33 1/2" high; right: 34" high.

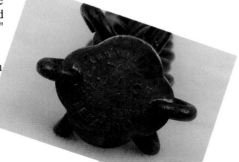

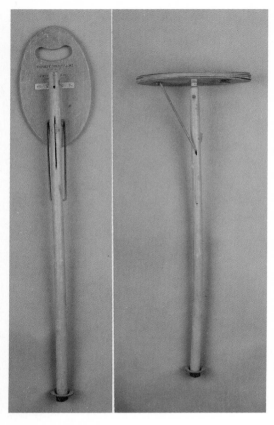

Yankee Snap Seat, New England Box Company, 31 1/2" high.

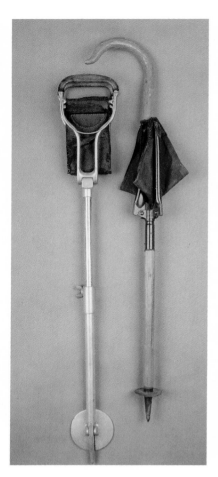

Two monopod seat canes. Left: folds out to make seat, 37 1/2" high closed, 32 1/2" high unfolded; right: crook handle with seat that folds out in three sections, 36 1/2" high.

Fold out seat cane with wicker seat, c. 1880, 35 1/2" high.

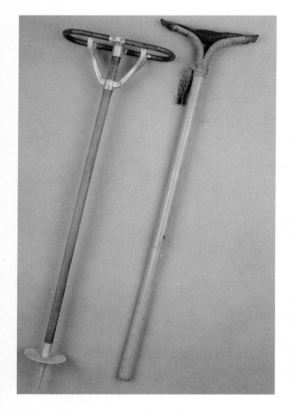

Two more seat canes. Left: folds out to be a one legged seat, 36 1/2" high folded shut, 32" high unfolded; right: always a seat, "ES-TIK Co. Hollywood" printed on bottom of the leather seat, 33" high.

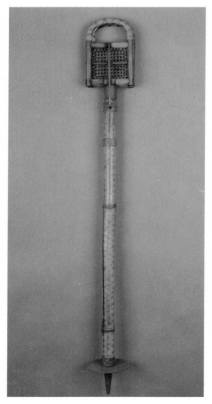

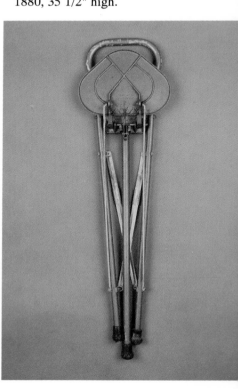

Fold out seat cane with leather seat, Wilson Turfrider, Wilson Sporting Goods Co., 41 1/4" high.

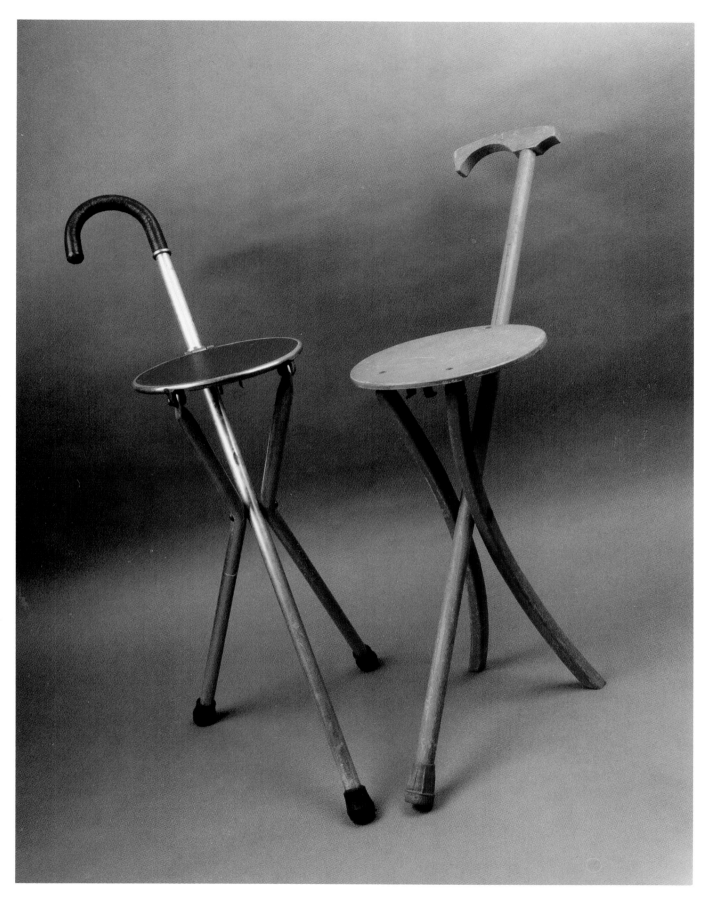

Two fold out seat canes. Left: of aluminum by Tirion Tripod, 34" high; right: wooden, 35 1/4" high.

Traveling Canes

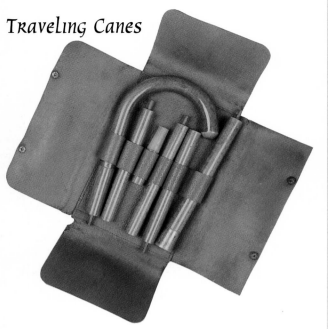

Traveling cane in a case, four shaft segments screw together and two options for handles are available (one straight handle and one crook handle), c. 1910. When closed, the package measures 10 3/4" x 7" x 1".

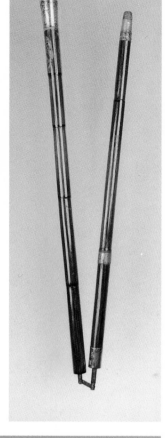

Silver handled traveling cane marked A. O. Fox on top, with three silver mustache shaped decorations on the shaft, unscrews and folds in half, 33 3/4" high.

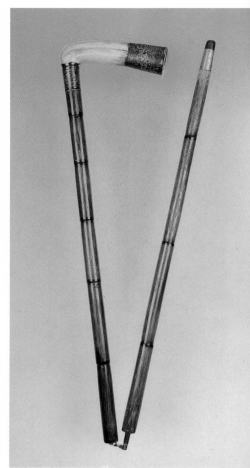

Bone and silver on partridge wood shaft, different mechanism, when unscrewed joint is twisted allowing two halves to lie flat next to each other, 36" high.

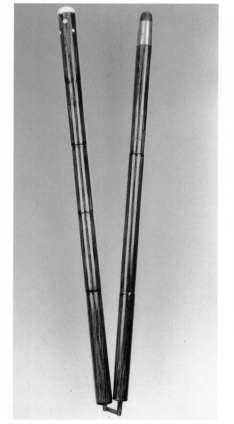

Ivory tip with ivory inlay into a step partridge wood shaft, this traveling cane unscrews and folds in the center, c. 1890. 35 1/4" high.

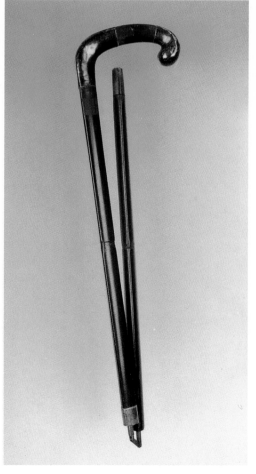

Traveling cane with a triangular shaft, Sterling Silver bands, and a Sterling Silver end cap, 1890. 34" high.

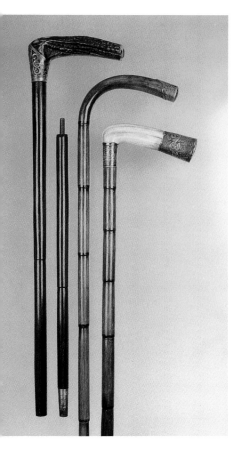

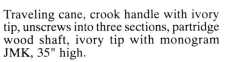

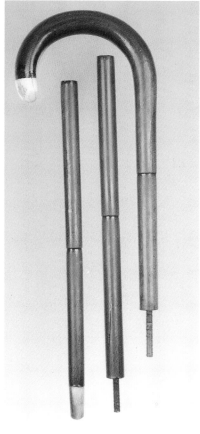

Three L handled traveling canes, the first is unscrewed with the parts laid side-by-side. Left: with stag horn, malacca, c. 1900, 33 3/4" high; center: silver on partridge wood, c. 1890, 34 3/4" high; right: bone and silver on step partridge wood, 36" high.

Traveling cane, crook handle with ivory tip, unscrews into three sections, partridge wood shaft, ivory tip with monogram JMK, 35" high.

Lighting Canes

Knob handled silver lighting cane, push up candle, handle flips back to reveal a light at the push of a button, 35 1/2" high.

Silver handled lighting cane with push up candle under a lid and an end lid for matches, 36" high.

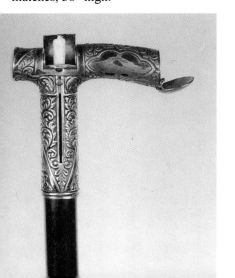

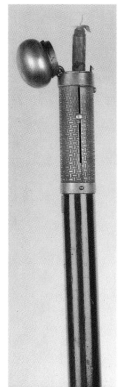

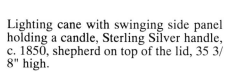

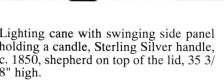

Lighting cane with swinging side panel holding a candle, Sterling Silver handle, c. 1850, shepherd on top of the lid, 35 3/8" high.

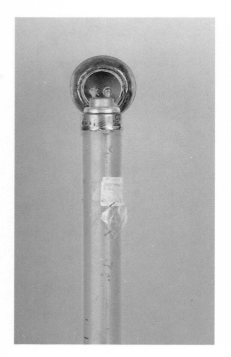

Scarce silver topped lighter cane, malacca shaft, 33 1/2" high.

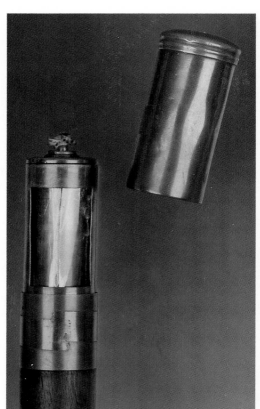

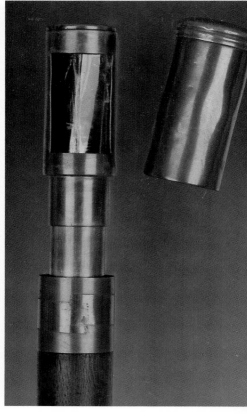

Lantern cane with unscrewing brass handle and isinglass lens, c. 1780, 36 1/4" high.

Old wick and oil lamp in a opening dog's head handle on a malacca shaft, 33 1/2" high.

Four lighting canes with lighting handles in different colors, orange, yellow, amber and red. Range in height from 35" to 36 3/4" high.

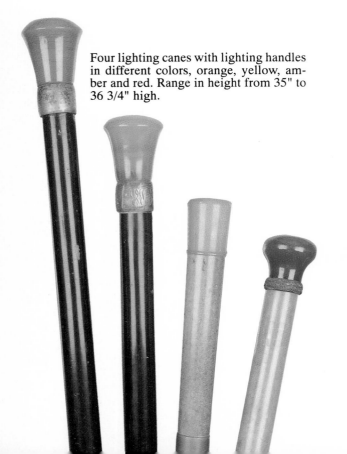

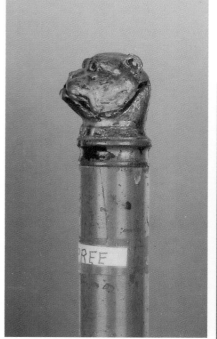

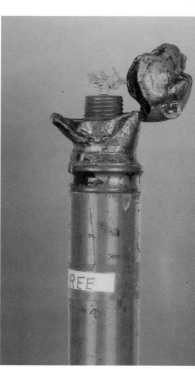

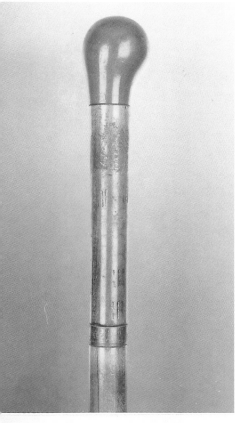

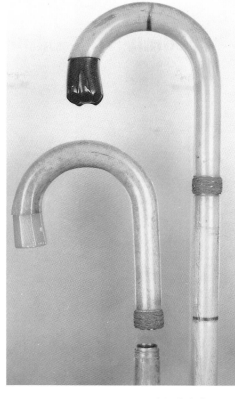

Two crook handled canes with lighting tips in orange and red, both with faceted tips. Lower: 37" high; upper: 36 1/2" high.

Three crook handled lighting canes with rounded lighting ends. Top: 36" high; center: 36 1/2" high; right: 37" high.

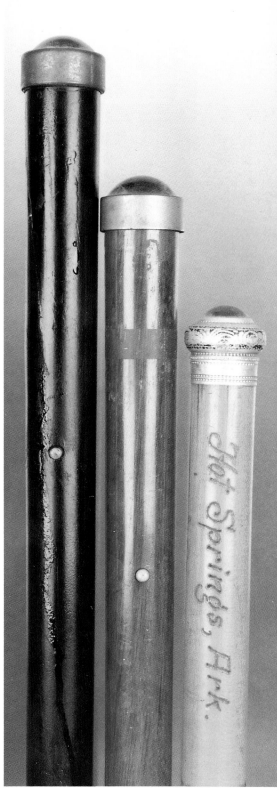

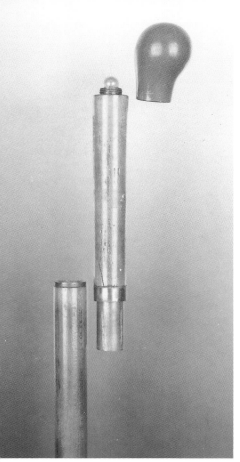

Pistol grip lighting cane with the flash-light in the handle, 36 1/2" high.

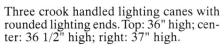

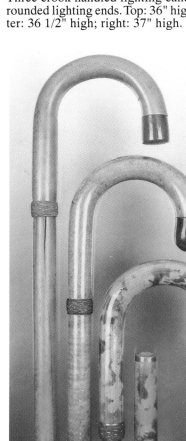

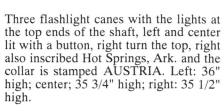

Three flashlight canes with the lights at the top ends of the shaft, left and center lit with a button, right turn the top, right also inscribed Hot Springs, Ark. and the collar is stamped AUSTRIA. Left: 36" high; center; 35 3/4" high; right: 35 1/2" high.

Canes for the Blind

Automatic Canes

Religious Canes

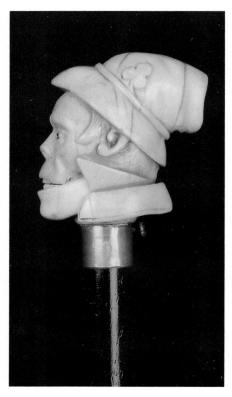

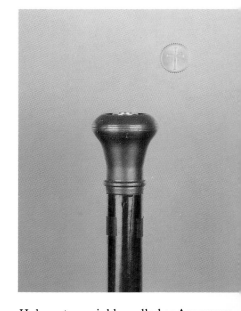

Holy water sprinkler called an Aspergum, with cross on cap, brass handle on a very fine snakewood shaft, c. 1930, 35" high. An inner container pulls out and when the cap is unscrewed, a perforated top used to emit holy water is seen.

Four folding canes for the blind with red tips, varying in height from 42" - 53 1/4" high.

Ivory Irishman "Automatic", rare, glass eyes, shamrock hat, silver collar with hallmark, c. 1880. Lower jaw opens and closes by operating a push button on the shaft. This cane dates to the middle of the 19th century. 38" high.

Folk Art Gadget Canes

Canes of War

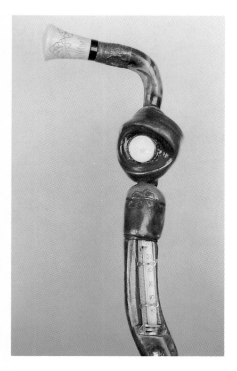

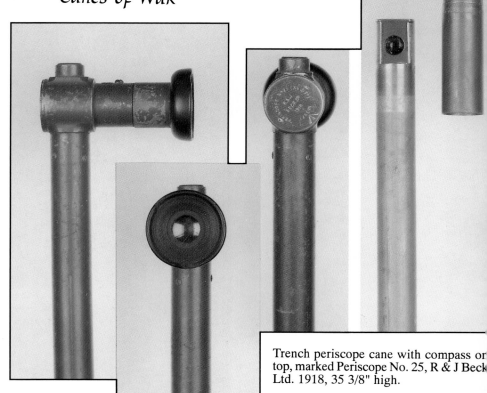

Folk art cane with compass and thermometer, 35" high.

Trench periscope cane with compass or top, marked Periscope No. 25, R & J Beck Ltd. 1918, 35 3/8" high.

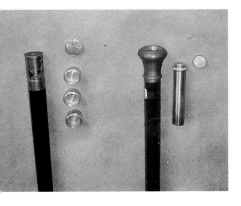

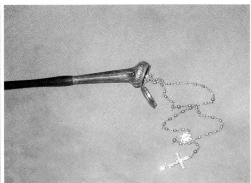

Left: cane for dispensing sacrament of Extreme Unction; Right: the Aspergum cane disassembled.

Rosary cane.

Spitting Canes

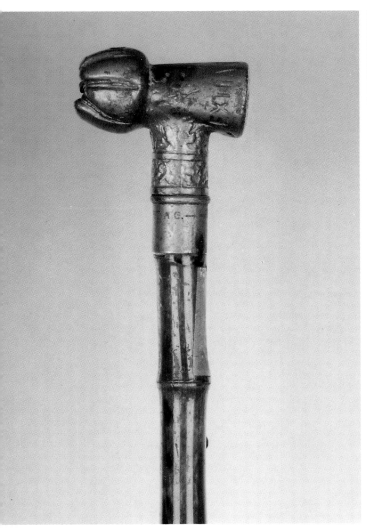

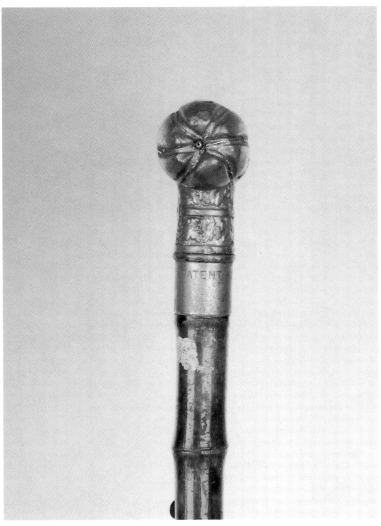

Odd spitting cane marked "EXTRA DRY," 34" high. Push button design described by the seller in Germany as a traveling salesman's cane to curtail his liquor intake by placing the left side in his mouth and spitting his intake therein.

Children's Canes

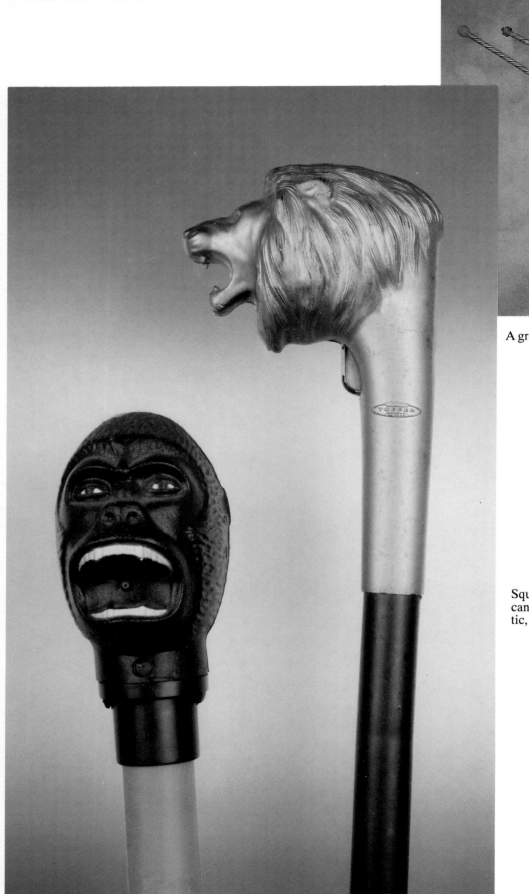

A group of childrens' cap-shooting canes.

Squirting gorilla and lion canes, the lion cane was produced by Topper. Both plastic, Gorilla 34" high, lion 30 1/2" high.

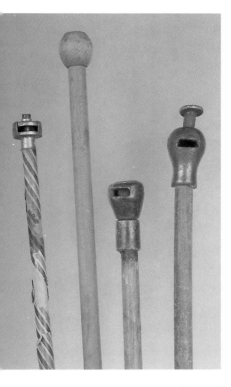

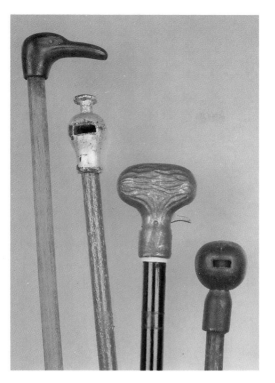

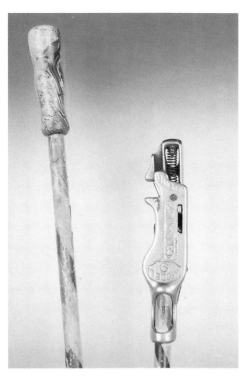

Four knob handled cap canes with small, single cap mechanisms, ranging from 24-32" high.

Four more cap canes, three with eagle heads and one with the firing mechanism in the handle which is in the shape of an explosion cloud, push the trigger up and the hammer drops from the other side of the handle, range from 29-33 1/2" high. These date from the early 1900s to 1920.

A different handle for these multiple cap firing canes by American called the Model 9 Repeater, 28" high.

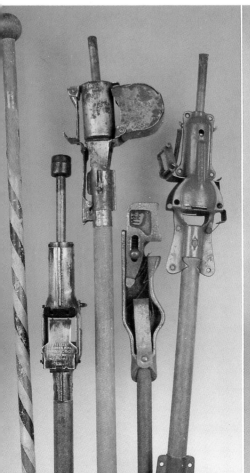

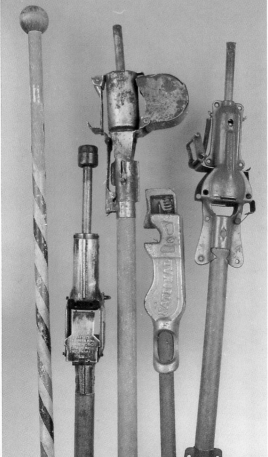

Bigger noise, firing more than one cap, holds a roll of caps, the second one in held a roll and was called an Automatic Torpedo Cane, first on left by Langson, third by National and the fourth is unnamed. range from 26 1/2" to 29 1/2" high. Dates from the early 1900s to 1920.

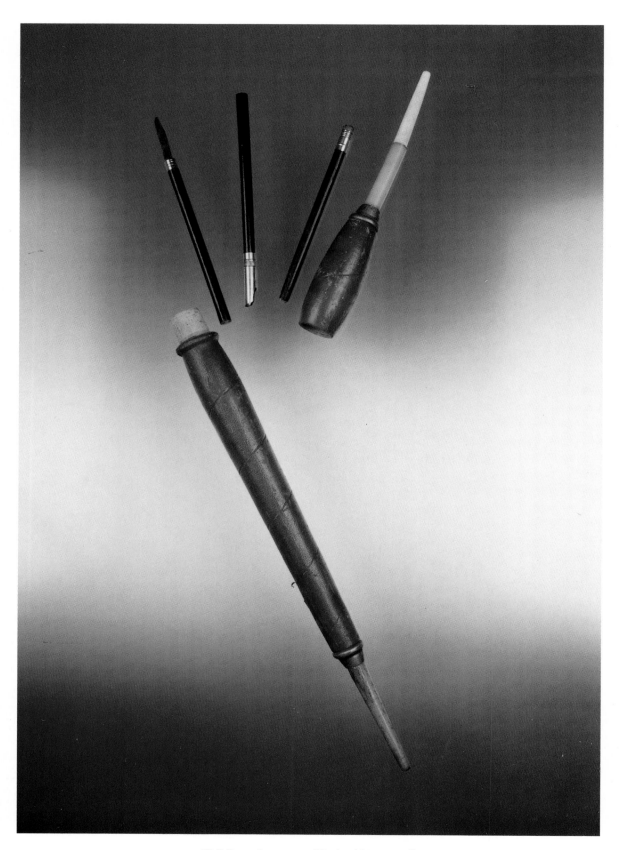

Child's gadget cane filled with a pencil
and a small knife to sharpen it. 19 1/2"
high.

Chapter 7
Memento Canes

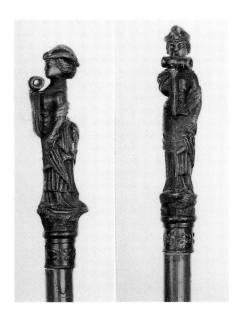

Anna E. Dickinson (1842-1932) cane. She was famous Civil War orator, author, playwright and lecturer on total abstinence, abolition of slavery, and women's suffrage. She was called the Joan of Arc of the Civil War. Anna E. Dickinson was also a splendid actress. 32 1/8" high.

Step malacca shaft with silver eyelets, c. 1790, silver handle with the name "John Sutter" (of Sutter's Mill, California where gold was discovered) engraved in the top, 35 1/4" high.

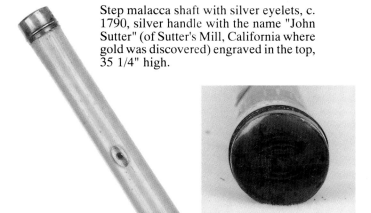

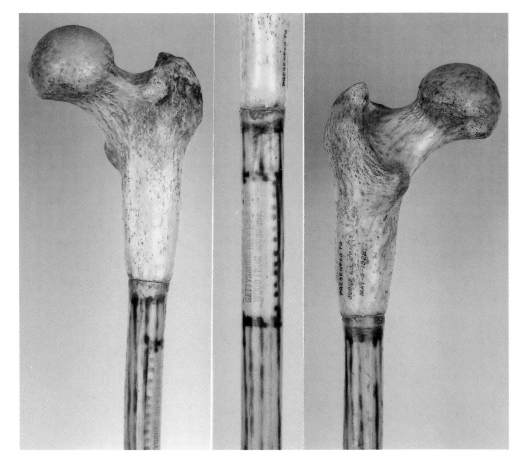

Cane of the American Civil War with the femur of a fallen soldier at Gettysburg. Obtained from a judge in Maine. The femur handle is marked "Presented to Judge L.L. Brigs, May 9, 1922." The shaft is marked "Gettysburg, July 1, 2, 3, 1863."

John Sutter, owner of Sutter's mill during the gold rush days.

Charter Oak Cane

Charter Oak: A white oak tree formerly stood in Hartford, Connecticut, in the trunk of which the Connecticut colonial charter was said to have been hidden in 1687. The tree was blown down in a storm on August 12, 1876. Its trunk was nearly 7 feet in diameter and its age was estimated at possibly 1,000 years.

Late in 1686, Sir Edmund Andros, royal governor of New York, was empowered by James II of England to create a Dominion of New England, consisting of the New England colonies. According to tradition, the charter disappeared during a meeting in 1687 when Andros demanded its surrender by colonial officials and it was concealed in the tree. Despite this incident, Connecticut submitted to the Dominion of New England, but the Dominion survived only two years.

I have a very old cane that has engraved on its silver eyelet the sole words, "Charter Oak."

Old Ship Relic Canes

It is said that the ship "Lawrence" which was Commodore Oliver H. Perry's flag ship in The War of 1812 on the Great Lakes is memorialized by more canes than all the other warships put together. It was launched in May of 1813 at Presque Isle Harbor, near Erie, Pennsylvania. It was named after Captain James Lawrence, commander of The Hornet known for his immortal order, "Don't give up the Ship" as he died at sea in an heroic battle. The flag ship Lawrence was 110 feet long. On September 10, 1813 the Lawrence was far in the lead of a fleet of nine ships when it engaged the British at Putin Bay and before its own ships could rescue it, the Lawrence was so badly damaged that Perry sped immediately for Erie to prevent her sinking. But the battle was won and Perry sent out the message. "We have met the enemy and they are ours. Two ships, two brigs, one schooner and one sloop." This touched off a nationwide acclaim and celebration.

I have such a cane with this declaration in silver. The ship was later purposely sunk for preservation and raised again two times, the last being in 1876 when it was exhibited at the Philadelphia Centennial Exhibition. Walking canes made from its timbers were sold at $2.00 a piece.

John Wilkes Booth Cane

John Wilkes Booth assassinated President Abraham Lincoln, our 16th President, on Good Friday, 1865. Within hours of the president's death, collectors were gathering relics and memorabilia of America's greatest tragedy. Not only anything worn and everything owned by or associated with the revered president, but even items owned or used by the assassin. So I was once offered and bought the above cane which was carried by John Wilkes Booth. Whether it is authentic, I do not know - there may be many similar canes just as there are of Charlie Chaplin's stick, but it certainly looks like the one which is pictured being held by Booth. It is a delicate stick, with a gold crutch handle and very short - as Booth was a small man. Two framed pictures came with the stick and the comparison of this cane with the one held by Booth is most remarkable.

John Wilkes Boothe cane with Boothe photos showing this cane, c. 1860, 31 1/2" high.

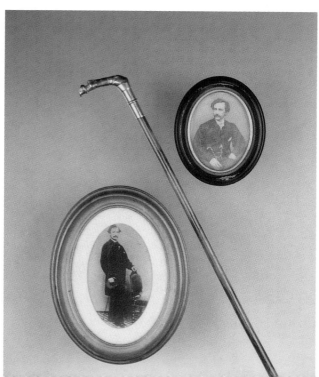

Pitcairn Island Cane

A cane carved by Ivan Christian of Pitcairn Island in the South Seas, South Pacific is a most desirable collectible. He was a descendant of Fletcher Christian, an officer on board the British ship Bounty. The handle of the cane I have has a black insertion in the middle of the surface, which is a piece of the Bounty rudder. Fletcher Christian led the mutiny against Captain William Bligh in 1789 and set Bligh and his 18 loyal men adrift in a small boat near the Fiji Islands in April 1789. Christian took the Bounty back to Tahiti where he left some mutineers who were later captured by the British. With eight shipmates, six native men, and twelve native women he sailed to Pitcairn, a rocky island only 3 miles square and with no fresh water. He burned and sank the Bounty on January 23, 1790 to prevent any of his group from leaving and to keep their island hideaway a secret.

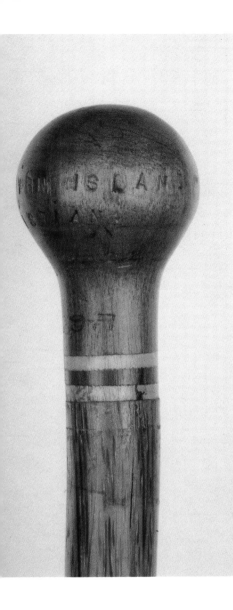

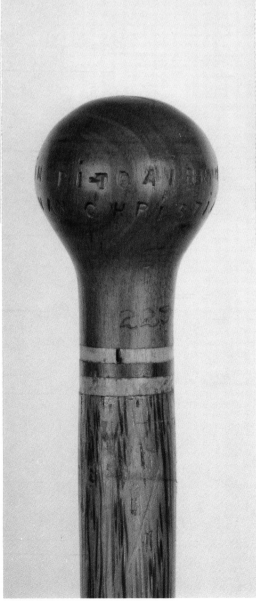

Wooden knob handle cane carved by Ivan Christian from Pitcairn Island, a small piece of the Bounty's rudder is inserted in the top of the knob, 35 1/4" high.

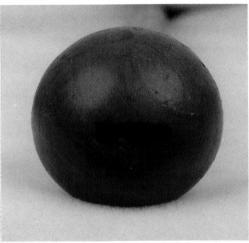

Rudder fragment from the Bounty.

Having no water but rain water to drink and no animals except a few goats, their assumed island paradise soon became a prison. Few ships would stop there as they had to anchor two miles out and risk heavy swells in a rowboat to reach the island. The population increased. In 1939 it numbered 215, but would be decimated every few years by ptomaine poisoning, lockjaw, measles, etc. All they had to trade were oranges and canes which they made from wood on uninhabited Henderson Island 100 miles away. They could not grow any potatoes or vegetables as large swarms of black rats ate up everything before the natives could pick it. I fortunately have one of their canes and it is displayed herein. The relic of the Bounty rudder in the cane is like a modern reliquary.

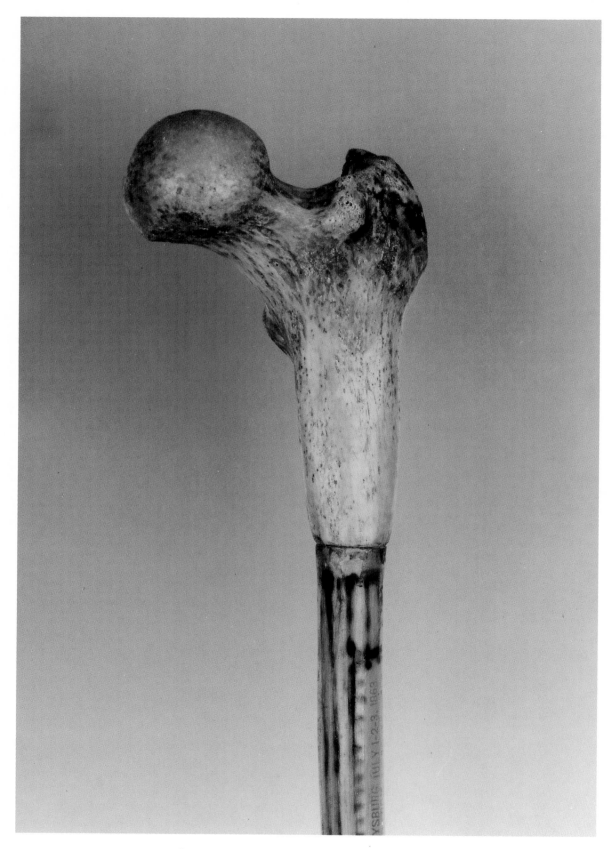

Cane of the American Civil War. The handle was made from the femur of a fallen soldier at Gettysburg. Obtained from a judge in Maine. The femur handle is marked "Presented to Judge L.L. Brigs, May 9, 1922." The shaft is marked "Gettysburg, July 1, 2, 3, 1863."

Chapter 8
Conversing About Canes

There is a story about Uncle Sam's Umbrella Shop in New York City, written originally by Jay Williams, in True Magazine in December of 1956. This shop was founded in 1866 and dealt only in canes and umbrellas. At the time of this story, the shop was owned by Norman Simon, who was a collector himself. I would visit his shop on every trip to New York City and even if I bought nothing, Norman enjoyed conversing about canes he had sold to famous persons and those originally owned by the elite which he still possessed.

Large caribou, straight antler handle on a polished diamond willow branch originally owned by a missionary bishop in Alaska, c. 1900. 38" high.

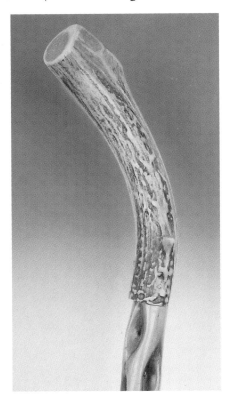

He was a kind and considerate man to and with collectors. One day, close to closing time, a young man came in and asked for a special cane to be made for him. It was to be made of ebony and have a 3 inch sterling top.

Though Norman had none fitting this exact description, he found the handle of one and the shaft of another that could be combined, but it would take some work. The young man pleaded and said he needed it that night and would wait for it. When it was finished — long after closing hours, the young man was overjoyed and thanked Norman profusely. It was then that Norman saw the man didn't look like a cane wearer. He asked why a young man needed such an elegant evening stick and with such alacrity. "It's not for me but for my father," the youth said. "He came to this country 40 years ago and always said that the mark of a successful man was a walking stick. He had the one he wanted all picked out in his mind and described it frequently - ebony with a three inch sterling handle. So now, he's got it. He died last night and we are going to bury it with him."

It was not unusual for a cane owner to be buried with his favorite cane or canes. The custom was established in prehistoric times, was common among the Egyptian Pharaohs and the American Indians, all of whom were buried with their most precious weapons and artifacts. In cane lore, we read about the burial of canes with their owners. I presently have a cane from Peru that is the same as those taken from early graves as shown in the museum in Bolivia. Mine was made in the early 1600s soon after the Spanish conquest as it has a cross amongst other medals hanging from the handle and all the accouterments are in solid silver on a wooden shaft. The silver is so old it is as black as ebony.

"It is recorded that the Justice of Norfolk directed in his will that he was to be buried in full dress suit and bag-wig and his trusty cane in his right hand."

In the Daily Chronicle of London 8/11/1913, we read:

"A gruesome walking stick was that used by the late Mr. Moberley Bell, so long manager of the "Times." It was a plain stout stick, mounted with a bone of his own body. When a correspondent in Alexandria he was crossing a railway line and caught the heel of his left foot between the points. A train was approaching and by desperate effort he wrenched himself free. But he so injured his ankle that an operation was necessary and one of the joint bones had to be removed. This he had mounted as the handle of the walking stick which he used to counteract the limp his accident had left him."

In more modern times, although almost 100 years ago, King Edward was said to have had over 2000 sticks, according to Cassell's Mag of 4/1909 in "Relics Dear to Royalty," by Constance Beerbohn.

I have a photostatic copy of a large collection of British newspaper clippings about canes from a most authoritative source — The British Patent Office from 1902 to 1930 — telling the yearly story of the cane amongst the people who attracted newspaper attention. Many, many human interest news items - like the 1918 story where a judge passed sentence on a young thief who had stolen a cane from a man who prized it highly (because it was given to him by the King of Spain on his last visit to England). "He, the judge, had forgiven the boy for stealing the stick, and had given him 10 cents to bring it back, but he had neither returned the money nor the stick."

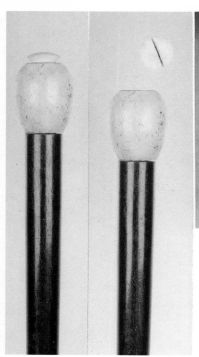
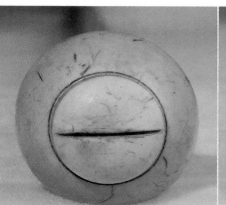
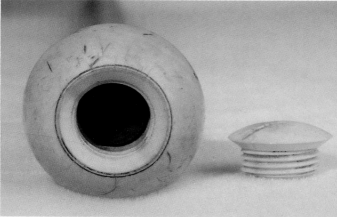

Bone knob handled compartment cane with screw off top, ebony shaft, c. 1900, 36 1/2" high.

The James Greenleaf Whittier

In the Daily Chronicle 10/29/1915, it was reported that the walking stick as we know it at present gained popularity in France during the 18th Century when it came to be carried by rich people who had no right to wear a sword. This carrying of a walking stick was regarded as a democratic triumph over the nobility who refused the commoners the right to wear the sword.

Many of the newspaper comments in the British patent office files mention Churchill's canes and their variety. Other clippings relate that in 1927 Berlin not only imposed a tax on women's bobbed hair and silk stockings, but also decided to tax walking sticks used by women. Of course, every new use for a new type of cane is filed in these records including, in 1927, that a pedestrian attached a horn to a cane to use in crossing congested streets; in 1930 in France a lady was caught smuggling dope in a hollowed out cane to the value of several thousand pounds; and in 1903 a cane was made by threading 10,923 used penny-postage stamps on a steel rod under pressure, placing the threaded stamps on a lathe tapering and finally varnishing the cane, all without any glue. On October 12, 1923 an item from the Valley of the Kings in Egypt tells how two canes, one all gold and the other all silver were found and unwrapped from their crumbling black linen in King Tuts tomb.

Sticks like umbrellas are frequently lost or forgotten on trains and the story is told of a well-known British peer whose umbrellas and sticks all bear a gold band with the damning inscription "Stolen from Lord _____." (May 28, 1925-Graphic).

All collectors of canes should read the fine article entitled, "Man and His Walking Stick" which appeared in the Gentleman's Magazine in 1898, written by R.A. Redford for the early history of the cane — especially its popularity starting in the 16th Century and on through the 17th and 18th Century in England.

Canes were always used as part of one's attire or as an aid to walking on difficult terrain. It was alleged and frequently repeated that in the jungles of Africa an ape or monkey was seen always in an upright position and carrying a beautiful cane with a fine silver handle. A hunting party was organized to search for him and surprisingly such a monkey was seen, but he escaped up a very tall tree, adroitly carrying his precious cane between his legs as he climbed. As there was no other way to apprehend the monkey, he was shot. On close examination, the cane was discovered to have been owned by a long lost and missing missionary. The question arose, did the monkey or ape attack and kill the missionary and then ape the missionary using his cane to walk or had he found the bright shiny silver tool and adapted it to walk upright more easily.

James Greenleaf Whittier was the best known and most beloved American poet of the 19th Century. His masterpiece "Snowbound" was a national best seller in the 1860s. Born in 1807, he lived to 1892. He was a rabid abolitionist. He was against slavery in every shape or form and wrote many verses condemning it. He edited the "Pennsylvania Freeman," a small newspaper championing his cause and dedicated to the abolition of slavery. An angry mob burned the building where the paper was printed. From wood salvaged from his building and Pennsylvania Hall, adjacent thereto and spared, a cane was made and presented to Whittier as a souvenir. So moved and inspired was the poet that he wrote a poem entitled, "Lines Written on Receiving an Elegant Walking Stick Manufactured from a Portion of the Wood of Pennsylvania Hall Which the Fire Spared." The poem was subsequently shortened to "The Relic" and it is always included in any anthology of the poet's works. It sets out magnificently his pleasure with the walking stick and his hallowed appreciation for it and the liberty he conceived it to represent. It is alleged he would use his cane to tap out the meter for his poetry even when mentally composing verses while attending religious services in the Friends Meeting House.

Here is one of the few outstanding poems ever dedicated to a walking stick:

"The Relic"

Written on receiving a cane
wrought from a
fragment of the wood-work of
Pennsylvania
Hall which the fire had spared.

Token of friendship true and tried,
From one whose fiery heart of youth
With mine has beaten, side by side,
For Liberty and Truth;
With honest pride the gift I take,
And prize it for the giver's sake.

But not alone because it tells
Of generous hand and heart sincere;
Around that gift of friendship dwells
A memory doubly dear;
Earth's noblest aim, man's holiest
thought,
With that memorial frail inwrought!

Pure thoughts and sweet like flowers
unfold,
And precious memories round it cling,
Even as the Prophet's rod of old
In beauty blossoming:
And buds of feeling, pure and good,
Spring from its cold unconscious wood.

Relic of Freedom's shrine! a brand
Plucked from its burning! let it be
Dear as a jewel from the hand
Of a lost friend to me!
Flower of a perished garland left,
Of life and beauty unbereft!

Oh, if the young enthusiast bears,
O'er weary waste and sea, the stone
Which crumbled from the Forum's
stairs,
Or round the Parthenon;
Or olive-bough from some wild tree
Hung over old Thermopylae:

If leaflets from some hero's tomb,
Or moss-wreath torn from ruins hoary;
Or faded flowers whose sisters bloom
On fields renowned in story;
Or fragment from the Alhambra's crest,
Or the gray rock by Druids blessed;

Sad Erin's shamrock greenly growing
Where Freedom led her stalwart kern,
Or Scotie's "rough bur thistle" blowing
On Bruce's Bannockburn;
Or Runnymede's wild English rose,
Or lichen plucked from Sempach's
snows!

If it be true that things like these
To heart and eye bright visions bring,
Shall not far holier memories
To this memorial cling?
Which needs no mellowing mist
of time
To hide the crimson stains of crime!

Wreck of a temple, unprofaned;
Of courts where Peace with Freedom
trod,
Lifting on high, with hands unstained,
Thanksgiving unto God;
Where Mercy's voice of love was
pleading
For human hearts in bondage bleeding!

Where, midst the sound of rushing feet

And curses on the night-air flung,
That pleading voice rose calm and sweet
From woman's earnest tongue;
And Riot turned his scowling glance,
Awed, from her tranquil countenance!

That temple now in ruin lies!
The fire-stain on its shattered wall,
And open to the changing skies
Its black and roofless hall,
It stands before a nation's sight,
A gravestone over buried Right!

But from that ruin, as of old,
The fire-scorched stones themselves
are crying,
And from their ashes white and cold
Its timbers are replying!
A voice which slavery cannot kill
Speaks from the crumbling arches still!

And even this relic from thy shrine,
O holy Freedom! hath to me
A potent power, a voice and sign
To testify of thee;
And, grasping it, me thinks I feel
A deeper faith, a stronger zeal.

And not unlike that mystic rod,
Of old stretched o'er the Egyptian
wave,
Which opened, in the strength of God,
A pathway for the slave,
It yet may point the bondman's way,
And turn the spoiler from his prey.

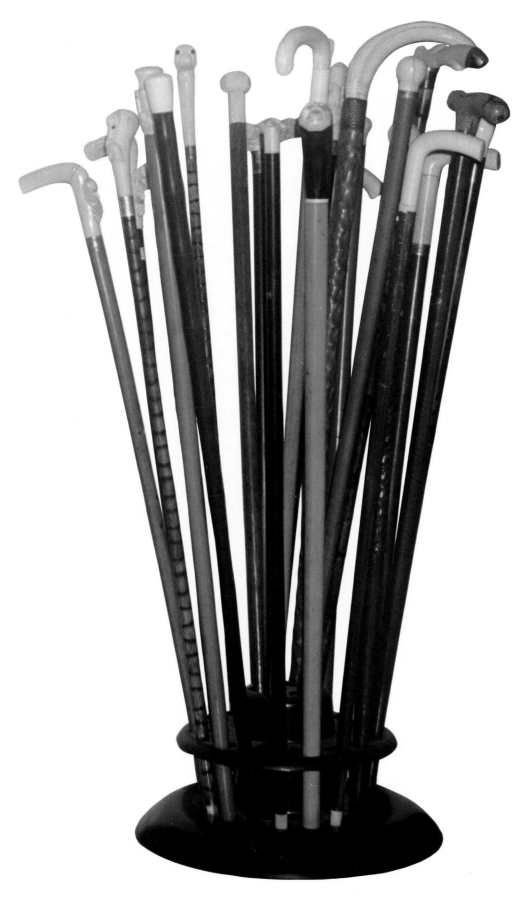

288

Chapter 9
Collecting Tips

Sources for Canes

Periodicals for cane collectors:

<u>The British Stickmakers Guild.</u>
Quarterly
c/o Eileen Dye
104 Pakefield St.
Lowestoft, Suffolk, NR33 OJS England
(Be sure to order all the back issues)

<u>Der Stocksammler</u>. Originally semi-annually, now yearly in German, English and French, edited by Youssef and Insa Kadri. They also own a cane shop and can supply hard to find antique sticks. He is a renowned authority on all types of ivory. Their firm is:
Injuka-Kunst
Mainzerstrasse, 15, D-80804
Munich, Germany
(049) 89-364-325.

<u>The Cane Collectors Chronicle</u>. This is a most informative quarterly on what is current in the field with articles by famous collectors and other experts. It gives news of the latest auction prices.

Other fine dealers in canes having large stocks on hand are:

Henry and Nancy Taron
Tradewinds Antiques
24 Magnolia Avenue
Manchester-by-the-Sea, MA 01944
USA
(508) 768-3327

<u>Michael German Antiques</u>
38 B Kensington Church Street
London, W8 4BX England
011-44-171-937-2771

<u>M.S. Rau, Inc.</u>
Attn. Bill Rau
630 Royal Street
New Orleans, LA 70130-2116 USA

<u>Charles A. Manghis</u>
Historian, Scrimshander and fine repairer of and
dealer in Scrimshaw canes
P.O. Box 46
Wakefield, MA 01880 USA
(617) 245-2225

<u>M.G. Segas</u> (for the rarest and finest canes)
Galerie 34
34 Passage Jouffray 75009 (pres Musee Grevin)
Paris, France
(1) 47,70,89,65

Magazines in which to advertise for canes:

<u>The Antique Trader</u>
P.O. Box 1050
Dubuque, IA 52004 USA

<u>Maine Antique Digest</u>
P.O. Box 1429
Waldoboro, Maine 04572-1429 USA

One must not forget the local flea markets, the best and largest of which are:

<u>Brimfield's</u> of Brimfield, Massachusetts
(413-245-9556)
Usually three times a year. In 1995, it is open May 10-14, July 12-16 and September 6-10. This is one of the largest in the country, always having about 450 dealers.

<u>Portobello Road</u>, London, England - miles of antique shops spreading five and six across the road and into each building on the sides.

<u>Bermondsey Road</u>, London, England

<u>The Fleamarket</u> in Rome, Italy

For ivory, fossil ivory and fossil oosick and related materials for repairing canes, write to:

<u>The Boon Trading Company, Inc.</u>
562 Coyote Road
Brinnon, WA 98320 USA
(206) 796-4330
This company also sends instruction sheets on how to cut and preserve ivory, etc.

Repairs to Canes and Secrets of the Trade

Many times a fine cane has a dented handle and needs repair. To remove a handle from a stick, steam from the spout of an old steam kettle will loosen the glue. Vinegar applied to the joint will also work, but one must put masking tape on the wood close to the joint to prevent spoiling the finish of the wood.

Usually on very old canes, the handle is attached with old horse glue, which came in sheets and was melted in a glue pot over a flame. This was then poured into the hollow cane handle and the shaft forced in. As the glue dried it made a good bond. With age, however, the glue might crack and one can hear the pieces inside rattle as one shakes the cane handle.

To remove this handle, it is best to keep turning the handle around as it is being held over a <u>candle</u> flame. Be careful to resist the impulse to use a stronger flame as from a gas torch. This can melt the handle too, so use only the candle. Soot may form on it, but this wipes off. Continue turning the handle to spread the heat and gradually the handle will, of its own accord, slide off. Once the handle has had its dents hammered out, it can be reapplied using the same glue reheated. Better still to replace a handle, melt out the old glue and mix quick drying plaster of paris or plastic wood powder with water, fill the handle and then push in the top of the shaft.

Now to repair the dented metal handle. Usually the silver and gold straight handles are very thin metal and frequently the dents can be pushed out by internal finger pressure once all the glue is removed from the inside of the handle. If more pressure is needed, a rounded top wooden stick can be used, while the handle is seated upside down on a rubber mat. Just move the rounded stick around and the dents should disappear. Deeper dents can be hammered out, hammering the outside of the handle which is held over the rounded top stick. Still more deeply scarred handles can sometimes be repaired by filling them 4/5 with water, placing a wooden or metal covering over the open end, taping it down, and then placing the whole cane handle in a clamp to keep the top firmly on. Now place the entire contrivance in the deep freeze. The expansion of the water should pop out the small dents and even some larger ones.

Another way to remove dents from a straight or pear shaped handle is to place the handle upside down on a rubber mat, fill it with 1/2 inch fine sand, insert a broad-headed instrument such as a large nail or spike head side down on the sand, and pound the other end of the instrument with a hammer as you twist and turn the instrument head in the various crevices under the sand. This will not work, however, where the dent is over very deeply engraved designs as it will obliterate the designs also.

Should there be a small dent in a wooden shaft, it can sometimes be swelled out by placing a wet cloth over the dent and rubbing a hot laundry iron over it lightly. The steam generated should swell the indentation to its former level.

To repair a large fracture or dent in an ivory shaft or cane handle, first clean out the crack or dent and then use white Devcon epoxy as a filler. This comes in two tubes, one contains Resin and the other tube contains the hardener. On a clean, dry, glossy sheet of cardboard (but be sure its glossy so it does not absorb the epoxy) press out one strip of epoxy & sprinkle with a little yellow ocher dry pigment. This is obtainable from any artist supply shop. After it is well mixed, add an equal strip from the hardener tube and mix both together. Keep adding more yellow ocher by pin head amounts until the right color is obtained to match the ivory being repaired. Fill this into the fracture or dents, let dry and then file and sand down the excess. No visual evidence of the defect should remain.

On black ebony, use the same procedure, but add lamp black powder instead of the ocher and you will get a perfect result. With other colored woods, other dry colored pigments should be used.

To straighten crooked cane shafts, first heat the cane at the crooked bend with a hot air gun or a hair dryer at the top setting, or use a gas flame, until the cane shaft is quite hot. Great care must be taken not to make a finish blister, which results if too much heat is applied too rapidly. Then bend the cane over the edge of a flat table with the bend to be straightened set just over the edge of the table. While one hand holds the cane down on the table, the other pushes the canes other end down so the table edge centers on the outer side of the bend to be straightened. This will always work.

When straightened, spray the cane with cold water from a plant sprayer to cool off the heated cane.

Many an antique cane is lessened in the eye of the purist collector because it has a modern thin thimble-like ferrule. I prefer making my own ferrule which I can put on the real antique cane if I can't find an old, less valuable cane with a good old ferrule that I can remove and use. This is very easy to do because I make it look exactly like the old cane makers did - not the factory jobs - but the old independent cottage-worker.

One need merely take a brass tube of the proper diameter as the bottom end of the cane, cut off a 3 inch piece of the tube, and flare out one end that will fit over the cane, giving the ferrule a cone-like appearance. Then take a steel rod of the proper diameter carried by any hardware store, cut off about 1 1/2 inches and, on a lathe, trim one end of the steel to make a shoulder with a male extension. This is then epoxied into the brass tube and onto the cane.

One thought needs explanation. Frequently in sales catalogues it is mentioned that the item is "ebonized." This is misleading because to the uninitiated it conveys the impression that the cane is made from the rare black (or reddish-black) ebony. Ebony is a most desirable shaft on a cane, but an ebonized cane means merely that it is made of any wood, but blackened by paint or in some other way to look like ebony.

How to Display a Cane Collection

I believe a collection of fine canes should be displayed as objects of beauty. Accordingly, I have the canes in many cane holders or old umbrella stands. These are made of brass, wood, an elephant's foot, elongated picture frames, and old navy leather cannon-powder holders and are distributed in various rooms as accent pieces. I am always on the lookout for different containers for my enormous collection.

I have also made several upright stands that hold 80 canes apiece. These fit right against the wall and take up little room. They are made of five 2 inch x 6 inch boards, each 3 feet long and are glued together in step fashion.

Each board has 16 holes, 1 inch in diameter, 5 inches deep and 1 1/2 inches apart drilled on its top side to hold the canes. The holes are so staggered that a cane on the second row appears between the first and second on the first row, etc.

This is an easy way to display 80 canes in one assembly and is very easy to make. Three or four against a wall will cover the wall and display a great number of canes without using much space.

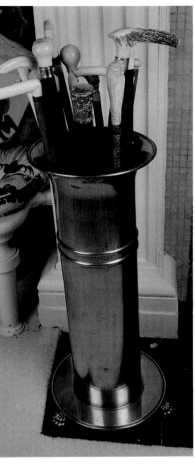

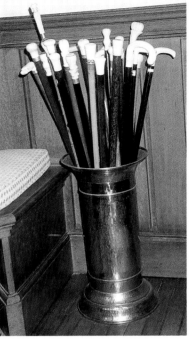

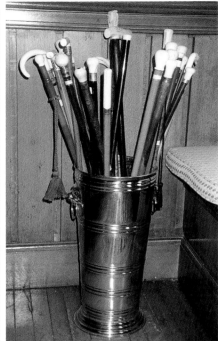

Canes displayed in brass holders.

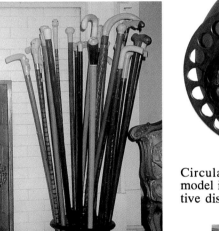

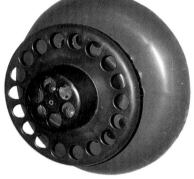

Another fine holder is an elongated hanging picture frame. Slanted pegs are glued into holes on the sides of the frame and then canes are laid horizontally across two pegs, one at each end.

Some collectors use low ceramic pots about 15 inches to 20 inches high, but to keep the canes from falling sideways from a preferred upright position, they fill the pots 3/4 full with sand and shove the sticks deeply into it.

Circular plastic holder and a similar model in use. This creates a very attractive display.

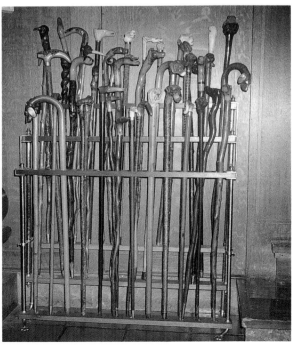

Wooden cane holders, a stand and a barrel.

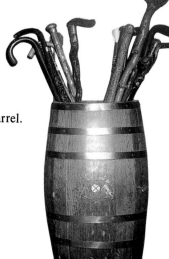

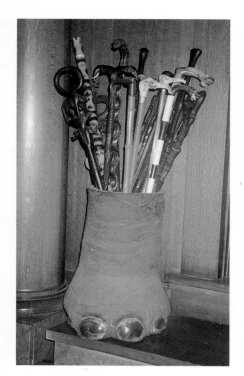

An elephant's foot cane holder.

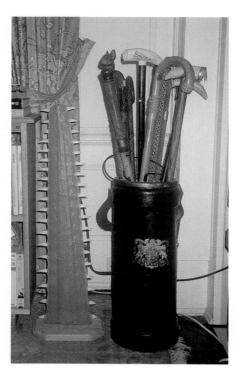

An old navy leather cannon-powder holder makes a unique and attractive cane stand.

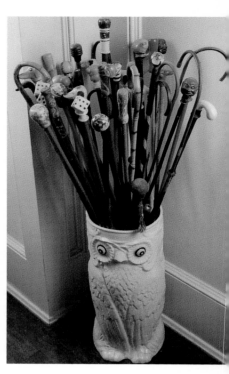

Some collectors also use ceramic containers to display canes.

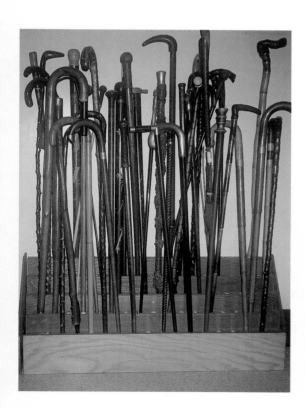

An upright stand of my own making, capable of holding up to 80 canes.

Another fine holder is an elongated hanging picture frame.

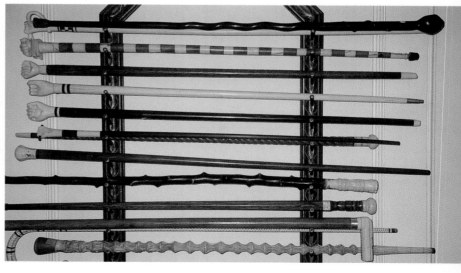

Appendix

Patents

The U.S. patent office in Washington, D.C. (branches of which can be found in the libraries of most large cities) and those of any other country, can give more exact information about a subject than any other source. Patent applications require witnesses and if a patent is granted, an official document certifies it as an original and useful invention.

It is not generally known that not only is the patent office a wonderful source for information on canes - giving the whole history of the cane from the date of the origin of that particular patent office - but each patent office maintains a yearly file of newspaper clippings on ideas that attract public notice and each item is cut out, dated, and filed. To obtain a patent one must claim that his idea is new and original among other things, i.e., it must never have been published before. I have applied for some patents and was surprised when I received from the U.S. Patent Office a whole set of clippings showing that my particular ideas had been written up in magazine articles 30 years before my application and, therefore, was not new or original. What could be a better source for information on any items if one knows how to go about finding it? Fortunately, with a law office in Washington, D.C. I was able to spend every weekend I was in Washington at the U.S. patent office researching canes, walking sticks, staffs, weapons, etc. all of which could lead to one original patent and information on a cane that could never be found elsewhere. In Detroit, Chicago and Cleveland, all being industrial centers, the public library has a patent section where all patents of the U.S. are filed and available for research.

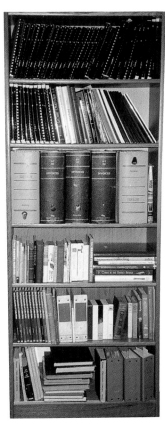

The top two rows of this bookshelf contain my copies of patents from the United States, Great Britain, and Germany. The top of the bookshelf and the third row contain additional source materials; the bottom three shelves hold my books and periodicals on canes and walking sticks.

For years I haunted the records of the patent office in Washington and in these large libraries of Detroit, Chicago, and Cleveland, searching out each patent ever issued on a gadget cane. I did the same in London, England and had it done for me by lawyer associates in Germany. I have garnered over 1700 patents on canes, each of which pictures the cane and identifies it with great precision and detail. I have had all these patents bound into 38 thick volumes:

8 volumes of U.S. cane patents since 1841
18 volumes of Great Britain cane patents since 1808
12 volumes of German cane patents since 1890

I have made my own index of all these 1700 patents, listing in chronological order the name of the inventor, the patent subject, its official number and the date the patent was granted. I have then compiled in alphabetical order a subject listing of all the patents with a reference to the page in the patent index where this patent may be found.

Many writers have come to my home to copy and use this source material for their own books on canes.

Rather than belabor this book with an over abundance of canes and with pictures of all the patented canes, I enclose my two indexes of the latter so that other serious collectors and students may utilize them. Every imaginable cane is included in this index. If more detail is required, one need merely write or phone the Patent and Trademark Office, Washington, D.C. 20231, (202) 703-557-4636. Should you wish the detailed patent, give the name of the inventor, subject and date of issue, and number of patent and enclose $3.00 for each copy of a patent ordered.

PATENT INDEXES FOR THE UNITED STATES, GREAT BRITAIN, AND GERMANY

Subject Index of United States Cane Patents

Anti Slip Canes
Attachments for Hanging, Locking and Carrying Canes
Attachments to Canes for Carrying Objects, Bags, etc.
Balloon Canes
Baton
Billiard Cue Cane
Blind Man's Canes
Brush Walking Stick
Burglar Alarm Cane
Camera and Tripod Canes
Campaign Cane, see also Flag and Pennant Canes; Sound Producing Cane
Chair, Stool and Table Canes
Collapsible Canes
Crutch and Invalid Canes and Attachments Thereto
Duplicate or Single Cane Combination
Electric Canes
Elevating Cane
Eye Glass Cane
Fan Canes and Umbrellas
Ferrules and Tips for Canes
Fishing Rod Canes
Flag and Pennant Canes
Garment Rack Walking Stick
Handles - Materials of and Construction of (Non Containers)
Handle Recepticals as Containers for Carrying Rubbers, Overshoes, Garments
Hat or Parasol Cover Cane
Head Rest Canes
Hearing Aid Canes
Illuminating and Reflecting Canes
Leash Stick
Life Saving Cane
Liquid Containing and Spraying Canes
Luggage Carrying Cane
Magician's and Theatrical Canes
Magnifying Canes (Telescope, Microscope, Opera Glass)
Map Canes
Materials of and Construction of Canes
Measuring and Surveying Canes and Supports
Musical and Music Stand Canes
Ownership Indicator Cane
Physician's Canes
Pick-up, Retrieving, Grasping and Holding Canes
Picture Case and Cane Combination
Purse and Vanity Canes (Handbag, Coin, Purse, etc.)
Recording Canes
Scent Detector Cane
Shock Absorbing Canes
Smoker's Canes (Pipes, Lighters, Cigar and Cigarette Humidor Match Safes)
Sound Producing Canes (Cap exploding, Torpedo, Whistling, Popping, etc.)
Sunshade Cane
Thermometer Cane
Toy Canes (Also see Sound Producing Canes)
Umbrella Canes
Watch Cane
Weapon Canes - Gun Canes
Weapon Canes - Sword, Knife, and other Canes
Weapon Canes, Billy Club, and Clobbering and Striking Canes
Whip Canes

Index of United States Cane Patents

Anti Slip Canes:

..Anti-slipping tip for canes or crutches, #990,006, April 18, 1911, J. H. Reading
..Sand carrying anti-slip cane, #1,050,124, January 14, 1913, J. C. Greeno
..Non-slip attachment for canes, #1,215,256, February 6, 1917, M. M. Dawson
..Anti-slipping cane, #2,005,507, June 18, 1935, W. E. Russell, et. al.

Attachments for Hanging, Locking and Carrying Canes:

..Ribbon-retainer for umbrella and cane handles, #213,022, March 4, 1879, J. Wright
..Handle for cane to hang same, #250,328, November 29, 1881, G. W. Hughes
..Ribbon and banner holder for canes, #394,509, December 11, 1888, J. G. Rahner
..Hanging attachment for canes, #485,806, November 8, 1892, C. A. Rudyard
..Umbrella handle for suspending same, #526,184, September 18, 1894, J. Gilbert
..Umbrella attachment-tassel cord, #809,551, January 9, 1906, Margaret A. Brunner
..Attachment for supporting or suspending umbrella, #971,173, September 27, 1910, G. D. Corey
..Umbrella attachment for suspending same from clothing, #1,032,199, July 9, 1912, T. C. Frederiksen
..Loop attachment for umbrella, #1,068,428, July 29, 1913, O. N. Hall
..Locking attachment for umbrellas and canes, #1,120,092, December 8, 1914, F. Seeber
..Lock handles for canes, etc., #1,136,125, April 20, 1915, I. M. Grodin
..Carrying-loop for folding umbrellas, #1,208,488, December 12, 1916, M. J. Coleman
..Loop for umbrellas and canes, #1,293,526, February 4, 1919, H. C. Overlin
..Umbrella handle attachment to hold same on table, etc., #1,329,915, February 3, 1920, L. B. McKenzie
..Means of carrying W. S., #1,498,287, June 17, 1924, E. Newman
..Umbrella carrier (strap handle), #1,520,070, December 23, 1924, H. P. Nelson

Attachments to Canes for Carrying Objects, Bags, etc:

..Cover holder for umbrellas, #926,483, June 29, 1909, J. M. L. Groby
..Umbrella fastening means for bags, #1,755,209, April 22, 1930, J. R. Danner
..Hook attachment for canes to carry objects, #1,758,379, May 13, 1930, J. F. Shaw

Balloon Canes:

..Balloon cane, #918,973, April 20, 1909, P. J. Creque
..Balloon cane, #1,567,322, December 29, 1925, Paul Jones

Baton, #2,450,545, October 5, 1948, R. K. Foster

Billiard Cue Canes:

..Billiard cue cane, #122,218, December 26, 1871, Charles A. Bogert
..Billiard cue walking cane, #298,111, May 6, 1886, W. G. Morse

Blind Man's Canes:

..Blind man's walking aparatus, #1,177,582, March 28, 1916, F. Murphy
..Signal cane for blind or crippled, #1,542,894, June 23, 1925, P. P. Langner
..Wheeled canes for blind, #2,445,942, July 27, 1948, G. B. Dusinberre
..Canes for blind persons, #3,029,828, April 17, 1962, I. H. Kravitt
..Blind man's walking cane, #3,158,162, November 24, 1964, R. C. Reel
..Directional obstacle detecting cane for the blind, #3,158,851, November 24, 1964, W. A. Ruthven
..Walking cane for disabled and blind, #3,223,099, December 14, 1965, C. C. Hagwood, Sr.

Brush Walking Stick, #343,012, June 1, 1886, W. E. Coster

Burglar Alarm Cane, #292,389, January 22, 1884, J. B. Van Zandt

Camera and Tripod Canes:

..Tripod cane, #414,903, November 12, 1889, J. F. Godillot
..Tripod cane, #464,999, December 15, 1891, W. E. Schneider
..Camera etc., tripod cane, #473,357, April 19, 1892, F. Servus
..Camera tripod cane, #513,058, January 16, 1894, B. Bahmer
..Tripod cane, #630,220, August 1, 1899, C. J. W. Hayes
..Telescopic tripod cane, #648,123, April 24, 1900, C. P. Goerz
..Tripod cane, #657,947, September 18, 1900, W. H. MacGill
..Camera support cane, #673,482, May 7, 1901, R. W. Shipway
..Tripod cane, #806,522, December 5, 1905, W. F. Clark
..Camera support cane, #825,006, July 3, 1906, G. S. Russell

Campaign Cane, see also Flag and Pennant Canes; Sound Producing Cane

..Campaign cane with light and pennant and whistle, #1,824,449, September 22, 1931, Agnes Sjoberg

Chair, Stool and Table Canes:

..Combined cane and chair, #33,073, August 20, 1861, C. H. Dascomb
..Improved convertible cane and stool, #34,096, January 7, 1862, J. Wade
..Combined seat and cane, #40,823, December 8, 1863, C. H. Dascomb

..Umbrella cane and seat, #96,848, November 16, 1869, G. Sweeny
..Stool cane, #126,767, May 14, 1872, C. G. Young
..Stool cane, #151,585, June 2, 1874, J. H. Gray
..Cane and seat, #176,122, April 11, 1876, E. Matteson
..Stool cane, #177,025, May 2, 1876, J. Smith
..Seat cane, #181,802, September 5, 1876, R. W. Smith and C. Jacoby
..Stool cane, #182,869, October 3, 1876, W. D. Taber
..Cane and camp stool, #194,175, August 14, 1877, D. B. Reynolds
..Cane and stool, #194,484, August 21, 1877, W. H. Truesdell
..Seat cane, #208,428, September 24, 1878, J. W. Smith
..Camp stool cane, #236,670, January 18, 1881, L. Burnham
..Picnic chair cane, #268,897, December 12, 1882, H. M. Houston
..Camp chair cane, #280,843, July 10, 1883, S. N. McGaughey
..Chair cane, #382,308, May 8, 1888, J. H. Kamerer
..Umbrella cane and camp stool, #384,790, June 19, 1888, M. Schiff
..Camp stool cane, #389,810, September 18, 1888, H. Hendrickson
..Stool cane, #391,901, October 30, 1888, W. Leisner
..Stool cane, #410,021, August 27, 1889, A. B. Purlingtin
..Stool, fan, drinking cup, and whistle cane, #412,379, October 8, 1889, W. Flam and A. B. Brandt
..Camp stool cane, #413,962, October 29, 1889, G. B. Putnam
..Stool cane, #436,176, September 9, 1890, H. Hendrickson
..Stool cane, #444,621, January 13, 1891, A. Schneider
..Table cane, #450,603, April 14, 1891, O. N. Kuhl
..Stool cane, #484,334, October 11, 1892, R. T. More
..Stool cane, #486,074, November 15, 1892, F. Benoit
..Seat cane, #489,294, January 3, 1893, C. Eframson
..Stool cane, #490,416, January 24, 1893, E. L. Sutton and C. R. Reed
..Stool cane, #493,285, March 14, 1893, J. A. Nixon
..Stool cane, #494,303, March 28, 1893, J. A. Nixon
..Stool cane, #497,617, May 16, 1893, W. Ward
..Stool cane, #498,487, May 30, 1893, E. C. Phillips
..Stool cane, #499,719, June 20, 1893, O. P. Dabney
..Stool cane, #504,326, September 5, 1893, A. L. Chapman
..Stool cane, #533,539, February 5, 1895, J. M. Kincade
..Stool cane, #510,747, June 11, 1895, J. P. H. Lane
..Seat cane, #558,187, April 14, 1896, G. A. Lewis
..Umbrella cane, #189,084, April 3, 1877, M. M. Copp
..Stool cane, #591,549, October 12, 1897, J. H. A. Behrens
..Folding chair cane, #617,641, January 10, 1899, N. Christianson
..Stool cane, #636,074, October 31, 1899, C. G. Skoog
..Seat cane, #642,954, February 6, 1900, N. Bois
..Stool cane, #651,360, June 12, 1900, J. O. Kapp
..Stool cane, #686,006, November 5, 1901, J. H. McConnell
..Table cane, #688,482, December 10, 1901, A. H. Peterson and J. H. Reford
..Seat cane, #713,114, November 11, 1902, E. LaForce
..Camp stool cane, #723,382, March 24, 1903, J. Halin

..Stool cane, #725,960, April 21, 1903, Charles W. Heog and Charles A. Klise
..Chair cane, #731,291, June 16, 1903, R. C. Dulin
..Stool cane, #757,776, April 19, 1904, Nola FeRussell
..Stool cane, #763,166, June 21, 1904, M. F. Dougherty
..Folding stool cane, #767,245, August 9, 1904, C. S. Rogers
..Stool cane, #767,246, August 9, 1904, C. S. Rogers
..Seat cane, #768,882, August 30, 1904, F. H. Morse
..Stool cane, #771,165, September 27, 1904, J. Manderson and R. Coombs
..Seat cane, #779,449, January 10, 1905, A. Wagner
..Stool cane, #787,166, April 11, 1905, E. C. Garden
..Seat cane, #794,833, July 18, 1905, J. Adamson
..Stool cane, #799,172, September 12, 1905, P. Linder
..Stool and umbrella cane, #803,187, October 31, 1905, H. H. McNamara
..Stool cane, #807,039, December 12, 1905, J. H. Martin
..Stool cane, #817,324, April 10, 1906, W. R. Jones
..Stool cane, #859,500, July 9, 1907, J. T. Kerr
..Camp stool cane, #952,335, March 15, 1910, M. Killian
..Chair cane, #952,366, March 15, 1910, J. J. Sheeham
..Stool cane, #980,159, December 27, 1910, J. O. Kapp
..Stool cane, #984,292, February 14, 1911, J. J. Paris
..Seat cane, #1,157,604, October 19, 1915, C. Vernet
..Stool cane, #1,282,105, October 22, 1918, J. M. Mowry
..Stool cane, #1,381,845, June 14, 1921, V. Kolchinsky
..Seat, saw cane, #1,456,304, May 22, 1923, L. Fritschka
..Stool cane, #1,545,054, July 7, 1925, W. W. Leister
..Seat cane, #1,828,144, October 20, 1931, W. Jasinski
..Walking stick seat, #1,863,457, June 14, 1932, H. D. Stevens
..Seat cane, #1,957,033, May 1, 1934, J. Silverman
..Stool cane, #1,997,142, April 9, 1935, A. A. Hanson
..Stool cane, #2,225,114, December 17, 1940, E. T. Haskins

Collapsible Canes:

..Collapsible cane, #1,336,638, April 13, 1920, F. Kutwicz
..Collapsible cane, #1,396,372, November 8, 1921, F. Kutwicz
..Collapsible rod, #3,669,133, June 13, 1972, J. Hyman
..Sectional or collapsing cane, #2,593,026, April 15, 1952, G. A. Hawkins

Crutch and Invalid Canes and Attachments Thereto:

..Convertible walking stick and crutch, #768,452, August 23, 1904, G. J. Hennessey
..Crutch cane, adjustable, #869,128, October 22, 1907, W. Autenrieth
..Crutch cane, adjustable, #869,682, October 29, 1907, W. Autenrieth
..Walking stick crutch, #989,463, April 11, 1911, R. R. Wilde
..Forearm rest walking cane, #1,244,249, October 23, 1917, E. Schlick
..Crutch cane, #1,400,394, December 13, 1921, Albert E. Warry
..Supporting and guiding cane (wheel on base), #1,527,239, February 24, 1925, G. J. Vaughan,

et. al.
..W. S. attachment for crippled, #1,547,046, July 21, 1925, J. A. King
..Self Supporting cane of invalids, #1,802,323, April 28, 1931, T. Aulmann
..Glider cane for invalids, #2,244,869, June 10, 1941, H. A. Everest et al.
..Article carrying attachment for crutches, #2,311,049, February 16, 1943, H. G. Hedden
..Crutch cane, #2,408,604, October 1, 1946, T. B. Brickson
..Crutch cane, #2,409,365, October 15, 1946, T. Lamb
..Crutch attachment, #2,423,635, July 8, 1947, F. H. Blum
..Package carrying crutch attachment, #2,553,730, May 22, 1951, C. W. Taylor
..Walking aid (crutch with containers), #2,580,088, January 1, 1952, J. C. Burkett
..Combined cane & crutch, #2,590,607, March 25, 1952, B. A. Grimball
..Collapsible invalid walkers, #2,906,148, November 15, 1960, C. E. Murcott
..Door Brace Cane, #786,755, April 4, 1905, F. Grey
..Duplicate or Single Cane Combination, #1,375,912, April 26, 1921, J. T. Huddle

Electric Canes:

..Galvonic battery cane to induce current thru palm, #202,094, April 9, 1878, G. P. Clarke
..Electric cane, #287,170, October 23, 1883, A. and A. Roovers
..Electric cane, #465,949, December 29, 1891, A. W and A. H. Roovers
..Electric cane, #484,618, October 18, 1892, S. D. Smith
..Electric cane, #578,471, March 9, 1897, W. N. Sherman
..Electric cane, #639,690, December 19, 1899, W. N. Sherman
..Electro-magnet cane to move metallic toys, #1,347,382, July 20, (?), W. W. Karro

Elevating Cane:

..Cane to stand on to elevate person, #2,127,976, Augu6t 23, 1938, P. Y. K. Howat

Eye Glass Cane, #143,248, September 30, 1871, C. K. Devey

Fan Canes and Umbrellas:

..Parasol and fan cane, #30,213, October 2, 1860, J. T. Eichberg
..Fan cane, #265,955, October 17, 1882, W. H. Fuller
..Fan cane, #285,530, September 25, 1883, W. Verbeck
..Fan cane, #524,678, August 14, 1894, M. Forst
..Fan attachment for umbrella, #610,358, September 6, 1898, K. E. Landau
..Electric fan for umbrellas, #1,148,332, July 27, 1915, S. Onyskow

Ferrules and Tips for Canes:

..Ferrule for cane, #2297, October 11, 1841, J. Bell
..Ferrules for canes, umbrellas, etc., #153,125, July 14, 1874, O. M. Smith
..Anti-slipping tip for canes or crutches, #990,006, April 18, 1911, J. H. Reading
..Cane and umbrella tip protector, #1,007,730, November 7, 1911, A. Pozzi
..Non-slip attachment for canes, #1,215,256, February 6, 1917, M. M. Dawson
..Adjustable rubber pad ferrule for canes, #1,372,517, March 22, 1921, F. King
..Adjustable resilient tip for canes, #1,568,423, January 5, 1926, Charles Sifferlen
..Anti-slipping cane, #2,005,507, June 18, 1935, W. E. Russell, et. al.

..Cane tip, #2,590,052, March 18, 1952, J. G. W. Struits

Fishing Rod Canes:

..Umbrella, whip, fishrod, cigar, pipe and match cane, #87,213, August 7, 1888, D. Crowley
..Fishing rod cane, #465,254, December 15, 1891, M. O. Felker
..Fishing rod cane, #475,852, May 31, 1892, J. H. Edgerly
..Fish rod cane, #1,285,679, November 26, 1918, L. Glowacki
..Fishing rod cane, #1,324,554, December 9, 1919, J. Kozlowski
..Fish rod cane, #1,336,088, April 6, 1920, T. Poremba
..Fishing implement cane, #1,442,813, January 23, 1923, J. W. Lobit

Flag and Pennant Canes:

..Flag cane, #169,918, November 16, 1875, W. R. Park
..Cane flag, #173,330, February 8, 1876, W. R. Park
..Flag cane, #389,806, September 18, 1888, J. E. Hale
..Flag cane, #390,961, October 9, 1888, J. F. Hair
..Flag cane, #470,873, March 15, 1892, W. A. Chapman and E. Gash
..Flag and whistle cane, #477,359, June 21, 1892, E. Gash
..Flag cane, #479,590, July 26, 1892, E. Gash
..Flag cane, #484,446, October 18, 1892, J. H. Nikirk
..Flag or map cane, #490,722, January 31, 1893, O. C. Pugh
..Flag or map cane, #498,187, May 23, 1893, O. C. Pugh
..Flag cane, #523,293, July 17, 1894, N. Smith
..Flag cane, #614,277, November 15, 1898, J. Schumm
..Flag cane, #696,957, April 8, 1902, J. W. Freeborn
..Flag cane, #706,501, August 5, 1902, A. Sjobero
..Horn and flag cane, #741,373, October 13, 1903, LeRoy Robertson
..Flag and torch with protective umbrella cane, #746,880, December 15, 1903, LeRoy Robertson
..Spring roller flag cane, #764,997, July 12, 1904, F. A. Finch
..Spring rolling flag cane, #772,408, October 18, 1904, E. E. Ely
..Flag or pennant cane, #880,047, February 25, 1908, W. S. Smith
..Flag cane, #1,219,386, March 13, 1917, C. T. Fernadez
..Swagger stick (pennant or color bearer), #1,577,627, February 24, 1925, W. Brewer
..Pennant holder walking stick, #1,060,133, April 29, 1913, W. A. Schmelz
..Cane with flag, #2,977,965, April 4, 1961, S. Lewis

Garment Rack Walking Stick, #1,270,973, July 2, 1918, M. Rosenwasser

Handles — Materials of and Construction of (Non Containers):

..Handle for canes, #30,225, October 2, 1860, Harvey and Ford
..Cane handle, #57,367, August 21, 1866, H. Nitzsche
..Improvement in bone handles for canes, #66,586, July 9, 1867, J. Harvey (reissued)
..Cane and umbrella handle, #150,945, May 19, 1874, G. Edme
..Cane handle-(horn usage)-,#232,085, September 7, 1880, M. Sternheimer
..Bell shaped handle for canes, #729,353, May 26, 1903, G. B. Keplinger
..Adjustable umbrella handle (straight or augular), #1,600,046, September 14, 1926, S. J. Goldwin

..Detachable handle for canes and umbrellas, #1,066,433, July 1, 1913, M. L. Marx
..Adjustable handle for novelty cane, #2,146,495, February 7, 1939, L. H. Amdur
..Ornamental implement handle, #2,684,682, July 27, 1954, H. N. Hudes, et. al.

Handle Recepticals as Containers for Carrying Rubbers, Overshoes, Garments, etc:

..Box handle for canes, #331,095, November 24, 1885, L. Steinberger
..Cane head receptical, #368,077, August 9, 1887, B. F. DuBois
..Receptical handle for cane and sunshade, #370,459, September 27, 1887, F. Faasen
..Utensil head for canes (to hold matches, striker, mirror, photographs, etc.), #383,598, May 29, 1888, M. Stiebritz, A. Miller
..Swing cover for cane top receptical, #412,550, October 8, 1889, A. B. Simon
..Brush in handle cane, #450,041, April 7, 1891, T. Russell
..Umbrella handle receptical, #921,023, May 11, 1909, J. Stern
..Cane for carrying water-proof garment, #1,591,333, July 6, 1926, S. C. Neidlinger
..Umbrella handle to carry overshoes, #1,859,627, May 24, 1932, Mabel Marsh
..Container handle (rubbers) for umbrellas, #1,931,078, October 17, 1933, J. E. McWilliams
..Umbrella handle to carry rubbers therein, #2,044,251, June 16, 1936, J. E. McWilliams
..Umbrella handle for holding rubbers, etc., #2,220,900, November 12, 1940

Hat or Parasol Cover Cane, #2,111,257, March 15, 1938, E. Wittcoff

Head Rest Canes:

..Head rest cane, #418,806, January 7, 1890, T. S. Minniss
..Head rest cane, #432,759, July 22, 1890, T. S. Minniss
..Head rest cane, #433,016, July 29, 1890, T. S. Minniss

Hearing Aid Canes:

..Auricle cane, #246,228, August 23, 1881, G. G. Smith
..Ear trumpet cane, #258,171, May 16, 1882, H. Waldstein
..Electric hearing aid cane, #311,180, January 27, 1885, L. Ehrlich

Illuminating and Reflecting Canes:

..Cane-illuminating walking staff, #24,718, July 12, 1859, Ansel Cain
..Cane, and umbrella, and lantern, #70,506, November 5, 1867, H. Beebe
..Cane and lamp combined, #71,460, November 26, 1867, T. Crossley
..Gas burner illuminating cane, #203,559, May 14, 1878, Le R. W. Rood
..Lamp cane, #251,843, January 3, 1882, J. Draper
..Illuminating cane with candle, #360,814, April 5, 1887, G. Muller
..Lighting cane, #373,049, November 15, 1887, O. H. Byring
..Match containing and lighting cane, #486,131, November 15, 1892, W. S. Sharpneck
..Lamp walking stick, #518,590, April 24, 1894, F. Deninger
..Torch cane, #577,879, March 2, 1897, O. F. Packard
..Gas light cane, #610,478, September 6, 1898, E. N. Dickerson
..Flag and torch with protective umbrella cane, #746,880, December 15, 1903, LeRoy Robertson
..Campaign cane-transparent head illuminated from within, #879,640, February 18, 1908, G. Hockenberry
..Illuminating novelty cane, #1,051,370, January 21, 1913, T. Hertz
..Umbrella with signal light, #1,795,268, March 3, 1931, Isidor Thomases
..Cane to illuminate figure in handle, (political cane), #1,908,662, May 9, 1933, F. A. Geier
..Signal indicator (stop) cane for pedestrians and invalids, #2,041,334, May 19, 1936, Louis Hage
..Illuminating cane to flash intermittently as cane connects ground or continuously, #2,144,558, January 24, 1939, G. A. Smith
..Illuminating cane to light way, #273,624, September 19, 1939, G. Dyer
..Protective signal walking stick with reflectors, #2,198,082, April 23, 1940, F. R. Harty
..Illuminating cane for support and signaling or to light up picture therein, #2,245,349, June 10, 1941, Frank Lombardi
..Illuminating cane and umbrella handle, #2,259,443, October 21, 1941, Frank A. Geier
..Reflective warning cane, #2,269,029, January 6, 1942, H. R. Lounsbery
..Illuminating cane (from bottom), #2,271,190, January 27, 1942, C. V. Giaimo
..Illuminating umbrella, #2,372,471, March 27, 1945, A. L. Campbell
..Umbrella with light on top, #2,507,919, May 16, 1950, F. J. Mazzeo
..Light reflecting cane (safety cane), #2,561,228, July 17, 1951, A. E. Richey
..Illuminating cane with cigarettes & lighter, #2,597,172, May 20, 1952, J. Parker
..Combined walking cane & light, #Des 207,764, May 23, 1967, E. Lozo

Leash Stick, #2,322,897, June 29, 1943, A. Van Den Bogoerdi, Jr.

Life Saving Cane, #1,443,121, January 23, 1923, N. T. Fogg

Liquid Containing and Spraying Canes:

..Perfume container handle for cane, #108,218, October 11, 1870, A. Wanner
..Liquid containing cane with suction mouth piece, #255,299, March 21, 1882, T. V. Keam
..Attachment to cane to remove liquid therein by suction, #268,838, December 12, 1882, F. G. and B. C. Stidger
..Perfumery charged cane, #295,359, March 18, 1884, E. R. and H. A. Cowles and M. Osborn
..Liquid recepticle cane, expressed by pushing button, #344,966, July 6, 1886, H. and L. Irvan
..Flask and drinking cup cane, #395,224, December 25, 1888, J. E. Hale
..Trick walking cane (water sprayer), #2,385,091, September 18, 1945, B. V. Lukowitz
..Trick walking cane, water squirter, #2,438,014, March 16, 1948, B. V. Lukowitz
..Spraying cane, #2,508,104, May 16, 1950, T. O. Dickensheets

Luggage Carrying Canes:

..Cane-simulating luggage carrier, #2,932,526, April 12, 1960, R. A. Campbell
..Combined walking stick & wheeled carrier for baggage, #2,812,950, November 12, 1957, D. E. Holloway

Magician's and Theatrical Canes:

..Magician's disappearing cane, #264,058, September 12, 1882, S. K. Bayley
..Trick sword (no cane), #714,534, November 25, 1902, W. Thomas
..Rain-making theatrical umbrella, #1,020,071, March 12, 1912, H. Askin

Magnifying Canes (Telescope, Microscope, Opera Glass):

..Cane and telescope combined, #80,324, July 28,

1868, G. W. Wilson
..Microscope, compass, spy glass, thermometer cane, #195,949, October 9, 1877, J. Pool
..Telescope cane, (opera glass), #223,706, January 20, 1880, J. B. Chandley and W. Wilson
..Opera glass cane, #266,473, October 24, 1882, S. Helfgott
..Telescope and cane, #1,473,527, November 6, 1923, E. Thimgren

Map Canes:

..Flag or map cane, #490,722, January 31, 1893, O. C. Pugh
..Flag or map cane, #498,187, May 23, 1893, O. C. Pugh
..Map or chart cane, #2,251,579, August 5, 1941, Frank D. Rugg

Materials of and Construction of Canes:

..Paper or other disc cane, #324,093, August 11, 1885, J. Dierks and T. B. Kail
..Composition cane, #442,048, December 2, 1890, E. Hofel
..Composition cane, #712,804, November 4, 1902, W. W. Jones
..Method of finishing canes, #797,505, August 15, 1905, I. Eisenstein
..Wire wound cane, #924,880, June 15, 1909, W. Bimblich
..Meshed wire cane, #947,984, February 1, 1910, L. Auverson
..Disk horn cane on steel rod, #1,522,427, January 6, 1925, C. Farruggio
..Cane construction wood inlays, #1,701,866, February 12, 1929, A. Soriente
..Cane construction, different colored woods, #1,791,939, February 10, 1931, A. Soriente
..Method and apparatus for making glass cane, #1,977,956, October 23, 1934, L. D. Soubier
..Method for making hollow metallic cane, #2,006,429, July 2, 1935, J. C. Anderson
..Cane... shell cane, #2,392,083, January 1, 1946, R. R. Dumbleton
..Cane construction, #2,642,884, June 23, 1953, G. A. Henderson, et. al.

Measuring and Surveying Canes and Supports:

..Slide gage cane, #448,016, March 10, 1891, R. Fuchs
..Gage cane, #505,385, September 19, 1893, G. W. Bowen
..Rule cane, #516,513, March 13, 1894, T. E. Tracy
..Railroad track gage cane, #670,297, March 19, 1901, H. Rittenhouse
..Combined walking cane & surveying instrument support, #2,548,711, April 10, 1951, W. Embrey
..Military interval swagger stick, #2,923,063, February 2, 1960, L. D. Hansen

Musical and Music Stand Canes:

..Music stand cane, #50,460, October 17, 1865, J. David
..Portable music stand (cane), #77,940, May 12, 1868, D. M. White
..Music-book stand cane, #150,162, April 28, 1874, A. Iske
..Combined music stand and walking cane, #185,425, December 19, 1876, W. Brand
..Music stand cane, #120,880, November 14, 1871, W. C. James
..Music supports (cane), #194,698, August 28, 1877
..Harmonica cane handle, #196,827, November 6, 1877, W. H. Rice
..Harmonica cane, #232,179, September 14, 1880, M. A. Gilman
..Music stand cane, #245,020, August 2, 1881, W. H Rushforth

..Music stand cane, #257,980, May 16, 1882, W. H. Rushforth
..Music stand walking cane, #263,667, August 29, 1882, J. G. Roberts
..Music rack cane, #330,922, November 24, 1885, O. B. Pierce
..Musical walking stick, #370,496, September 27, 1887, M. Seliger
..Whistle cane, #398,213, February 19, 1889, H. Atkinson and G. W. Hull
..Fife containing cane, #401,061, April 9, 1889, P. Pilson and J. Ploudre
..Music stand cane, #448,185, March 10, 1891, E. Harders and M. P. Fleischman
..Music rack cane, #478,460, July 5, 1892, H. W. Potter
..Music stand cane, #553,867, February 4, 1896, J. Mueller
..Music stand cane, #645,527, March 13, 1900, J. Latourell and E. A. Fischer
..Musical cane, (campaign horn, etc.), #894,512, July 28, 1908, D. A. Lohr
..Music rack and cane, #956,336, April 26, 1910, L. D. Gaughenour
..Musical instrument cane, #956,504, April 26, 1910, D. Pinelli
..Musical instrument cane (ukelele or guitar), #1,611,563, December 21, 1926, M. Rothman

Ownership Indicator Cane, #893,519, July 14, 1908, C. F. Kellom

Physician's Canes:

..Physician's medicine cane, #26,721, January 3, 1860, S. T. Trowbridge
..Medicine case cane, #139,020, May 20, 1873, M. Osborne
..Medicine case and stethoscope cane, #156,456, November 3, 1874, R. G. English

Pick-up, Retrieving, Grasping and Holding Canes:

..Extensible cane for lowering funeral vault covers, etc., #341,715, May 11, 1886, A. H. Allen
..Ticket holder cane, #382,823, May 15, 1888
..Grapple cane, #465,222, December 15, 1891, K. A. E. Ulbricht
..Holder cane, to hold hats, gloves, etc., #610,870, September 13, 1898, J. Quigley
..Swagger stick with hook for grasping, #1,339,162, May 4, 1920, J. M. Callahan
..Swagger stick with hook, #1,339,257, May 4, 1920, J. M. Callahan
..Pick-up walking stick, #1,905,076, April 25, 1933, L. Van Sciver
..Pick-up cane, #2,346,038, April 3, 1944, W. H. Mason
..Utility cane (picker-upper) for handicapped persons, #2,836,188, May 27, 1958, L. Jordan
..Litter retrieving cane, #2,861,835, November 25, 1958, J. J. Smith
..Combination cane & retriever, #3,093,402, June 11, 1953, E. L. Sisson

Picture Case and Cane Combination, #86,991, February 16, 1869, H. D. McGeorge

Purse and Vanity Canes (Handbag, Coin, Purse, etc.):

..Omnibus cane, to hand fare to drivers, contains 3 cent pieces, #19,765, March 30, 1858, S. W. Francis
..Brush and comb cane, #237,027, January 25, 1881, R. Lamb
..Coin discharging cane, #362,886, May 10, 1887, E. W. Furrell
..Toilet case cane, #367,224, July 26, 1887, I. L. Myers
..Coin counter and match safe cane, #394,327, December 11, 1888, J. M. Basinger
..Coin recepticle cane, #880,419, February 25, 1908, W. A. Swaren

..Coin holder umbrella handle, #907,049, December 15, 1908, E. Herold
..Vanity case handle for parasols, #1,129,730, February 23, 1915, D. Reich
..Hollow handle with hand cords and coin purse, #1,380,213, May 31, 1921, R. Kamenetzky
..Handbag cane, #1,526,246, February 10, 1925, W. Simek
..Vanity cane, #1,579,622, April 6, 1926, E. T. Rasmussen
..Container handle (vanity) for umbrella or cane, #1,593,162, July 20, 1926, H. L. Diehl, et al.
..Handbag cane, #1,653,024, December 20, 1927, W. Simek
..Ladies compact in parasol handle, #1,762,869, June 10, 1930, R. A. Kratochwill
..Umbrella and parasol handle with compact, #1,827,862, October 20, 1931, Emil Weber
..Bag carrying cane, #1,838,986, December 29, 1931, A. Callender
..Vanity gear shift knob, #1,993,938, March 12, 1935, G. W. McDonald
..Walking stick and bag, #2,210,493, August 6, 1940, F. A. Lisi
..Beach stick, to hold articles, #2,509,074, May 23, 1950, G. Reiley
..Combined staff & beach bag, #2,582,904, July 6, 1954, J. F. Divine
..Utility handle for umbrellas, (compact & coin container), #3,245,421, April 12, 1966, K. Braun, et. al.

Recording Canes:

..Diary cane (or notebook cane), #489,385, January 3, 1893, R. W. Meily and G. W. Buchanan
..Baby history and recorder, #1,996,553, April 2, 1935, M. M. Scully

Scent Detector Cane, #2,007,324, July 9, 1935, H. M. Budgett

Shock Absorbing Canes:

..Elastic pressure walking cane, #340,738, April 27, 1886
..Cane attachment (shock absorber), #788,541, May 2, 1905, A. Kunkel
..Adjustable resilient tip for canes, #1,568,423, January 5, 1926, Charles Sifferlen
..Washer and shock absorbing cane, #1,058,333, January 27, 1914, A. D. Goetz
..Shock absorbing cane, #2,899,968, August 18, 1959, L. L. Reichenbach
..Adjustable resilient walking cane, #2,802,479, August 13, 1957, S. L. Hickman

Smoker's Canes (Pipes, Lighters, Cigar and Cigarette Humidor Match Safes):

..Compartment cane (pipe, cigars, tobacco and matches), #82,949, October 13, 1868, L. G. Heylin
..Cane pipe, #190,859, May 15, 1877, N. L. Hirsch and W. M. Ettinger
..Match-safe cane top, #233,676, October 26, 1880, L. Helman
..Spittoon cane, #240,806, May 3, 1881, M. L. Baxter
..Combined cane, cigar cane, pipe bowl, etc., #253,011, January 31, 1882, D. Crowley
..Pipe case cane, #275,100, April 3, 1883, J. P. Weaver
..Cigar case cane, #295,654, March 25, 1884, D. Lee, Jr.
..Cigar, etc., container cane, #325,198, August 25, 1885, D. Crowley
..Cigar and cigarette case cane, #368,823, August 23, 1887, G. B. Fowler
..Cigar and cigarette container cane, #372,177, October 25, 1887, S. Simmons
..Umbrella, whip, fishrod, cigar, pipe, and match cane, #387,213, August 7, 1888
..Cigarette and match cane, #391,123, October 16, 1888, G. H. Coursen

..Pipe in a cane, #395,426, January 1, 1889, G. H. Coursen
..Seat and pipe cane, #429,234, June 3, 1890, W. Flan
..Tobacco pipe tube cane, #457,160, August 4, 1891, H. Lillenberger
..Firemaking cane (tinder lighter), #476,015, May 31, 1892, J. J. Him
..Hooka (smoking pipe) cane, #690,655, January 7, 1902, Syed Ali Mohammed Khan
..Tobacco pipe cane, #1,013,776, January 2, 1912, I. Hoffman
..W. S. cigarette lighter, #1,651,418, December 6, 1927, A. T. Steventon
..Cigar etc., lighter cane, #1,660,830, February 28, 1928, I. Caesar
..Cigar etc., lighter cane, (at bottom), #1,662,102, March 13, 1928, I. Caesar
..Cigar lighter cane, #1,719,458, July 2, 1929, A. R. Visitacion
..Cigar and cigarette carrier in cane, #1,806,709, May 26, 1931, J. Rosinsky
..Container cane for cigarettes, etc., #1,809,746, June 9, 1931
..Pryophoric lighting cane, (for cigars, etc.), #1,930,501, October 17, 1933, L. V. Aronson
..Umbrella cane with cigarette cane, cigarette lighter, light, drinking cup, magnifying glass, and camera support, #2,214,300, September 10, 1940, George C. Henderson

Sound Producing Canes (Cap exploding, Torpedo, Whistling, Popping, etc.):

..Toy-cartridge exploder cane, #159,107, January 26, 1875, J. B. McHarg
..Toy cap exploder, #190,481, May 8, 1877, W. G. Fischer
..Detonating toy cane, #209,768, November 12, 1878, J. McConnell
..Pop gun cane handle, #233,613, October 26, 1880, M. A. Gilman
..Toy cartridge exploder cane, #377,359, February 7, 1888, J. B. McHarg
..Torpedo cane, #401,810, April 23, 1889, H. P. Young
..Detonator cane, #426,423, April 29, 1890, G. D. Adams
..Flag and whistle cane, #477,359, June 21, 1892, E. Gash
..Torpedo exploder cane, #605,685, July 5, 1898, A. Riecke
..Sounding toy cane, #650,048, May 22, 1900, L. Knott
..Torpedo cane, #688,157, December 3, 1901, F. Caples
..Magazine torpedo cane, #696,956, April 8, 1902, J. H. Fox
..Magazine torpedo cane, #704,310, July 8, 1902, J. H. Fox
..Torpedo cane, #709,095, September 16, 1902, J. S. Judy
..Toy gun cane, #704,648, July 15, 1902. F. H. Jury
..Magazine torpedo cane, #709,457, September 23, 1902, J. B. Allen
..Magazine cap exploding cane, #723,218, March 17, 1903, J. R. Stanley and F. S. Howard
..Sounding cane, #726,854, May 5, 1903, J. L. Brink
..Magazine torpedo cane, #732,587, June 30, 1903, H. Rese
..Magazine torpedo cane, #738,379, September 8, 1903, D. D. Weisell
..Horn and flag cane, #741,373, October 13, 1903, LeRoy Robertson
..Magazine torpedo cane, #761,309, May 31, 1904, C. W. Leslie, Dec'd.
..Torpedo cane, #767,440, August 16, 1904, P. R. Roberts
..Repeating torpedo cane, #773,635, November 1, 1904, J. H. Fox
..Whistling push down parade cane, #778,346, December 27, 1904, H. W. Wylie
..Detonating cane, #796,834, August 8, 1905, G. H. Fisher

..Repeating torpedo cane, #801,567, October 10, 1905, H. H. Bernhard
..Repeating torpedo cane, #810,386, January 23, 1906, R. Bean
..Repeating torpedo cane, #840,425, January 1, 1907, J. H. Bevington
..Torpedo cane, #842,061, January 22, 1907, R. Bean
..Repeating detonating cane, #850,354, April 16, 1907, A. and N. Del Grande
..Repeating detonating cane, #850,353, April 16, 1907, A. and N. Del Grande
..Repeating torpedo cane, #876,683, January 14, 1908, R. Bean
..Cane for exploding caps, #926,307, June 29, 1909, C. V. Wertz
..Torpedo cane, #879,572, September 1, 1908, R. Bean
..Sound producing cane (squeeze ball), #953,586, March 29, 1910, R. C. Bolles
..Popgun cane, #1,924,957, August 29, 1933, Melville L. Orr
..Torpedo firing cane, #1,955,338, April 17, 1934, J. A. Mars
..Sound producing walking stick, #2,055,845, September 29, 1936, Pasquale Marinacci
..Whistling cane by pressing against ground, #2,183,975, December 19, 1939, R. H. Savage
..Whistling cane by pressing against ground, #2,193,644, March 12, 1940, E. H. Pitney
..Cricket cane (toy making clacking noise), #2,610,441, September 16, 1952, J. E. Unger
..Electronic sound producing cane, #3,435,153, March 25, 1969, C. D'Amato

Sunshade Cane, #1,618,065, February 15, 1927, J. D. Davis

Thermometer Cane:

..Cane and thermometer, #72,539, December 24, 1867, J. L. Reber

Toy Canes (Also see: Sound Producing Canes):

..Cane head (toy, animal or bird head), #79,208, June 23, 1868, A. Cooke
..Cane with bouncing ball up and down shaft, #847,066, March 12, 1907, F. L. Hall
..Bouncing cane, #1,513,380, October 28, 1924, E. R. Dumbolton
..Novelty cane for rotating it's bottom, #2,087,222, July 13, 1937, E. A. Matthews
..Amusement cane for jumping over, #2,181,979, December 5, 1939, A. F. Schaeffer
..Combination umbrella & water pistol, #3,038,483, June 12, 1962, L. Altsheler

Umbrella Canes:

..Umbrella and cane combined, #5500, April 11, 1848, S. Wright
..Umbrella and cane combined, #5553, May 9, 1848, I. Hammond
..Cane umbrella, #18,500, October 27, 1857, H. Crosby, Jr.
..Combined umbrella and cane, #53,778, April 10, 1866, P. T. Brownell
..Cane and umbrella combined, #73,074, January 7, 1868, G. Bockstaller
..Combined umbrella and cane, #97,559, December 7, 1869, A. Smith
..Umbrella cane, #139,295, May 27, 1873, T. R. L. Chevers
..Umbrella cane, #138,726, May 6, 1873, E. Wright
..Umbrella cane, #157,070, August 24, 1875, J. N. Colby and J. E. Coffin
..Umbrella cane, #158,092, September 28, 1875, T. Harris and A. Kindermann
..Umbrella cane, #169,406, November 2, 1875, J. Boyd
..Umbrella cane, #182,025, September 12, 1876, A. Kindermann and T. Harris

..Umbrella cane, #189,084, April 3, 1877, M. M. Copp
..Umbrella cane, #195,492, September 25, 1877, T. F. Darcy
..Umbrella cane, #196,592, October 30, 1877, A. Mungle
..Umbrella cane, #241,312, May 10, 1881, M. A. Dees
..Umbrella cane, #253,897, February 21, 1882, G. T. Smith
..Umbrella cane, #293,830, February 19, 1884, H. A. Whiting and W. J. Winghart
..Umbrella cane, #358,412, February 22, 1887, G. F. Seaver
..Cane umbrella, #368,407, August 16, 1887, J. McCormick
..Umbrella cane, #376,870, January 24, 1888, W. H. G. Ellis
..Umbrella cane, #386,078, July 10, 1888, J. McCormick
..Umbrella, whip, fishrod, cigar, pipe, and match cane, #387,213, August 7, (?), D. Crowley
..Umbrella cane, #442,491, December 9, 1890, C. H. Morgan
..Umbrella cane, #453,194, June 2, 1891, S. J. and J. Knox
..Umbrella cane, #489,351, January 3, 1893, R. Waples
..Umbrella cane, #500,051, June 20, 1893, W. B. Blake
..Umbrella cane, #506,289, October 10, 1893, E. Weber
..Umbrella cane, #506,289, October 10, 1893, Ernest Weber
..Umbrella cane, #517,315, March 27, 1894, R. Waples, Jr.
..Umbrella cane, #531,878, January 1, 1895, R. N. Smith
..Umbrella cane, #536,223, March 26, 1895, C. H. Morgan
..Umbrella cane, #541,844, July 2, 1895, E. C. Geneux
..Umbrella cane, #572,983, December 15, 1896, E. E. Greene
..Umbrella cane, #579,162, March 23, 1897, A. G. Moyer
..Umbrella cane, #580,397, April 13, 1897, W. P. Hiscock
..Umbrella cane, #588,595, August 24, 1897, J. H. Nolan
..Umbrella cane, #629,460, July 25, 1899, J. R. Nagell
..Umbrella cane, #661,990, November 20, 1900, H. Hugendubel
..Umbrella cane, #647,288, May 14, 1901, R. Waples, Jr.
..Umbrella cane, #741,678, October 20, 1903, R. Kronenberg
..Umbrella cane, #752,740, February 23, 1904, J. P. Wilkins
..Umbrella cane, #807,035, December 12, 1905, J. and H. Landes
..Umbrella cane, #1,023,686, April 16, 1912, F. E. Siggins
..Umbrella pouch, #2,289,134, July 7, 1942, R. O. Loria
..Combined umbrella handle & receptacle, #2,312,041, February 23, 1943, H. A. Lillie
..Illuminated umbrella, #2,372,471, March 27, 1945, A. L. Campbell
..Umbrella with light on top, #2,507,919, May 16, 1950, F. J. Mazzeo
..Umbrella stick, #2,989,968, June 27, 1961, H. G. Vogel
..Combination umbrella & water pistol, #3,038,483, June 12, 1962, L. Altsheler

Watch Cane, #409,267, August 20, 1889, J. W. Allen

Weapon Canes — Gun Canes:

..Revolver cane, #12,328, January 30, 1855, A. O. H. P. Schorn
..Breach-loading walking stick gun, #17,915, August 4, 1857, I. Buckman

..Cane gun, #19,328, February 8, 1858, J. F. Thomas
..Muzzle-loading firearm-improvement in walking stick guns, #19,674, March 28, 1858, R. R. Beckwith
..Rifle cane, #28,160, May 8, 1860, A. Crow
..Muzzle-loading firearm cane gun, #29,676, August 21, 1850, A. Davis
..Combined cane, umbrella, pistol, dagger and campstool combined, #63,552, April 2, 1867, D. Morrison
..Cane gun, #104,087, June 7, 1870, W. H. Werner
..Cane gun, #125,460, April 9, 1872, A. Karutz
..Umbrella, sword and gun cane, #146,054, December 30, 1873, F. Eckstein
..Cane gun, #170,684, December 7, 1875, C. Melaye
..Magazine cane gun, #189,305, April 10, 1877, M. Daigle
..Gun cane, #329,430, November 3, 1885, E. D. Bean
..Cane gun, #349,864, September 28, 1886, F. A. Wardwell
..Cane gun barrel, #380,975, April 10, 1888, E. D. Bean
..Gun cane, #426,373, April 22, 1890, J. Frick
..Gun cane, #517,438, April 3, 1894, R. F. Cook
..Gun cane, #518,546, April 17, 1894, O. Janke
..Gun cane, #547,117, October 1, 1895, N. G. Hanson
..Pistol barrel cane, #584,222, June 8, 1894, J. A. Hammer
..Gun cane, #610,675, September 13, 1898, E. H. Ericson
..Cane gun, #628,142, July 4, 1899, E. H. Ericson
..Rifle cane, #969,672, September 6, 1910, H. Tarvardian
..Gun cane, fish rod and umbrella, #1,283,015, October 29, 1918, F. Yung
..Cane gun, #1,320,493, November 4, 1919, S. and F. Pelc
..W. S. Machine gun, #1,474,292, November 13, 1923, H. Renard
..Gun cane, #1,569,700, January 12, 1926, F. S. Bernabe
..Gun cane, #1,613,593, January 4, 1927, B. B. Walker

Weapon Canes — Sword, Knife, and other Canes:

..Sword cane, #8,346, September 9, 1851, S. A. Hudson
..Whip cane with clasp knife handle, #308,017, November 11, 1884, E. M. Turner
..Umbrella cane w/sword, #360,544, April 5, 1887, P. Verrier and J. E. Bonnevaux
..Sword container cane—for carrying blade of dress sword, #384,584, June 12, 1888
..Weapon cane (knife blades caused to project up and down sides of shaft) #857,047, June 18, 1907, K. Gehrer
..Sword cane, #350,249, October 5, 1886, E. Holman
..Tool or dagger cane, #889,035, May 26, 1908, W. T. Newsom
..Knife in handle, and flashing cane, #1,509,157, September 23, 1924, P. Leano
..Knife (switch blade) cane, #1,624,591, April 12, 1927, R. Fleming

Weapon Canes, Billy Club, and Clobbering and Striking Canes:

..Flying head weapon cane, #396,027, January 8, 1889, W. M. Carpenter
..Billy cane, #566,306, August 25, 1896, L. Goldsmith

Whip Canes:

..Cane whip, #79,691, July 7, 1858, Sallada and Pearson
..Cane and whip, #98,664, January 11, 1870, C. L. Bushnell

..Cane whip, #109,297, November 15, 1870, C. L. Bushnell
..Socket-joints for whip canes, #162,605, April 27, 1875, J. A. Bechler
..Cane whip, #169,485, November 2, 1875, O. H. Saxton
..Whip cane, #256,061, April 4, 1882, L. C. Seltzer
..Whip cane, #266,166, October 17, 1882, T. R. Lawhead
..Whip cane with clasp knife handle, #308,017, November 11, 1884, E. M. Turner
..Whip cane, #319,689, June 9, 1885, W. Fish
..Whip cane #344,757, June 29, 1886, R. M. Thomas
..Whip cane, #375,485, December 27, 1887, O. Godward
..Umbrella, whip, fishrod, cigar, pipe and match cane, #387,213, August 7, 1888, D. Crowley
..Whip cane, #459,081, September 8, 1891, M. O. Felker
..Whip cane, #482,895, September 20, 1892, M. O. Felker
..Whip cane, #696,705, April 1, 1902, M. A. Allen
..Whip cane, #741,219, October 13, 1903, H. H. Brandes
..Whip cane, #815,458, March 20, 1906, J. R. Morris

Subject Index of British Cane Patents

Index of British Cane Patents

Advertising Canes:

..Advertising printing cane, #6295, May 10, 1886, T. M. Potter and T. Allen
..Ad-carrying hooks on cane, #5651, April 17, 1888, J. Brown
..Printing cane for ads on pavement, #12277, June 22, 1893, H. Battams and T. Sichel
..Advertising table W. S., #1531, January 23, 1901, A. H. Paterson and J. H. Reford

Anti Slip Canes:

..Protruding point cane (anti-slip), #10293, June 17, 1891, A. Lowitzki
..Non slip W. S. tip, #132,935, April 15, 1919, J. T. Akerman

Attachments to, and Canes for Carrying Parcels:

..W. S. with strap for carrying parcels, #22722, November 27, 1893, H. M. Boehmer
..Attachment to hold objects, #22896, November 13, 1901, W. Batchelor
..Parcel carrier (clip) attachment to W. S., #12742, June 1, 1907, A. H. Atkins
..W. S. with bag, #2549, February 1, 1910, E. A. Clark
..W. S. with parcel carrier attachment, #8898, June 16, 1915, R. J. Moffat
..Parcel carrier attachment for W. S., #130,810, August 28, 1918, J. A. Martin
..Hand truck W. S., #153,710, August 29, 1919, G. Beechley
..Bag and wheel W. S. (carrying device), #229,513, March 21, 1924, C. B. Sheridan

..W. S. with hooks for carrying objects, #247,668, November 21, 1924, J F. Shaw
..Luggage trolly W. S., #789,849, February 28, 1956, D. E. Holloway

Attachments to Suspend Cane from Person, etc:

..Attachable to person cane, #15133, October 22, 1888, A. D. Vlies
..Attachable to belt cane, #1543, January 29, 1890, P. A. Martin
..W. S. suspender to attach to person, #8352, April 25, 1893, A. W. Abbott
..Attachments for carrying W. S., #15500, August 14, 1894, J. J. Osborn
..Attachment for W. S. to person, #5821, March 16, 1896, J. G. H. Percy
..Attachment to attach W. S. to person, #24,407, November 2, 1896, W. E. Munro
..Attachment to suspend W. S., #9l53, May 1, 1899, J. Muller
..Attachment to suspend W. S. from objects, #9546, May 6, 1899, C. L. E. Busse and F. R. Kugnel
..Attachment to suspend W. S., #22482, November 10, 1899, E. S. Rooyen and J. S. Lewy
..Hanging-up hooks for W. S., #25175, December 19, 1899, J. Muller
..Attachment to suspend W. S., #13854, July 8, 1901, W. F. Oxley
..Attachment for suspending W. S., #17892, September 7, 1901, F. Cowburn
..Attachment to suspend W. S. from person, #16307, July 22, 1902, E. Currie
..Attachable to person W. S., #12148, June 10, 1905, A. L. Procter
..Attachable to person W. S., #4065, February 19, 1906, T. P. Blake and W. C. V. Harwood

Back Support Cane, #4202, April 2, 1885, P. Bathermel

Barometer and Thermometer Canes:

..Thermometer W. C., #1388, May 7, 1872, L. Engel
..Mercury Barometer in W. S., #288, February 1, 1859, T. P. Purssglove
..Almanak or thermometer cane, #799, March 31, 1864, M. Kurts
..Yard stick and mine temperature taker, #101,448, April 9, 1916, A. G. Gulliford

Bicycle Canes:

..Bicycle W. S., #19887, November 4, 1892, A. Viada Viladesau
..Bicycle tire pump W. S., #24800, December 20, 1894, M. Muller
..Cycle support W. S., #9511, April 27, 1903, R. Benesch

Billiard Cue W. S., #1741, June 17, 1870, T. Greenwood and J. Fabian

Boot Cane:

..W. S. for pulling off boots, #8956, April 15, 1909, Count F. von Taxis

Brush Cane:

..Shoe and clothes brush W. S., #224,737, December 10, 1923, L. D. Spyropoulos

Calendar Canes:

..Perpetual calendar W. S., #334, January 27, 1876, J. Fissethaler
..Calendar rings W. S., #821, February 14, 1883, A. E. Maudslay
..Perpetual calendar cane, #14726, October 29, 1887, T. H. D. Gilen
..Date calendar W. S., #8786, April 6, 1897, H. H. Lake

Collapsable, Folding, and Telescoping Canes and Umbrellas:

..Telescopic handle, perfuming agent, #1452, June 11, 1862, J. F. Kain
..Telescopic W. S., #922, March 26, 1872, Barnes Richards
..Folding W. S. for pocket, #400, February 3, 1873, J. H. Weber and J. Roy
..Telescopic umbrella (To Shorten for Packing), #6458, March 25, 1899, N. Foley
..Collapsible W. S. for packing, #23445, October 29, 1903, C. Ford
..Breakdown W. S. (3 pieces), #3052, February 14, 1905, E. A. Mitchell
..Collapsable umbrella cane, Method of Mfg., #20799, October 2, 1908, R. Genck
..Breakdown W. S. to carry surgical dressings, #27215, November 26, 1912, A. Hemrich
..Collapsable W. S., #184,548, May 31, 1921, F. Kutwicz
..Folding W. S., #296,653, April 19, 1928, E. Spitznagel
..Collapsable umbrella cane, #316,794, September 1, 1928, T. Fuchs
..Telescopic cane for invalids of diff. heights, #685,781, April 26, 1951, Concentric Mfg. Co.
..Collapsable W. S., #1,182,285, May 25, 1967, C. C. Olson

Camera Stands and Tripod Canes:

..Sketching easel W. S., #1672, April 16, 1881, A. J. Welsby
..Camera tripod cane, #12855, September 27, 1884, W. Watts
..Tripod cane, #14801, October 15, 1888, G. C. Inkpen
..Tripod cane, #4082, March 8, 1889, F. Shrew
..Camera tripod, #15530, October 3, 1889, R. W. Boyd, et. al.
..Camera stand, #1155, January 22, 1890, W. R. Baker
..Camera tripod cane, #2043, February 7, 1890, A. G. Rider
..Camera cane, #13686, August 14, 1891, A. Campbell
..Camera stand cane, #16377, September 13, 1892, E. C. Ouvry
..Camera tripod cane, #12163, June 23, 1894, W. J. Pickersgill
..Camera tripod cane, #5017, March 9, 1895, A. M. Morrison
..Telescopic camera stand cane, #19367, September 26, 1899, C. P. Goerz
..Camera stand W. S., #16282, September 13, 1900, R. W. Shipway
..Camera stand cane, #20180, November 9, 1900, R. W. Shipway
..Camera case, #17810, August 13, 1902, E. Kronke
..Camera stand cane, #21383, October 1, 1902, R. T. Glascodine
..Camera stand W. S., #8058, April 7, 1903, G. Geiger
..Camera stand cane, #5680, March 8, 1904, J. Bicker
..Camera stand W. S., #14462, July 13, 1905, G. S. Russell
..Camera tripod cane, #2473, January 3, 1907, W. Burton
..Camera stand W. S., #6121, April 24, 1915, H. Rottenburg
..Tripod W. S., #138,094, January 20, 1920, H. E. Hollinger
..Camera stand W. S., #172,380, August 31, 1920, L. D. Wright
..Camera support W. S., #321,007, September 11, 1928, Newman and Guardia, Ltd.
..Camera stand W. S., #370,648, April 8, 1931, F. H. Owens
..Kinematographic apparatus cane (camera stand), #687,588, June 7, 1950, Paillard Soc.

Caricature Cane (Handle in Shape of People), #4581, March 28, 1887, H. Workman

Caricature Face W. S. to Smoke Cigars, #7666, April 25, 1900, G. Grabosch

Carriage Key or Corkscrew Cane, #1888, June 19, 1869, J. Brooker

Coin Receptacle Cane, #12333, September 12, 1887, E. A. Olivieri

Corkserew Canes:

..Carriage key or corkscrew cane, #1888, June 19, 1869, J. Brooker
..Alarm whistle cane, door fastener, key, corkscrew, #29472, December 13, 1897

Dog Canes:

..Dog leader cane, #14812, October 15, 1888, H. M. Bryans
..Dog lead cane, #4351, February 21, 1907, A. F. Bell
..Dog leash W. S., #26249, November 23, 1911, G. L. Jones
..Dog fight stopping cane (pepper container), #11927, May 17, 1911, L. G. Roberts
..Dog lead W. S., #12505, May 29, 1913, F. Sandall

Door Fastening Canes:

..W. S. for securing or fastening doors, #2392, August 28, 1862, G. Cooke
..Alarm whistle cane, door fastener, key, corkscrew, #29472, December 13, 1897

Electronic and Magnetic Canes:

..Magnetic cane, #4153, October 26, 1875, J. Cole
..Electronic cane for health shocks, #1509, March 29, 1882, J. Hicksson
..Magnet cane, #21752, October 7, 1902, H. Saward et. al.
..Medical cane: electric and magnetic, #24951, November 17, 1904, T. Cook
..Electrotheropeutic cane, #259,689, July 23, 1925, E. N. Snowden
..Electrotheropeutic cane, #259,892, July 23, 1925, E. N. Snowden

Elevating Canes:

..Step-up or elevating cane (viewing stand), #262, January 5, 1898, A. Rust
..Foldable step W. S., #1,443,760, November 22, 1973, T. A. L. Apperly

Eye Glass Canes:

..Eye glass cane, #3031, February 20, 1889, G. G. Bussey
..Eye glass cane, #29019, December 23, 1911, W. Bilinski

Exercising Canes:

..Walking stick exerciser, #3346, August 24, 1878, E. G. Brewer
..Exercising W. S., #5960, March 14, 1903, R. F. Henning

Fan Canes:

..Fan parasol, #1459, April 22, 1873, F. Delmos
..Fan and umbrella W. S., #1897, May 11, 1878, E. Edmonds
..Pneumatic fan W. S., #27382, December 11, 1902, J. V. D. Blavetti

Fence Spreader Cane:

..Seat cane and wire fence spreader, #868,541, September 19, 1958, I. S. C. Rose

Ferrules and Tips of Canes:

..Ferrules, #919, April 6, 1871, J. Hughes
..Ferrules, #2602, October 3, 1871, F. S. Stoney
..Ferrules, #2936, November 1, 1871, W. R. Lake
..Ferrules, #688, February 25, 1875, T. O. Jones
..Ferrules, #616, February 15, 1876, T. Warwicks
..Ferrules, #3414, August 30, 1876, J. J. Bennett
..Ferrules, #875, March 5, 1877, A. M. Clark
..Ferrules, #4203, November 9, 1877, R. Harrington
..Ferrules and mfg, thereof, #4641, November 11, 1880, G. G. Lusher
..Ferrules, #2261, May 13, 1882, W. H. Beck
..Ferrules, #5760, May 11, 1885, W. Fearnley
..Ferrules, #13655, November 10, 1885, J. Ashdown
..Ferrules, #14125, November 18, 1885, J. Ashdown
..Ferrules, #17816, December 27, 1887, C. P. Hawley
..Ferrules, #7137, May 14, 1888, A. Gilmour
..Ferrules, #8405, June 8, 1888, J. Lund
..Novelties Ferrules, #17849, December 6, 1888, J. G. Hopgood
..Ferrules, #170, January 4, 1889, J. Emmett
..Ferrules, #5552, April 1, 1889, W. Marten
..Ferrule, adjustable length, #9095, June 1, 1889, F. Strasser
..Ferrules, #6388, April 26, 1890, J. H. May
..Ferrules, #15653, October 3, 1890, F. W. Schroder and S. Culp
..Ferrules, #17353, September 29, 1892, H. Laughlin
..Ferrules, #7063, April 6, 1893. D. Broucher
..Ferrules, #18452, October 3, 1893, R. Cunliffe
..Ferrules, #12568, June 28, 1894, W. P. Thompson
..Ferrules, #19715, October 17, 1894, T. Pounds
..Ferrules and cases for cane umbrellas, #9087, May 7, 1895, E. H. Hirsh
..Ferrules, #19631, October 19, 1895. T. Mutton
..Ferrules, #24348, December 19, 1895, W. J. Fox
..Ferrules, #13798, June 23, 1896, W. H. Glover
..Ferrules, #4220, February 16, 1897, A. H. Barton and W. Beaves
..Ferrules for canes, #5661, March 8, 1898, W. Lederle
..Ferrules, #24569, November 28, 1905, T. H. Collingbourne
..Ferrules for W. S., #16353, July 16, 1907, H. W. Lake
..Removeable ferrules to shorten and pack W. S., #3955, February 17, 1910, A. D. Robbins
..Ferrules, #5560, March 5, 1910, H. J. Frost and H. Bradwell
..Ferrules, #25451, November 30, 1910, R. A. Moxhay
..Ferrules, #1509, January 19, 1912, J. H. Bent
..Ferrules, #5109, February 28, 1913, P. Muschiol
..Ferrules, #125,340, December 16, 1918, W. Haslam
..Ferrule, #141,966, June 23, 1919, W. L. W. Wikley
..Ferrule shock absorber with spring, #141,593, August 22, 1919, W. F. Fanning
..Ferrules, #614,949, T. Lamb

Fishing Canes:

..Fly rod fishing cane, #23710, October 17, 1912, P. G. Mould
..Tent and fishing pole W. S., #190,884, November 29, 1921, J. Holroyd, et. al.
..Fishing rod W. S., #214,973, April 26, 1923, S. E. Sands
..Fish rod cane, #381,909, June 27, 1932, C. Grandjean

Foot Rest W. S., #20876, September 21, 1896, Baron von Hammer-Purgetall

Gardening and Pruning Canes:

..Pruning cane, #4732, March 11, 1884, R. W. Cowen
..Pruning saw cane, #18350, November 14, 1890, J. J. Holzapffel
..Gardening cane (weed killer), #9555, May 19, 1892, J. Brooke
..Weed extractor W. S. #191,646, February 28, 1922, C. E. West
..Planting device W. S., #235,111, February 12, 1925, M. Bonneault

Gas Detecting W. S. for Miners, #4488, November 4, 1879

Golfing Canes:

..Golf club cane, #17918, October 20, 1891, J. Buchanan
..Golf club cane support, #10188, May 28, 1892, R. Anderson
..Golf club support cane, #3770, February 21, 1894, K. W. Hedges
..Golf club support W. S., #23563, December 4, 1894, C. S, Good
..Golf club cane with removeable heads, #10867, May 13, 1903, A. M. Robertson
..Golf club W. S., #15892, July 10, 1913, M. J. Cooper
..Golf cane, #325,677, January 31, 1929, H. Hartley
..Golf ball pick up W. S., #682,885, June 12, 1951, Fordham Pressing Ltd.

Grain Sampling W. S., #2378, June 7, 1876, W. Brookes

Handles (Bending, Construction Materials and Method of Mfg):

..Tortishell handles, #187, January 25, 1855, B. Samuel
..Handles (glass, ivory, horn, etc.), #714, March 30, 1855, E. V. Neale and T. Dawson
..Handles (Indea rubber), #875, April 19, 1855, J. H. Johnson
..Handles, #2981, November 30, 1857, S. Solomon
..Handles, #2667, November 25, 1858, R. H. Hess
..Handles (method of straightening), #2066, September 10, 1859, A. Smith
..Handles, #308, February 4, 1860, J. Smith
..Materials for handles, #253, January 31, 1862, D. Littlehales
..Handles, #870, March 28, 1862, R. Lublinski
..Handles, #1600, May 28, 1862, C. Cohen
..Handles (Jambees canes), #2043, July 17, 1862, M. Kurts
..Handles (method of bending), #3092, November 18, 1862, J. Raphel
..Handles, #3142, November 22, 1862, M. Mishores
..Bending ends of partridge canes, #3022, December 2, 1863, R. Lublinski
..Handles (method of bending wood), #561, March 5, 1854, W. Dangerfield
..Handles (method of bending), #682, March 10, 1864, J. Jones and R. D. Jones
..Detachable handles, #2823, November 12, 1864, C. S. Cadman
..Handles, #1682, June 23, 1865, M. D. Rosenthal and S. Gradenwitz
..Handles (imitation ivory), #3310, December 22, 1865, M. D. Rosenthal and S. Gradenwitz
..Handles (plastic, imitation ivory), #536, February 18, 1868, W. E. Newton
..Enamelled heads of canes, #1534, May 11, 1868, A. Boucher
..Handles (rajah root imitation), #2168, July 17, 1869, J. Bernstein
..Handles at angles, #1334, May 10, 1870, J. Dangerfield
..Handles (skin covered), #1736, June 17, 1870, C. A. Bleuemel
..Knobs for W. S., #1362, May 20, 1871, A. V. Newton
..Handles and Ferrules for W. S., #2064, August 4, 1871, G. T. Bousfield

..Crystal handles, #1582, May 5, 1874, T. O. Jones
..Handles, method of affixing, #2285, July 1, 1874, W. Clissold
..Enamel (Niello) work on handles, #2997, September 2, 1874, C. L. Lustig
..Handles-ornamenting, #4356, December 17, 1874, A. M. Clark
..Knobs from W. S. to tripod, #937, March 13, 1875, W. Morgan-Brown
..Ornamenting handles, #3181, September 10, 1875, W. Clissold
..Handles-papier mache, #494, February 7, 1876, J. Watson
..Handles-graining and ornamenting wood, #2517, June 17, 1876, C. A. Bluemel
..Handles, "Tip Cap", #237, January 18, 1878, A. Dittrock
..Handles, #3219, August 14, 1878, R. Church
..Handles for canes, #1022, March 14, 1879, A. G. Airon
..Handles for canes, #4978, December 5, 1878, W. E. Gedge
..Handles-machinery for mfg., #2581, February 2, 1884, B. Acton
..Handles, #4772, March 12, 1884, J. Howell and J. W. Anderson
..Handles, #411, January 12, 1885, C. Norton
..Handles, #5984, May 15, 1885, J. Knight
..Handles, #312, January 8, 1886, E. Hahn
..Method of bending handle and machine for, #299, January 6, 1892, F. S. Metz
..Handles, #19017, October 22, 1892, H. A. Ollivant.
..Wedge for attaching handles, #1334, January 22, 1893, W. H. Brown
..Handle-method of attaching removeable handle, #3595, February 18, 1893, T. Clark
..Handles, #12452, 1896, E. Cadoret
..Handles-making of plastic, #3412, February 14, 1896 L. F. A. Magdolf
..Handles, #20954, September 22, 1896, E. Taylor
..Interchangable handles, #24,889, November 6, 1896, A. C. Hirsh
..Handgrips for W. S., #28,426, December 12, 1896, J. K. Pogue
..Handle for canes, #10013, April 22, 1897, J. Melson
..Handles for seat sticks, #21604, September 21, 1897, O. Von Saal
..Metal head for W. S. and process for making, #16165, August 8, 1899, I. Mayer
..Handles, composition, #17878, September 5, 1899, G. Bestwick
..Handles of W. S. mfg. method, #10037, May 31, 1900, J. J. Westerdick
..Handles, method of attaching to J. S., #22778, December 13, 1900, R. Hadden
..Removeable handles, #674, January 10, 1901, E. Knottusch
..Handles-veneering process, #7037, April 3, 1901, G. Hugendubel
..Handles-construction, #9951, May 14, 1901, J. Melson
..Handles, method of bending, #20563, October 14, 1901, R. Moddan
..Handles, formula and process for moulding, #24406, November 30, 1901, F. A. Brausil
..Handles, method of construction in attaching, #16985, July 31, 1902, H. Whitaker and H. Ebenrett
..Handles, method of construction, #19702, September 9, 1902, A. E. Wale
..Handles-for watches or pictures, #12581, June 3, 1903, S. Ruhmann
..Handles, coating with metal, #12582, June 3, 1903, M. Polack
..Handles, filling with alum to dent proof, #13308, June 13, 1903, A. Richter
..Handles, construction by electrolysis, #24211, November 7, 1903, C. von Hofe

..Handles, removeable and replaceable and method of attachment, #11737, May 21, 1904, W. I. Cushion, et al.

..Handles, removeable and construction of, #19980, September 16, 1904, A. A. Revel

..Handles and process from celluloid, #22245, October 15, 1904, T. Didier

..Handles, process for filling (says alum n. g.), #11609, June 2, 1905, A. Richter and T. Gluck

..Handles, process for filling and construction, #11845, June 6, 1905, A. Richter

..Handles-detachable and interchangable, #845, January 12, 1906, J. B. Rosenstein

..Handles, tool for making #20997, October 5, 1908, Walker Brothers

..Handles, caps for canes, #26234, December 4, 1908, C. F. Gaunt

..Handles, process for mfg., tubular handles, #1442, January 20, 1909, Soc. H. Lapointe, et cie.

..Handles, process for coating, #8022, April 3, 1909, R. G. Wahlen and C. Wahlen

..Handles, #15465, June 28, 1910, P. Lorne

..Handles, plaited with cane, #1695, January 23, 1911,. S. Brown

..Handles, method of covering with fabric, #4636, February 23, 1911. F. W. Bussell

..Handle design as "V", #170,777, November 29, 1920, Cooper and Sons, Ltd.

..Handles-design, #206,452, May 16, 1923, P. R. Manger

..Handles, method of construction, #304,517, March 29, 1928, H. R. Lee

..Handles, method of growing and forming, #473,999, May 5, 1936, H. C. Hack

..Knobs-method of attaching to W. S., #550,003, July 15, 1941, F. Conham

..Handle ornamentation, #769,114, May 3, 1955, H. P. Gordon

..Handles (metal), #1638, July 11, 1956, R. Harrington

..Handle design for invalids, #1,135,512, May 15, 1967, E. C. Bennett

..Illuminated W. S. handles, #1,209,952, November 30, 1967, C. Chester

..Handles, method of making out of sections, #1,188,042, October 11, 1968, Airfix Plastics Ltd.

..W. S. crutch with lowering and raising handle, #1,314,342, November 14, 1969, Premier Lamp and Engineering Co. Ltd.

Hearing Aid Canes:

..Hearing aid cane, #7694, May 4, 1891, J. W. Cousins

..Hearing aid cane, #9975, May 14, 1901, H. G. Wieder and J. Hupfeld

Heating Canes:

..Stove in W. S. handle, #25347, November 11, 1896, D. M. B. H. Dundoland

..W. S. with annular water heater, #12596, June 12, 1908, R. C. Sayer

Hollow Cane:

..Souvenir cane-hollow for chocolates, #11740, May 23, 1902, M. R. Regan

Hunting Cane:

..Aiming pole and camp stool cane, #16444, August 16, 1899, G. Becker

Illuminating and Reflecting Canes (Candles, Electric, etc.):

..Lighting cane, #2421, September 1, 1862, W. Clark

..Lamp cane, #40, January 6, 1858, E. Gourdin

..Illuminated W. S., #3462, September 2, 1876, E. G. Brewer

..Candle lamp W. S., #47, January 4, 1882, A. M. Clark

..Match and candle cane, #5051, April 5, 1887, G. Miller

..Candle and match cane, #17270, December 15, 1887, F. J. Biggs

..Lamp cane, #12721, July 27, 1891, H. Diffetot

..Lighting and illuminating cane, #13345, August 7, 1891, Brierly

..Electric light W. S., #97, January 2, 1892, H. Levi

..Lamp cane, #8928, May 11, 1892, R. Von Horvath and F. Uzell

..W. S. with sight hole and reflectors, #14472, 1892, J. Livtschak ..Candle holder W. S., #15166, August 23, 1892, A. Dohn

..Lamp cane, #8350, April 27, 1894, H. H . Leigh

..Lamp cane, #12137, June 22, 1894, H. Newbold

..Miner's lamp W. S. #19710, October 21, 1895, R. Llewellyn

..Oil lamp W. S. to illuminate and to light lamps and cigars, #12167, June 22, 1895, J. D. Lawrence

..Electric lamp cane, #16804, August 3, 1898, C. Muller

..Electric lamp W. S., #20214, November 9, 1900, T. Bergmann

..Electric lamp W. S., #23332, October 12, 1909, W. P. Thompson

..Lamp cane, #7440, March 24, 1911, O. Loeb and R. Loeb

..Lamp attachment for W. S., #101,585, March 24, 1916, T. Y. Unwin

..Electric lamp W. S., #130,491, August 21, 1918, A. R. Upward

..Lamp, pistol and bayonet W. S., #144,540, October 15, 1919, H. J. P. Renard and B. Demorteau

..Flashing light cane (as it strikes ground), #284,076, January 24, 1927, J. A. Mayhoe

..Lighting cane, #269,832, March 4, 1927, M. B. El-Araby

..Lamp cane, #339,082, December 20, 1929, E. J. Ellison

..Reflecting signal W. S. for use by pedestrians, #497,123, March 7, 1938, K. Schlapfer

..W. S. with lamp on bottom, #536,610, October 17, 1939, 1941, J. H. Bingham

..W. S. with lamp on bottom, #535,829, October 20, 1939, 1941, G. J. Berry

..W. S. with lamp on bottom, #536,373, October 20, 1939, 1941, A. D. Kaufman

..Reg. globe light W. S. for blind, #747,976, December 1, 1953, Z. H. Miller

..Lamp cane, #953,659, January 15, 1962, V. J. A. Bullock

..Illuminated shaft W. S., #1,142,842, February 21, 1966, H. W. Marks

..Illuminated W. S. handles, #1,209,952, November 30, 1967, C. Chester

..Flashing light W. S., #1,135,930, December 15, 1967, P. A. McGuffie

..Illuminated W. S., #1,270,457, June 24, 1959, Secretary of State for Defense

..Illuminated W. S., #1,391,700, April 11, 1972, C. Blazdell

..Inflatable Floats in W. S. for Swimming and Life Saving, #14268, June 27, 1903, C. Bieber

Invalid and Crutch Canes and Attachments Thereto:

..Invalid arm rest W. S., #15624, November 5, 1915, E. Schlick

..J. S. crutch, #l07,499, Cctober 10, 1916, A. Hunter

..Wheel guide blind man's cane, #132,152, January 9, 1919, G. C. Hooper

..Elbow crutch W. S., #141,590, August 12, 1919, A. E. Warry

..Reg. globe light W. S. for blind, #747,976, December 1, 1953, Z. H. Miller

..W. S. Wheeled feeler for blind, #1,009,293, June 1, 1964, M. McShepherd

..W. S. Crutch, #1,081,185, March 28, 1966, E. F. Exter

..Invalids W. S., #1,181,795, July 18, 1967, A. S. Seamark

..Tripod W. S. for invalids, #1,313,570, December 29, 1970, Humenics of Delaware, Inc.

..W. S. crutch with lowering and raising handle, #1,314,342, November 14, 1969, Premier Lamp and Engineering Co., Ltd.

..Crutch cane, #1,452,277, January 27, 1973, Zimmer Orthopedic Ltd.

Identification Labels and Plates for Canes:

..Name plates for W. S., #3001, November 28, 1861, S. A. Carpenter

..Name band box W. S., #2926, February 25, 1887, G. Barnley

..Metalic letters for W. S., #24160, December 15, 1893, E. and W. Bettis

..Address labels for W. S., #17045, September 25, 1900, C. H. Underwood

..Device for fixing labels on W.S., #26891, December 11, 1908, C. F. Gaunt

..Identification device for W. S., #363,261, April 14, 1931, T. R. Lulham

..Identification plate for W. S., #424,666, December 18, 1933, E. M. Hutchinson

..Insect Catching Net W. S., #26337, November 13, 1909, A. Weinland

Key Canes:

..Carriage key or corkscrew cane, #1888, June 19, 1869, J. Brooker

..Alarm whistle cane, door fastener, key, corkscrew, #29472, December 13, 1897

..Leg Rest W. S., #23779, December 9, 1914, G. E. Marshall

Length Adjustable Canes:

..Length adjustable W. S., #12502, October 2, 1886, V. Daniels

..Telescopic cane for invalids of diff. heights, #685,781, Concentric Mfg. Co.

Liquid Containing and Serving Canes:

..Liquid carrying W. S., #2410, October 15, 1856, B. J. Heywood,

..Liquid containing cane, #7863, May 29, 1888, A. H. Craig

..Tippling W. S., (drinker's cane), #1961, July 30, 1866, J. J. Wheeler

..Liquid and cup cane, #22848, December 31, 1891, H. Windmuller and M. Keffel

..Collapsable and liquid carrying cane, #1091, January 15, 1902, T. Leach

..Liquid container and cup W. S., #183,622, May 13, 1921, J. Purves

Locking Device on Canes to Prevent Their Theft:

..Locking device for W. S., #4545, March 9, 1900, E. L. Appleby

..Locking device for W. S. to prevent theft, #20853, September 28, 1903, L. Levinger

Map Canes:

..Map cane, #3802, September 26, 1878, W. A. Barlow

..Map and guide cane, #3366, March 10, 1886, T. P. Johnston

Materials and Construction and Ornamenting of Canes:

..Materials for making W. S., #2288, October 14, 1858, C. Cowper

..Ornamenting W. S., #1638, July 20, 1858, G. Wheatley

..Materials for covering and ornamenting W. S., #2661, October 31, 1860, T. G. Ghislin

..Materials for covering and ornamenting canes, #1157, May 8, 1851, J. Pickett

..Design for W. S., #2482, October 4, 1861, T. G. Ghislin
..Tubes to cover W. S. #1508, June 17, 1864, M. E. Bowra
..Material for W. S., #2371, September 15, 1866, J. Keystone
..Ornamenting sticks, #3641, November 30, 1868, R. A. Green
..Ornamenting canes, (carrying names, photographs, etc.), #112, January 30, 1870, J. Wright, et. al.
..Ornamenting wood, #1397, April 22, 1874, C. A. Bluemal
..Materials for W. S., #2566, June 26, 1879, E. C. T. Blake and W. Boggett
..Material for W. S., #4241, October 18, 1880, C. D. Obel
..Materials for canes (paper on steel shaft), #17447, December 19, 1887, J. H. Clymer
..Machine for spinning canes, #20978, December 31, 1889, J. Browning
..Method of making W. S. of leather, #5498, April 11, 1890, C. Sims
..W. S. Material, #15811, September 3, 1892, H. W. Boswell
..Materials and method of making W. S., #7389, April 13, 1894, J. E. Bousfield
..Method of making W. S., #2183, January 31, 1895, L. Sandberg
..W. S. Material-flocks and paper, #5596, March 3, 1897, P. W. H. Gray
..Construction of W. S., #8836, May 12, 1900, G. Rau
..Materials for W. S.-veneering metal rods, #873, January 14, 1901, L. Sandberg
..W. S. method of construction, #20140, 1902, E. Kronenberg
..Material and method of construction of W. S., #4951, February 27, 1902, E. and S. Sandhagen
..Colorng process for blackthorn canes, #118531 May 25, 1903, H. A. Acres
..W. S., construction of, #15573, July 14, 1903, W. W. Jones
..Whip cord cane (construction of), #4514, March 4, 1905, F. W. Parnell
..Materials for canes, composition, #22580, October 14, 1907, New Eccles Rubber Works
..W. S. with natural bark covering (french polish), #13820, June 7, 1910, J. Root
..W. S. design, #972,471, November 29, 1960, W. Schuster

Measuring, Level and Gauge Canes:

..Measuring tape W. S., #2671, July 31, 1874, R. Whitaker and A. Holden
..Slide rule cane, #4310, November 7, 1876, H. E. Newton
..Cane measuring to determine length needed W. S., #17472, November 30, 1888, J. W. Anderson
..Surveying cane (with spirit level), #14476, August 27, 1891, J. Trimming
..Rail gauge and level cane, #16033, September 7, 1892, W. P. Thompson
..Measuring staff W. S., #5526, March 14, 1899, F. W. Golby
..Horse measuring cane, #4427, February 25, 1903, E. Newman
..Surveying W. S., #177,440, May 31, 1921, R. and A. Seidler
..Weighing and measuring cane (level and clinometer), #280,953, November 19, 1927, M. Slotosch
..Tree measuring W. S., #571,337, April 5, 1943, P. Davey and R. C. W. Davey

Music Stand and Easel Canes (Also See Tripod Canes):

..Easel and music stand cane, #829, April 2, 1864, F. Potts and A. H. Green
..Sketching easel W. S., #1672, April 16, 1881, A. J. Welsby
..Music stand W. S., #5133, March 19, 1884, C. Spratt

..Easel or music stand cane, #6182, April 26, 1888, J. Fullwood
..Music stand cane, #9345, May 11, 1894, A. G. Wallis
..Music stand W. S., #13379, July 11, 1895, J. Thomas
..Music and camera stand, #3040, February 7, 1898, G. Burnett
..Music stand cane, #107,515, November 4, 1916, C. Hosking

Paper Knife W. S., #5194, December 19, 1879, G. H. R. Dobbs

Pen and Pencil Canes:

..Pencil holder cane, #12240, August 1, 1889, G. Dumenil
..Pencil cane, #15080, August 7, 1894, C. H. Dumenil and V. H. Brigg
..Pen and pencil W. S., #16624, July 26, 1902, F. Czilinsky
..Pencil and whistle W. S., #23079, November 25, 1914, C. A. J. Cook and W. A. Bigg

Periscope Canes:

..Periscope cane, #8579, April 3, 1897, J. E. Gayer
..Periscope W. S., #21438, November 27, 1900, W. Youlter
..Periscope W. S. (polemoscope), #26031, December 2, l908, N. Dickson
..Seat and periscope cane, #1,085,924, August 8, 1966, E. R. Hill and C. Davis

Physicians Canes:

..Doctor's disinfecting cane handle, #178, January 19, 1872, D. A. Doudney and H. O. Adams
..Phials in handle of W. S., #4622, October 21, 1881, E. Edwards
..Breakdown W. S. to carry surgical dressings, #27215, November 26, 1912, A. Hemrich

Pick-up Canes:

..W. S. with pliers (long arm), #2909, February 6, 1909, C. A. F. Fennell
..Pick-up cane, #998,788, July 2, 1964, A. J. Colbert
..Pick-up cane, #356,341, June 20, 1930, C. E. F. Crombie
..Pick-up cane, #11219, July 1, 1891, K. A. E. Ulbricht

Picture and Locket Canes:

..Pictures in W. S. handles, #2563, August 30, 1869, L. Goldberg
..W. S. with portraits, #20810, October 30, 1894, A. Penn
..Locket W. S., #11611, August 11, 1915, W. Scaife

Prospecting Canes:

..Gold prospecting cane, #12987, September 8, 1888, E. C. Noar
..Prospecting cane with boring tool, #7606, March 30, 1909, H. Menzel

Scooter Cane, #174,175, October 18, 1920, W. M. F. Sherwood

Serpent Cane (toy), #7441, May 8, 1884, W. M. Campbell

Smoker's Canes (For Matches, Lighters, Cigars, Cigarettes, Pipes, Snuff, etc.):

a) Cigar and cigarette canes;
..Cigar and match container W. S., #5139, December 15, 1879, H. Ciotti
..Cigarette and match dispenser, #15345, November 25, 1886, A. J. Willis

..Cigar cane, #4016, March 17, 1887, S. Simmons
..Cigar humidor cane, #13836, October 12, 1887, A. M. Clark
..Pipe, cigar holder, etc., Cane, #2335, February 2, 1895, Windmuller
..Smoker's cane-cigar, cigarettes and matches, #24093, December 16, 1895, W. Daniels
..Cigar and match container and producer W. S., #22673, October 5, 1912, T. D. Scott
..Cigarette, etc., swagger stick W. S., #23176, November 27, 1914, J. H. Faulkner
..Cigarette case and lighter cane, #168,287, June 7, 1921, O. Singer
..Cigarette case etc., W. S., #187,849, November 1, 1921, O. Singer
..Cigar and cigarette container and lighter W. S., #246,299, July 31, 1925, A. T. Steventon
..Cigarette case W. S., #309,777, June 13, 1928, E. M. F. Decobert

b) Match and lighter canes for cigars, cigarettes and pipes;
..Pipe lighter and illuminator, #4206, December 4, 1875, W. R. Lake
..Matchbox W. S., #26, January 2, 1878, N. H. Holding
..Matchbox, etc., W. S. #2634, July 1, 1878, N. H. Holding
..Cigar and pipe lighter cane, #512, January 12, 1886, W. Walton
..Cigar and pipe lighter cane, #410, January 11, 1887, W. Walton
..Match, etc., cane, #2048, February 10, 1888, J. W. Anderson
..Smoking pipe and match cane, #15443, October 26, 1888, G. H. Coursen
..Match lighting surface on W. S., #7986, May 14, 1889, W. H. Marston
..Matchbox in cane, #6843, May 3, 1890, E. E. Wood
..Match box cane, #10352, June 18, 1891, T. Clark
..Match delivering (lit) cane, #16215, September 24, 1891, F. Wallis
..Lighter for cigars and pipes in W. S., #973, January 18, 1892, J. Wetter
..Clip on match lighting surface for cane, #18396, October 14, 1892, J. Badger
..Match box and cigar cutter W. S. #20260, October 27, 1893, W. R. Corke
..Match box W. S., #23427, December 5, 1893, C. H. Dumenil
..Match box, etc., W. S., #1962, January 28, 1895, J. W. Anderson and J. Howell
..Band for W. S. to strike matches, #3140, February 10, 1903, T. Robinson
..Attachment for W. S. to strike matches, #27067, December 12, 1904, J. J. Scanlon
..Lighting appliance W. S., #10727, May 31, 1911, K. Redlich
..Cigarette lighter W. S., #313,365, August 15, 1928, E. R. Visitacion

c) Miscellaneous smoking canes;
..Cigar cutter, etc., W. S., #9535, April 25, 1902, C. F. Hoffmann
..Cigar perforation W. S., #7911, May 11, 1889, H. P. Hodges
..Smoker's case W. S., #4479, March 6, 1884, J. Jones
..Caricature face W. S. to smoke cigars, #7666, April 25, 1900, G. Grabosch

d) Pipe canes;
..Smoking pipe in W. S., #2750, November 21, 1856, S. Rothenheim
..Smoking pipe in W. S., #1085, May 14, 1858, J. Colgate
..Pipe cane, #2916, November 20, 1863, E. Pezold
..Tobacco pipe W. S., #1618, May 5, 1873, J. O. Spong
..Smoking pipe W. S., #2095, May 18, 1876, G. Grant
..Tobacco pipe cane, #15043, November 19, 1886, S. Wildeblood
..Smoking pipe and match cane, #15443, October 26, 1888, G. H. Coursen

..Smoker's cane, pipe, etc., #13497, July 12, 1894, W. P. Thompson
..Tobacco pipe cane, #16151, August 24, 1894, E. R. Jeschke
..Pipe, cigar holder, etc., cane, #2335, February 2, 1895, Windmuller
..Tobacco pipe (hookah) cane, #12692, June 21, 1901, S. A. M. Kahn
..Tobacco pipe, #14475, July 8, 1908, H. Guthmann
..Smoking pipe cane, #27134, December 4, 1911, I. Hoffman

e) Snuff box canes;
..Snuff box W. S., #17760, September 24, 1895, T. Wright
..Snuff compartments, etc., outside of cane, #7476, May 19, 1888, G. J. Lysaght

Sound Producing Canes:

..Knife and Whistle cane, #13351, August 7, 1891, J. J. Holtzapffel
..Alarm whistle cane, door fastener, key, cork screw, #29472, December 13, 1897
..Pencil and Whistle W. S., #23079, November 25, 1514, C. A. J. Cook and W. A. Bigg

Spring Canes:

..Spring balance W. S. (for weighing), #3187, March 6, 1886, A. G. Bartlett
..Coil spring to propel person cane, #13548, August 28, 1890, W. F. Norman
..W. S. with support tension device, #737,014, February 16, 1953, W. Schuster and V. Krause

Stool, Seat, Desk, Table and Bed Canes:

..Table W. S., #999, March 24, 1868, D. Lewis
..Seat Cane, #1661, April 28, 1877, L. Field
..Seat Cane, #1671, April 30, 1877, M. Burke
..Stool and table cane, #1316, April 2, 1879, J. W. Gray
..Stool cane, #4576, September 26, 1882, J. C. Mewburn
..Camp bed and stool cane, #12464, September 16, 1884, H. J. Maddan
..Seat cane, #13414, October 4, 1887, C. Lange
..Camp stool cane, #19836, December 10, 1809, A. Schneider
..Card table W. S., #7345, May 12, 1890, J. Swithenbank
..Stool cane, 14179, September 9, 1890, H. Hendrickson
..Table cane, #15205, September 25, 1890, O. N. Kuhl
..Card table W. S., #779, January 15, 1891, J. Swithenbank
..Reading desk cane, #1864, January 27, 1893, G. A. Biddell
..Stool cane, #5711, March 14, 1393, J. A. Nixon
..Seat cane, #9189, May 8, 1893, P. Hoffmann
..Stool cane, #9813, May 16, 1893, W. Ward
..Seat or desk cane, #20637, November 1, 1893, H. Bunting
..Seat cane, #21123, November 3, 1894, J. J. W. Behrens
..Seat cane, #24094, December 11, 1894, E. Keller
..Seat or table W. S. #13378, July 11, 1895, J. Thomas
Seat or table cane, #20831, November 4, 1895, W. P. Thompson
..Table W. S. #21471, September 29, 1896, W. Archdeacon
..Chair cane, #1893, January 23, 1897, J. H. A. Behrens
..Chair cane, #24411, October 21, 1897, M. Ruckdeschel and A. Mockel
..Campstool W. S., #11351, May 18, 1898, G. F. Redfern
..Stool cane, #20402, September 27, 1898, C. G. Skoog
..Stand and seat cane, #16282, August 10, 1899, H. J. Hudson

..Aiming pole and camp stool cane, #16444, August 16, 1899, G. Becker
..Camp stool cane, #2785, February 12, 1900, A. von Andrassy
..Campstool W. S., #22863, December 14, 1900, C. E. Burnap
..Camp stool cane, #10363, May 18, 1901, W. P. Thompson
..Table or seat cane, #16830, August 22, 1901, W. Mills
..Stool cane, #7077, March 27, 1903, J. Wood
..Seat cane, #11362, May 17, 1904, J. T. Preston and G. T. Lawson
..Seat cane, #14390, June 25, 1904, A. Wagner
..Seat cane, #16167, July 21, 1504, C. S. Rogers
..Seat cane, #27931, December 21, 1904, W. Spiegelberg
..Seat cane, #12445, May 29, 1907, W. Schocke
..Seat cane, #19503, August 30, 1907, A. Becke
..Seat cane, #9079, April 25, 1908, W. E. Lake
..W. S. seat, #7833, March 31, 1910, A. Frei
..Seat cane, #23303, October 23, 1911, C. G. Hanemian
..Seat cane, #25, January 1, 1912, F. B. Mitchell
..Camp stool cane, #24634, October 28, 1912, G. Gallewski
..Seat, stand and telescope etc., W. S., #337,135, October 28, 1929, Le Sueute
..Seat cane, #1,169,662, February 26, 1968, H. Kettler
..Stool cane, #12351, May 19, 1910, P. C. Vernet
..Seat cane, #6092, March 10, 1911, F. H. Christmas
..Table cane, #20646, March 5, 1912, S. S. Frank
..Stool cane, #21326, September 22, 1913, T. Glendenning
..Seat cane, #211,676, February 2, 1923, A. H. V. Williams
..Table or seat cane, #281,964, June 29, 1927, L. J. Brun
..Seat or footstool cane, #352,059, April 1, 1930, P. J. Le Sueur
..Seat cane, #381,285, August 15, 1931, P. J. Le Sueur
..Seat cane and wire fence spreader, #868,541, September 19, 1958, I. S. C. Rose
..Seat and periscope cane, #1,085,924, August 8, 1965, E. R. Hill and C. Davis

Surveying Canes:

..Surveying cane (with spirit level), #14476, August 27, 1891, J. Trimming
..Surveying instrument holder cane, #5535, March 21, 1892, G. Haussarman
..Surveying instrument tripod, #5724, March 19, 1894, L. J. A. ebber, et. al.
..Surveying cane, #1534, January 22, 1903, W. W. B. Hulton
..Surveying W. S., #177,440, May 31, 1921, R. and A. Seidler
..Surveyors marking cane, point out of ferrule, #220,089, May 15, 1923, R. O. McGown

Swimming Cane:

..Inflatable floats in W. S. for swimming and life saving, #14268, June 27, 1903, C. Bieber

Swivel for W. S. or Crutch, #23778, November 23, 1901, J. H. Hammond and W. Bridge Water

Telescope, Microscope and Opera Glass Canes:

..Gun, telescope, pen and ink, paper, pencil and drawing instruments, #3837, August 7, 1814, H. Kleft
..Opera glass W. S., #4181, September 28, 1881, L. M. Promis
..Opera glass holder W. S., #5654, November 28, 1882, A. J. Boult
..Gun or telescope cane, #4108, June 9, 1897, E. H. Ericson
..Telescope or opera glass W. S., #20756, September 19, 1906, W. H. Robinson and F. Ward

..Telescope in W. S., #9541, April 24, 1907, F. W. W. Baker
..Telescope aud microscope, etc., W. S., #18586, August 12, 1909, L. Wallmuller
..Field glass holder W. S., #181,457, March 10, 1921, D. E. Norton

Tent Pole Canes:

..W. S. as tent support, #7323, April 12, 1894, W. L. Wise
..W. S. as tent poIe, #23523, October 23, 1896, A. J. Nicholson
..Tent pole cane, #132, January 2, 1903, H. Dichtl
..Tent and fishing pole W. S., #190,884, November 29, 1921, J. Holroyd, et. al.

Theodolite and Tripod, #3616, October 21, 1874, G. Francis

Ticket Holding Cane, #3766, March 17, 1896, E. Mogel

Toy Canes:

..Toy air gun cane, #2672, October 3, 1862, W. Clark
..Air dart gun (toy), #2857, July 17, 1878, W. R. Davis
..Serpent cane (toy), #7441, May 8, 1884, W. M. Campbell

Trick Canes:

..Conjuring tricks W. S., #3298, February 14, 1899, J. A. Cumine and G. von Reinolts
..Puzzle W. S., #13663, July 1, 1899, A. G. A. Marness and R. C. Spurin

Umbrella Canes:

..Umbrella W. S., #3171, October 8, 1808, E. Thomason
..Umbrella in W. S., #3189, December 29, 1808, McGregor, M. and J. McForland
..Umbrella in W. S., #3228, April 19, 1809, P. B. Thomason
..Umbrella in W. S., #7735, July 13, 1838, A. Cochrane
..Umbrella in W. S., #13554, March 13, 1851, T. Dawson
..Umbrella W. S., #1635, July 9, 1853, T. Restall
..Umbrella W. S., mfg. of, #2503, November 28, 1854, T. Restall
..Umbrella W. S., #984, April 19, 1850, J. Wilis
..Umbrella cane, #2469, October 8, 1863, R. G. Watson and W. J. Kendall
..Umbrella cane, #2577, October 20, 1863, T. Restall
..Umbrella W. S., #40, January 6, 1864, J. I. and H. G. Tracy
..Umbrella cane, #1175, May 9, 1864, W. G. Haid
..Umbrella cane, #2205, September 9, 1864, T. Restall
..Rib band on umbrella W. S., #918, March 31, 1865, T. K. Mace
..Umbrella W. S., #1673, June 22, 1865, N. DeBecker
..Umbrella cane, #556, February 19, 1868, F. H. Renault
..Parasol W. S., #3781, October 12, 1877, F. Barrett
..Umbrella W. S., #4728, December 12, 1877, A. M. Clark
..Umbrella W. S., #359, January 29, 1878, H. J. Felton
..Umbrella W. S., #657, February 18, 1878, E. Gardner
..Umbrella W. S., #848, February 26, 1880, A. G. Henderson
..Umbrella with detachable W. S., #2910, July 14, 1880, W. L. Wise
..Umbrella W. S., #5784, December 5, 1882, J. T. Ford
..Umbrella cane, #5027, October 23, 1883, T. Hetherington

..Umbrella W. S., #5555, November 28, 1883, J. H. Johnson
..Umbrella cane, #13257, October 6, 1884, H. H. Lake
..Umbrella cane, #2179, February 17, 1885, L. A. Groth
..Umbrella cane, #4913, April 8, 1886, S. H. McKenzie
..Spring umbrella cane, #9152, July 14, 1886, A. C. Farrington
..Umbrella cane, #13887, October 29, 1886, T. A. Classan and J. Jampson
..Umbrella cane (pulls out and attaches to handle), #11626, August 26, 1887, W. P. Thompson
..Umbrella cane, #15823, December 18, 1887, G. Beech
..Umbrella cane, #9045, June 21, 1888, W. Phillips
..Umbrella cane, #10054, July 10, 1888, G. H. Rayner
..Umbrella cane, #20364, December 18, 1889, A. Pichler
..Umbrella cane (star frame), #5932, April 18, 1890, J. H. Rief and E. Weber
..Umbrella cane (collapsable outer shaft), #18464, November 15, 1890, C. H. 0. Strohback
..Umbrella cane, #11445, July 6, 1891, S. J. & J. Knox
..Umbrella cane, #472, January 9, 1892, K. Hall
..Umbrella cane, #5514, March 21, 1892, J. Greenwood
..Umbrella cane, #12195, June 30, 1892, M. Hartung and P. Adam
..Umbrella W. S., #7685, April 15, 1893, E. L. Downing
..Umbrella cane, #12629, June 27, 1893, H. H. Lake
..Umbrella cane, #13002, July 3, 1893, R. Waples, Jr.
..Umbrella cane with smelling salts and scents, #11720, June 16, 1894, J. Cook
..Umbrella W. S., #19979, October 19, 1894, T. Ashford
..Umbrella cane, #6235, March 26, 1895, C. H. Morgan
..Umbrella cane, #2757, February 6, 1896, F. Goldschmidt
..Umbrella W. S., #8422, April 21, 1896, R. Waples
..Umbrella cane, #22723, October 13, 1896, R. Waples
..Umbrella cane, #3340, February 8, 1897, G. Lund
..Umbrella cane, #10060, April 22, 1897, E. Hugendubel
..Umbrella cane, #19527, August 24, 1897, J. H. Nolan
..Umbrella cane, #21635, September 21, 1897, W. Hall and P. Leonard
..Umbrella cane, #26764, November 16, 1897, R. J. Edwards
..Umbrella cane, #23989, November 14, 1898, E. Hugendubel
..Telescopic umbrella (to shorten for packing), #6458, March 25, 1899, N. Foley
..Umbrella cane, #10320, May 6, 1903, R. Kronenberg
..Umbrella cane, interchangeable stick or umbrella, #1647, January 12, 1905, F. Joath
..Umbrella cane, #25272, December 5, 1905, F. Tooth
..Umbrella cane, #28224, December 11, 1906, J. B. Hall
..Umbrella cane, #4700, February 26, 1907, F. Bech
..Collapsible umbrella cane, method of mfg., #20779, October 2, 1908, R. Genck
..Umbrella W. S., #15418, July 1, 1909, I. M. Hoppenstand
..Umbrella cane, #24564, November 4, 1911, A. Scheibler
..Umbrella cane, #11187, May 13, 1913, E. Efflinger
..Umbrella cane, #29500, December 23, 1913, M. W. Hare
..Collapsable umbrella cane, #316,794, September 1, 1928, T. Fuchs

..Umbrella shape W. S., #462,135, September 4, 1935, F. B. Cornell
..Umbrella cane, #806,139, June 4, 1957, A. Kortenbuch, et. al.
..Umbrella W. S., #2974, November 3, 1962, H. Stallard

Vanity, Handbag and Purse Canes:

..Vanity cane, powder puff, needles and thimbles, #1379, April 15, 1875, W. L. Hosking
..Purse cane, #10152, June 15, 1891, T. W. Cox
..Vanity cane (toilet articles), #20303, November 10, 1892, A. J. Boult
..Vanity bag W. S., #335,455, December 2, 1929, W. Popp

Watch Canes:

..Solar watch in W. S. handle, #1551, June 25, 1853, A. Sandoz
..Watch cane, #5024, April 23, 1885, W. R. Lake
..Watch cane, #6226, April 28, 1887, F. Knoeferl
..Watch cane, #8341, June 7, 1888, C. A. Herzog
..Handles-for watches or pictures, #12581, June 3, 1903, S. Ruhmann
..Watch cane, #276,278, May 3, 1927, C. H. Lawton

Weapon Canes:

a) Gun canes;
..Gun, telescope, pen and ink, paper, pencil and drawing instruments, #3837, August 7, 1814, H. Kleft
..Percussion gun locks, #4861, November 12, 1823, John Day
..Gun cane, #1897, August 30, 1854, B. Meyers
..Gun cane with safety elevator, #1231, May 18, 1859, E. Charlesworth
..Gun cane, #1648, May 31, 1862, T. Lawden
..Air gun W. S., #2931, October 30, 1862, P. Giffard
..Toy air gun cane, #2672, October 3, 1862, W . Clark
..Gun canes, #1785, July 16, 1864, A. Wyley
..Gun cane, #2711, October 19, 1866, T. Restell
..Gun cane, #863, March 25, 1867, A. Wyley
..Gun cane (compressed air or gas cartridges), #21, January 3, 1872, P. Giffard
..Gun cane, #3917, December 24, 1872, A. M. Clark
..Gun cane (___power), #4825, December 13, 1871 A. M. Clark
..Air dart gun (toy), #2857, July 17, 1878, W. R. Davis
..Revolver and sword W. S., #1936, May 11, 1880, C. Jacquelin
..Revolver cane, #4146, October 12, 1880, A. J. Boult
..Gun cane, #13184, September 29, 1887, A. Lindner
..Gun cane, #17580, December 3, 1888, A. Lindner
..Gun cane (toy), #2025, February 5, 1889, J. Haywood
..Gun cane, #17532, October 14, 1891, A. C. Argles
..Gun cane, #22040, November 19, 1895, N. G. Hanson
..Gun or telescope cane, #14108, June 9, 1897, E. H. Ericson
..Gun cane, #14109, June 9, 1897, E. H. Ericson
..Gun cane, #25127, December 15, 1899, C. Ramus
..Gun cane (revolver), #921, January 13, 1902, G. Tresenreuter
..Gun rest W. S. and seat, #14105, June 22, 1904, T. Grunewald
..Gun cane and umbrella, #10882, May 9, 1906, H. Longenhan
..Gun cane, #26611, November 23, 1906, H. Renfors
..Pneumatic gun cane, #14447, June 22, 1907, J. Lucking

..Lamp, pistol and bayonet W. S., #144,540, October 15, 1919, H. J. P. Renard and B. Demorteau
..Shooting practice cane (trigger makes clicking sound), #333,935, May 23, 1929, A. S. Purdey

b) Sword, knife and other bladed canes;
..Sword cane, #3668, March 16, 1813, G. Dodd
..Spear cane, #3329, December 21, 1870, F. J. Walthew
..Revolver and sword W. S., #1935, May 11, 1880, C. Jacquelin
..Dagger in ferrule cane, #587, January 14, 1887, H. Marx
..Knife and whistle cane, #13361, August 7, 1891, J. J. Holtzapffel
..Weapon cane-moveable handle as halt or hand guard, #28702, December 30, 1903, W. Freh
..Sword cane (flickout), #158,482, April 29, 1920, T. H. Randolph
..Weapon and stool umbrella W. S., #18013, August 7, 1913, L. C. Jacquet
..Defense hand guard W. S., #411,759, December 5, 1923, F. Jung

c) Billy and black-jack canes;
.."Billy" canes, #17249, August 4, 1896, L. Goldsmith
..Rubber black jack cane, #2727, February 7, 1895, H. Krodik

Whip Canes:

..Buggy whip cane, #17815, December 27, 1887, O. Godward
..Whip cane (dog or riding) #19102, November 28, 1889, J. F. Young

Wire Cutting Canes:

..Grabbing or cutting W. S., #3970, March 20, 1886, A. M. Clark
..Wire cutter W. S. and riding crop, #5689, March 27, 1900, F. V. Dalton
..Barb wire cutting cane, #5322, March 2, 1914, C. C. Ellison

Wireless Receiving Cane, #229,356, August 20, 1923, A. Compere

Subject Index of German Cane Patents

Index of German Cane Patents

..Ferrule for canes, Ernst Romer, Neisse, #572479, March 2, 1933
..Ferrule with two interchangeable, jointed, anti-skip protectors, Otto Friedrich Heinrich, Leipzig, #694731, Feb. 19, 1919
..Cane ferrule, Carl Kessal and Carl Makoben, Lutjenburg (Ostholst.), #826,186, Nov. 11, 1950
..Flexible elastic ferrule for canes, Richard Stopford Higginbotham, Henderson,Aukland, New Zealand #1750 533, Sept. 5, 1955
...Anti-skid protective tip for crutches & canes, Karl Wolfel, Erbendorf, #1762 156, Dec. 3, 1957
...Anti-skid protective tip for crutches & canes, (All weather ferrule - a Moveable blade), Fritz Fischer, Celle, (Hann.) #1763 897, Jan. 22, 1958
...Hunting cane tip, Karl Keil, Nordingen (Bay.) 1779 507, Oct. 16, 1958
..Support umbrella with skid proof ferrules, Dipl.-Ing. Walter Massmann, Koln- Lindenthal, #1785 713 Jan. 24, 1959
..Multipurpose Ferrule, Joseph Bittner, Kempten (Allgau, #1789 699, March 10, 1959
..Crutch cane for disabled, with anti-skid bottom & warning blink light, Hans Schollhammer and Karl Scheiblener, Steyr (Austria), #1860 713, May 21, 1962
..Mountain cane with double ferrule, Hans Wolf, Munchen #1231 395, Oct. 22, 1965
..Skid-proof tip for mountain canes (double ferrule) Hans Wolf, Munchen, #1,963,894, Oct. 22, 1965
..Ferrule for canes, Ernst Herzog, Eschwege, #1,952,141, Aug. 16, 1966
..Ferrule with hard metal cone, Johann Egle, Irsee Uber Kaufbeuren, #1,957,815, Dec. 20, 1966
..Cane for sick with adjustable anti-skid device, Karl Weissenrieder, Neuhaus Uber Ravensburg, #1,967,349, March 31, 1967
..Anti-skid device for cane tips, Erhard & Leimer, K.G., Augsburg, #1,963,017, March 28, 1967
..Anti-skid cane with projections from rubber ferrule, Richard Schiller, Halfern, #1632 518 Jan. 8, 1968
..Rubber anti-skid device for canes with metal & pointed ferrules, Rudolph Hermann, Eggenfelden, #1993 635, April 22, 1968
..Buffer ferrule for canes, crutches, Gotz-Gerd, Kuhn, Harixbeck, #75 18 377, June 9, 1975
..Safety crutch cane with large springed ferrule, Holger Weber, Konstanz, #7821396, July 17, 1978
..Safety ferrule with retractable steel tips,Adalbert Georg Schramm, #7901543, Jan. 20, 1979
..Bottom part for safety canes, i.e., crutches, Helger G. Weber, Konstanz, #P29026526, Jan. 24, 1979, no details or drawings
..Protective rubber ferrules for canes & crutches, Eduard Riebauer, Stuttgart, #7922 100, August 2, 1979

Flag or banner canes:

..Cane with flag or banner, Gerhard Manusch, Aichach, #2003458, Jan. 27, 1970
..Multipurpose cane with billard cue, saw blade, flag, knife convertible to lance, or mountain climbing, etc., Chin-Tui Kuo, Taichung, Hsi Tun District Taiwan, #8130208, Oct. 16, 1981

Galoshes removal canes:

..Cane or umbrella with a device to put on or take off galoshes, Franz Graf von Taxis, Innsbruck, #226472, June 3, 1909

Gripping & pick-up canes:

..Pickup cane -cane with gripping appliance, Karl Albert Egon Ulbricht, Taubenheim, bei Meissen, #59435, March 13, 1891
..Crutch cane for disabled with attachments for pick up, & other purposes, Erna Kunze geb.

Scholer, Ernst Kunze and Siegfried Heinz, Wilden, #1,945,282, Oct. 1, l965
..Cane to pick up leaves, paper, etc. Zoll geb. Noe, Chista, Angermund, #7238236, Oct. 18, 1972
..Gripping cane, Erika Kunkel, geb. Schuler Frankfurt, #26 26544, June 14, 1976

Handles for canes; material, construction, method of manufacturing & bonding & uniting to shaft:

..Method of connecting handle on canes and umbrellas, F. Prager, Liegnitz, #16596, July 12, 1881
..Method of uniting handles on canes & umbrellas, C. F. Prager, Liegnitz, #22756, Dec. 5, 1882
..Removable cane handle, Hug Matadorff, Berlin, #49282, Jan. 13, 1889
..Spring cushioned handle for canes and umbrellas, Karl Johan Nilsson, Gadderas Orrefons (Sweden) #122952, Nov. 20, 1900
..Cane or umbrella elongating handle, Hermann Jack, Vienna, #   July 7, 1903
..Cross-cut reinforcement for cane and umbrella handles, which consist of two hollow parts, filled with Georg Rohde, Hamburg, #373304, March 4, 1921
..Safety device to protect handle from becoming loose, Rosenkaimer G.m.b.H., Leichlingen (Rhld) #1750 532, June 26, 1957
..Crutch handles for umbrellas & canes, Ernst. Ed. Deneke, Hamburg, #1758 2 65,Aug. 20, 1957
..Mechanism for interchangeable umbrella handles & ferrules, Albert R. Bursch, Koln, #1806 645, Nov. 4, 1959
..Cane with metal or plastic handle, Gunter Stengel, Eschwege, #1834 633, Jan. 13, 1961
..Spray-molded handle made of plastic, Kull K.G. Haan, #1991 651, Feb. 29, 1968
..Handle for canes, Sanitatshaus Paul Kowsky, Neumunster, #67 51912, July 24, 1968
..Cane with different handles, Hanns Bausenhart, Ulm/Donau, #68 13 589, Dec. 31, 1968
..Cane with individually designed knobs or handles, Ludwig Engelhardt, Mannheim, #7147879, Dec. 20, 1971
..Hiking cane with reformable grip, Joseph Zierhut, Augsburg, #7431522, Sept. 19, 1974
..Cane handle strap, C. Stiefenhofer, KG, Munich, #7705302, Feb. 22, 1977
..Cane or Umbrella handle, Hugendubel Co. Stuttgart, #7827952, Sept. 20, 1978

Handles with moving parts:

..Cane handle with moving parts - in shape of a skull, jaw and eyes and tongue move, Ernst Bolle, Berlin, #23871, March 8, 1883

Heating canes:

..Heating device for cane or umbrella handle, Carl W. Linder, Weyer, Rhld., #180961, July 23, 1905

Hunting canes:

..Cane changeable into a hunting chair with rifle support, Frederich Seeger and Dr. Leo Luben, #82806, Feb. 22, 1895
..Hunting seat cane containing a telephone instrument in its seat capable of making contact with overhead wires, Joseph Strecker, Grottkau, #204490, March 18, 1908
..Hunting seat cane, which can be transformed into a tree stand, Ludwig Hambek, Zierdorf, Nied. Osterr, #286577, June 18, 1914
..Aiming cane for hunting and military purposes, Anton Diemer, Staaken b. Spandau, #319449, June 15, 1918
..Seat cane and for tracking, mountaineering, aiming and hunting, Kurt von Kaneke, Bad Doberan, Mecklbg., and Carl Hermann Eichhorn, Rostook, #481826, May 8, 1928

..Hunting seat cane and aiming cane, Herman Muller, Berlin - Baumschulenweg, #611516, March 14, 1935
..Hunting seat and aiming cane, Hermann Wandrey, Landsberg, Warthe, #690071, Nov. 10, 1938
..Hunting cane with rifle support pulling upward out of handle and folding out, Joseph Hillemeyer, Neuhaus, Kr. Paderborn, #712919, March 16, 1939
..Walking and aiming cane, (entire cane splits lengthwise) Hans -Heinrich Hallensleben, Grohnde, (Kr. Hameln-Pyrmont) #834 724, Sept. 14, 1950
..Mountain & aiming cane, Dr. Roman Heyn, Dentist, Worms/Rhein, #67 52 987, Sept. 25, 1968
..Mountain & aiming cane, Dr. Roman Heyn, Dentist, Worms/Rhein, #69 14 496, Nov. 4, 1969
..Hunting & Mountain climbing cane or staff with aiming device seat carrier (removable) etc., Heinz Schmidke, Barkhausen, #7232343, Sept. 1, 1972

Illuminating canes: candles, electric light, etc.,

..Cane or umbrella handle containing a candle, Ernst Mogel, Dresden, #37004, Dec. 24, 1885
..Cane with incandescent light bulb in handle, Richard Von Horvath, Vienna, #59816, Jan 23, 1891
..Attachment on canes & umbrellas for the mechanical extraction of candles, & lighting of same, Valentine Landsberg, Berlin, #77785, May 11, 1893
..Cane with electric lamp in handle, Franz Oleschko, Wieschowa, Kr. Tarnowitz, Ob. Schl., #230600, Feb.15, 1910
..Cane with electrical lighting device, Gebr. Goldmann, Berlin, #263478, April 24, 1912
..Cane or umbrella with built-in electrical lamp and removable handle, Franz Krausze, Halberstadt, #260482, Aug. 24, 1912
..Electric light (that pops out of top of handle) for canes and umbrellas, Julius Morber, Berlin, #318852,Dec. 3, 1918
..Cane with electric lamp & battery in handle, Glas., and Konservenglas - Vertrieh, G.m.b.H., Leipzig, #384590, May 8, 1921
..Cane with electric light in handle & battery in staff, Arno Fleischhaver, Weimar, #402552, Jan. 18, 1923
..Cane with flashlight in handle, Joh. Hermann, Singer, Crimmitschau, Sa. #530240, May 25, 1930
..Cane with signal blink light, Joseph Stanek, Hausenstamm, #1751317, Sept. 1, 1955
..Light cane, Fa H. Grote, Hamburg, #1783337, Nov. 19, 1958
..Telescoping illuminating ladies umbrella, Julius Flick, Heilbronn/Neckar, #1807 621, Dec. 2, 1959
..Illuminating cane, (flashlight), Ludwig Blas, Munchen #1834 634, April 25, 1961
..Signal light cane for the disabled, Helmut Tkatz, Berlin -Charlottenburg, #1856 222, March 2O, 1962
..Crutch cane for disabled, with anti-slip bottom & warning blink light, Hans Schollhammer and Karl I Scheiblehner, Steyr (Austria) #1860713, May 21, 1962
..Lightable cane, Preduktion and Auswertung Eugen Von Bongart, Berlin, #1931 964, Nov. 16, 1965
..Lighting cane, Paul Otto Mross, Gelsenkirchen, Erle, #1954 125, Jan. 12, 1966
..Cane handle with lighting device, Helmut Starke, Langenberg, #1 955 064, Nov. 26, 1966
..Cane with light (on bottom), Helmut Tkatz, Berlin, #1 298 687, May 10, 1967
..Cane with built-in light to light end of cane itself, Stefan Maier, Aach., #1972 162, June 17, 1967
..Safety cane with lighted shaft, Manfred Kunzel,Pinneberg, #198 537, Jan. 1, 1968

..Interchangeable, automatic light & alarm knob (handle) for umbrellas & canes, Helmut Tkatz, Berlin, #66 01 622, March 12, 1968

..Cane with lighting device in shaft or handle, Helmut starke, Langenberg, #1991 652, April 17, 1968

..Cane with light in handle, Rudolf Lochner, Munich, #675 51513, Nov. 9, 1968

..Seat cane with light, stand, etc., Johannes - Filippou, Hamburg, #6921683, May 30, 1969

..Lightable cane, Hugo Hable, Regensburg, #6904 512, June 2, 1969

..Cane with lighting device at front & rear of cane handle & in interior of shaft, Schenk, Gerhard, Schenk geb. Laege, Elfriede, Berlin, #7301866, Jan. 16, 1973

..Cane light, Hans Guntner, Freilassing, #7305329 Feb. 13, 1973

..Cane with light at bottom & battery in handle, Michael Wagner, Herrenberg, #7310739, March 21, 1973

..Safety cane for disabled, with light on outside & inside shaft & special ferrule, Wilhelm Falkenstein, Zimmer, Mattias, #79 34 514, Oct. 15, 1974

..Blinking & signal light cane for blind, etc., Edmund Metze, Berlin, #75 07519, March 11, 1973

..Lighting cane for disabled, Willi Wodniczak, Iggersheim Aktenzeichen, #P2536651.2, Aug. 16, 1975

..Signal & lighting walking cane for the disabled, on bottom, Bernt Westarp, Wuppertel, #7604 457 Feb. 14 1976

..Cane with electric light in handle, Johannes Heggemann, Hoxter, # 7638 27 8, Dec. 7, 1976, & April 21, 1977

..Cane with electrical light, Maximillian Pritzl, Munich, #7638178, #2655215, Dec. 12, 1976

..Warning light cane for blind, Joseph Widmer, Rumlang (Switzerland), #77 09 703, March 28, 1977

..Cane with electric light in handle, Helmut Tkatz, Berlin, #P2719322, April 27, 1977, & Nov. 2, 1978

..Crutch cane with light, Hans Kuhne, Offenbach, #77 35 591, Nov. 21, 1977

..Device to produce light effects on textiles, clothing, & decorative materials (cane?), Heinz Pape, Munich, #P2949901.2, Dec. 12, 1979, No details or drawings

..Safety cane with built-in signal light, Jacob Puscher, Rosengarten, #81 30 275, Oct. 16, 1981

Invalid & crutch canes & attachments thereto:

..Crutch cane consisting of two articulated, jointed components, Hermann Praedel, Mikultschutz, #283037, Feb. 22, 1914

..Walking cane for war veteran, injured, and the blind, (contains a light), Otto Paufler, Philadelphia, Pa., U.S.A. #387717, Oct. 5, 1922

..Cane or crutch especially designed for the sight or walking disabled, Walter Wittke, Hamburg, #891602, Feb. 27, 1949

..Cane for disabled, Fritz Wening, Vreden (Westf.) #1754108. April 20, 1957

..Crutch cane for disabled, with anti-slip bottom & warning blink light, Hans Schollhammer & Karl Scheiblehner, Steyr (Austria), #1880 713, May 21, 1962

..Signal light cane for the disabled, Helmut Tkatz, Berlin, Charlottenburg, #1856 222, March 20, 1962

..Safety crutch cane, Max Emil Kasper, Wehr, #P 2 314 510, March 28, 1973, No details or drawings

..Wheeled cane for the disabled, Hubert Adolf Laufer, Harsewinkel, #7434514, Oct. 15, 1974

..Springed ice spear in ferrule for canes for disabled, Willi Klossek, Basse Aktenzeichen, #25494706, Nov. 11, 1975

..Walking support which can be adjusted lengthwise, Ortopedia Gmb H, Kiel, #P28228504, May 24, 1978, No details or drawings

..Walking support, John William Kennott Marsh, Fawkham, Dartford, Kent, United Kingdom, #P3010 901.4, March 21, 1980, No details or drawings

..Wheeled safety canes for the blind, Manfred Seichter, Hamburg, Aktenzeichen: P29075307, Anmeldetag: Feb. 26, 1979, Offenlegungstag: Sept. 4, 1980

..Bottom part for safety canes -crutches, Holger G. Weber, Konstanz, #P30 39324.9, Oct. 17, 1980 No details or drawings

..Ball bearing for walking cane, crutches, etc., Josef Lottner, Koln, P3102 868.3-35, Jan. 29, 1981

..Ball bearing for walking cane, crutch, etc. Josef Lottner, Koln, P3117 614.3-35, May 5, 1981

..Cane for hiking, strolling, or for the disabled, Gastroch - Stocke GmbH, Bad Sooden - Allendorf #82 07180, March 13, 1982

Lifting Canes:

..Cane with lifting device, May & Grammelspacher, Rastatt (Baden), #72531, Feb. 4, 1893

..Cane with lifting device, Wilhelm Beyer, Bielefeld, #71069, Dec. 23, 1892

Liquid carrying & dispensing & drinking canes:

..Syringe cane, Hugo Alisch, Berlin, #5683, Dec. 11, 1878

..Spray cane, Willie Trappen, Geldern, #8108813, March 26, 1981

..Seat cane with drinking device, Michael Flurscheim, Eisenwerk, Gaggenau in Gaggenau (Baden) #24515, March 7, 1883

..Safety closure for liquids on atomisers in cane handles, Robert Becker, Berlin, #33109, Nov. 15, 1884

..Syringe or squirt cane (tin handle), Eisenwerke Gaggenau, Flurscheim & Bergmann, Gaggenau (baden) #34124, May 20, 1885

..Liquid absorbing cane (for emptying drink glasses, etc., sucks up thru end of crook handle & stores in cane), Jon Karl Hausmann, Cochem, #42984, Oct. 14, 1887

..Cane capable of holding liquids and whose handle contains a drinking vessel, Hugo Windmuller and Max Keffel, Berlin, #64321, Dec. 20, 1891

..Cane with drinking vessel, E. Honold, Stolberg, (Rheinland) #63678, Feb. 9, 1892

..Hand operated device for the measured distribution of liquids (cane?), Friedrich Wehde, Bomlitz, #P2610724, March 13, 1976, No details or drawings

..Device for distribution of liquids, especially suited for blood tracks on the floor, Friedrich Wehde, Bomlitz, #P2649475, Oct. 29, 1976, No details or drawings

Locking devices & identifications on canes to prevent their theft or loss:

..Cane or umbrella handle with suspension device to hand same, Jacques Muller, Berlin, #109778, April 28, 1899

..Fastening device for attaching umbrellas & canes to pockets of clothing, etc., A. Werner, Dusseldorf, #120890, March 30, 1900

..Cane or umbrella handle with locking device, L. Barth, Jr., Leipzig, #131017, May 3, 1900

..Locks to attach to and for securing canes, and umbrellas, Wilhelm Bernhard, Frankfurt, a.M., #129732, May 9, 1901

..Locking handle to prevent loss or theft of umbrella or cane, Leopold Levinger, Nurnberg, #159586, Aug. 14, 1903

..Holding hook for umbrellas, canes, etc., which when in repose lies hidden in the cane, Franz Rothe, Langenleuba, Niederhain, S.A. #172743, Jan. 14, 1905

..Protective device against theft of umbrellas, canes, etc., Rudolf Lack, Olten, Schweiz,

#264171, Feb. 27, 1912

..Attachment to, for holding canes & umbrellas, Paul Thomke, Aleksandrowice b. Bielsko (Bielitz), Poland, #503168, April 28, 1928

..Rollup security chain & catch in cane handle to prevent loss thereof, Christoph Reiff, Frankfurt, a.M., #527111, July 2, 1930

..Security or protective device for cane or umbrella, Christoph Reiff, Frankfurt a.M., #549997, April 21, 1932

..Address tag for umbrellas and canes, etc., Carl Heinz Bruckhoff, Offenbach/Main, #1969 230, April 13, 1967

..Umbrella with identification on handle, Hugendubel Co. Stuttgart, #7336988, Oct. 13, 1973

Magnetic supporting or adhering devices for canes:

..Magnetic supporting or adhering device for canes, Arno Ehrhardt, Arno #78 30371, Oct. 12, 1978

Measuring guage, & level canes:

..Cane with slide caliper rule, (handle slides open) Fuchs, Biberach a.d. Riss. #53033, Dec. 29, 1889

..Compass cane for making circles, Paul Schiweck, Zessel b. Oels I. Schl. #114572, Jan. 31, 1900

..Thermometer cane, Johan Dixner, Stockholm, #139586, April 15, 1902

..Measuring stick cane, Wilhelm Nestle, and Herman Nestle, Dornstetten, (Wurtt.) #161039, July 28, 1904

..Cane with measuring device for measuring thickness of trees, Fritz Knobiel, Neu Sussemilken b. Alten Sussemilken, Ostpr- #32885, June 27, 1918

..Caliper, Compass, (Circle Making) & measuring cane, Reinhold Seidler, Oberrossau b. Mittweida i. Sa. #383807, May 22, 1921

..Cane slide rule, (for measuring logs) Heinrich de Jong, Bochum #28683, March 25, 1824

Medicinal cane:

..Tubular insert, containing medicine vials for canes, Amin Aaly al Omari, Berlin, Schweiz, #311240, Oct. 9, 1917

Miscellaneous unclassified canes:

..Cane, Friedrich Ulrich, Durnenzimmern bei Nordlingen #1936 122, Jan. 19, 1966

..Cane, Margareta Brandl geb. Henning, Bebra, #1 943 022, June 1, 1966

..Walking cane unit, Blasius Speidel, Jungingen, #P2360 067, Dec. 1, 1973, No details or drawings

Mountain climbing canes:

..Mountain cane which can be transformed into an ice pick or spade, Anton Schiebel, Wangen i. Allgau, #391028, July 1, 1922

..Tourist umbrella, which can be disassembled into an ice pick, etc., and packed in a knapsack, Rudolf Franz Ullmann, Vienna, #399970, July 26, 1926

..Seat cane and for tracking, mountaineering, aiming and hunting, Kurt von Kaneke, Bad Doberan, Mecklbg, and carl hermann Eichhorn, Rostook, #481826, May 8, 1928

..Multipurpose cane with billard cue, saw blade, flag, knife convertible to lance, or mountain climbing, etc., Chin-Tui Kuo, Taichung, Nsi Tun District Taiwan, #8130208. Oct. 16, 1981

Optical canes, binocular, telescope, etc.,:

..Telescope cane, Franz Hoen, Bulach, Switzerland, #253986, Nov. 14, 1911

..Handle doubling as binoculars for canes, umbrellas, etc., Wladyslaw Bilinski, Warsaw, #254562, Dec. 21, 1911
..Telescope cane (Optical) J.T.F. Conti, and A.P.J. Masson, Paris #272619, June 2, 1912
..Cane with built-in binoculars in handle, Ernst Katscher, Bremen, #514769, Dec. 12, 1929

Pen and ink cane:

..Pen and ink cane, Friedrich Bruckner, Frankfurt, a.M. #59469, Jan. 30, 1891

Plaques & Shields for canes:

..Plaque for canes, Arno Wallpach, Salzach/Osterreich, #1 951 233, Oct. 13, 1966
..Cane Shield (Nagel), Max Bohlinger, Kempton Allg. #69 06 614, Feb. 20, 1969

Radio canes:

..Radio cane with built-in microtransister with Battery (Germanium -Dioden) or Ferruginous Core with or without battery, Erwin Koch, Munchen, #1783 336, Dec. 12, 1958
..Radio cane with transistors, Erwin Koch, Munchen, #1830 126 Feb. 3, 1961
..Radio & loud speaker (battery operated) umbrella handle, Antonio Veggetti, Pforzheim, #80 13 541, May 20, 1980

Raincoat cane:

..Cane containing a raincoat, Walter Grunwald, I and Erna Grundwald, geb. Stade, Riesenburg, Westpr., #458915, May 18, 1927

Riding crop cane:

..Cane or riding crop, Metallechlauchfabrik, Pforzheim, vorm. HeH. Witzehmann, G.m.B.H., Pforzheim #252533, Dec. 10, 1910 9

Saw canes:

..Cane saw, Gerhard Janensch, Charlottenburg, #364544, Dec. 7, 1921
..An extendable cane with a saw on end, Hans Friemann, Gaisthal, Oberpfalz, #477338, Sept. 22, 1928 35

Seat canes:

..Seat cane, Robert Sieber, Zeitz #6989, Feb. 9, 1879
..Cane hunting seat, Gottlieb van Meenen, Koln, a.Rh. #10968, March 12, 1880
..Umbrella cane able to be elongated to serve as a support, Felix Prager, Liegnitz, #13873, Oct. 19, 1880
..Seat cane, Julius Unger, Cannstatt, (Wurttemberg) #21613, May 31, 1882
..Hunting and travel seat cane, G. Heinze, Langenoels, bei Lauban, #20413, June 8, 1882
..Folding Campstool cane, Wilhelm Walcker, Paris, #22107, Oct. 3, 1882
..Improvement of previous seat cane #10,968, H. Emil Wurmbach, Herborn, an der Koln-Giessener Bahn, #23824, Dec. 10, 1882
..Seat cane with drinking device, Michael Flurscheim, Eisenwerk, Gaggenau in Gaggenau (Baden) #24515, March 7, 1883
..Hunting and travel seat cane, G. Heinze, Langenoel s bei Lauban, #24521, April 10, 1883
..Hunting seat cane, Johs Olshausen, Hamburg, #25228, July 1, 1883
..Cane which can be used as a four-footed chair with back rest, Sigmung Scharfberg and Heinrich Sanft, Berlin, #26861, Oct. 25, 1883
..Seat cane, Carl Friedrich Queiser, Ziegenhain, (Provinz Hessen-Nassaul #27103, Nov. 15, 1883

..Hunting seat cane, Otto Schulz, Plagwitz bei Leipzig, #29428, June 1, 1884
..Combination camp bed & came chair cane, Anton Luger, Vienna, #31869, Sept. 16, 1884
..Seat cane, Franz Fischer, Berlin, #31142, Nov. 2, 1884
..Seat cane, Wilhelm Bachmann, Nurnberg, #31684, Nov. 5, 1884
..Hunting seat cane, Ferdinand Alff, Taben a.d. Saar, #40973, April 6, 1887
..Umbrella seat cane, C. Steiner, Leipzig, #40975, April 16, 1887
..Seat cane, C.F. Winter, Cudowa Kreis Glatz, #44777, Jan. 3, 1888
..Combination cane, Carl Luckat, Berlin, #49568, Oct. 14, 1888
..Seat cane, Franz Graf Zedtwitz, Liebensteine, bei Eger, #63550, Oct. 2, 1891
..Seat cane, Paul Tumena and Albert Gerths, Barmen, #65149, Oct. 14, 1891
..Stool Cane, Engelbert Clever, Coln, a. Rh. #64757, Dec. 19, 1891
..Seat cane, Otto Schwartz, Munich, #66423, April 14, 1892
..Stool Cane, Heinrich Schmoll, Berlin #74563, Feb. 7, 1893
..Height adjustable hunting seat cane, Oscar Nauen, Koslin, #75220, Nov. 5, 1893
..Hunting cane with vertically adjustable seat, Emil Keller, Wetzlar, #80680, July 27, 1894
..Cane Changeable into a hunting chair with rifle support, Frederick Seeger and Dr. Leo, Luben, #82806, Feb. 22, 1895
..Seat cane, Matthaus Sewina, Breslau #86186, July 9, 1895
..Chair cane, Heinz, Behrens, Hamburg, #92845, Sept. 8, 1896
..Seat cane, Joseph Poralla, Beuthen, Oberschlesien, #94195, Jan. 1, 1897
..Chair cane, Max Ruckdeschel and Albin Mockel, Adorf, #97023, Aug. 22, 1897
.. Hunting seat cane, Hugo Berthold, Rothenfeldel b. Osnabruck, #106239, Nov.1, 1898
..Seat cane, Carl Oswald Beyer, Obernhau, i.S. #98206, Nov. 27, 1897
..Hunting cane which can be disassembled and whose handle can be used as a seat, Eduard Otto, Hohenlimburg I.W., #124484, Oct. 10, 1900
..Cane converting into a 3 legged camp stool, Edward Bonnes, Christiana, #126129, Nov. 28, 1900
..Folding campstool cane, Jay Kyle Sheffy, Chicago, USA. #125930, Dec. 21, 1900
..Hunting seat cane, C. Stolze and C. Sebbesse, Aschersleben, #127981, Jan. 26, 1901
..Seat cane, Heinrich Gerigk, Johannisburg, Ostpr. #132550, June 26, 1901
..Cane stool, M. Schaede, Saalfeld, A.S., #130357, July 21, 1901
..Hunting seat cane, Aschersleben, #129318, Sept. 15, 1901
..Hunting and tourist cane with a curved handle which when parted lengthwise can be transformed into a seat, Peter Meyer, Coln- Nippes, #175482, Jan. 17, 1904
..Seat cane, Gustav Adolf Strecker, Hamburg, #164444, May 25, 1904
..Hunting seat cane, with removable folding seat, Carl Jahn, Dusseldorf, #165912, Sept. 9, 1904
..Hollow stem seat cane holding its parts, George Starck, Weingarten, Rheinpf, #164808, Dec. 3, 1904
..Umbrella which can be transformed into a chair with back rest, Louis Hunke, Munster, I.W., #169047, March 22, 1905
..Folding three legged pocket or cane stool, Carl Erwin Bruchheuser, Coln. A. Rh. #169090, May 25, 1905
..Travel device useable as a cane, umbrella and Stool, Karl Bachle, Wiesbaden, #170410, June 16, 1905
..Hunting seat cane whose seat handle can be taken off or tightened, August Muller and Heinrich Muller, Witzenhausen, #176852, Sept. 14, 1905

..Seat cane, Johann Karl Kohler, Chorlottenburg, #190488, April 8, 1906
..Cane chair, Adolf Hauszmann, Waldheim, B. Tachau, i. Bohmen, #191679, Oct. 18, 1906
..Cane Stool, Stanislaw Pankowski, Krakow, #188196, Dec. 20, 1906
..Seat for hunting canes, Wilhelm Schocke, and Dr. Heinrich Schweiter, Cassel, #19279 1, Jan. 18, 1907
..Hunting cane seat, Armin Becke, Muhlhausen, i. Th. #199985, July 5, 1907
..Folding hunting seat cane, Wilhelm Schocke, cassel, #197558, Sept. 13, 1907
..Hunting seat cane, Heinrich Buszemeier, Brake, i. Lippe, #219013, Feb. 14, 1908
..Hunting seat cane containing a telephone instrument in its seat capable of making contact with overhead wires, Joseph Strecker, Grottkau, #204490, March 18, 1908
..Hunting seat cane, Gerhard Baron, Campenhausen, Sassenhof b. Riga, #204625, March 28, 1908
..Hunting stool cane, Ludwig Frauenstorfer, Mannheim, #212799, Nov. 24, 1908
..Cane Stool, Philipp Fuhr and Adam Werner, Laudenbach, Baden, #219853, Dec. 5, 1908
..Seat cane, Otto Koch, Berlin, #227831, May 18, 1909
..Seat cane, August Stauber, Zurich, #233694, Feb. 5, 1910
..Seat cane, Charles Vernet, Dinan, Cotes du Nord. #235678, April 27, 1910
..Hunting seat cane, Otto Koch, Berlin, #235272, May 18, 1909, July 21, 1910 & May 17, 1924
..Hunting cane with claw handle, whose halves can be opened into a seat, Peter Meyer, Coln-Nippes, #244176, May 10, 1911
..Camp Stool cane, Gotthard Nauke, Czerwicka, O-Schl. #239848, Nov. 29, 1911
..Seat cane with a simultaneous driving momentum of the seat braces, Wilhelm Hensche, Elberfeld, #264693, June 9, 1912
..Seat cane, Charles Jaquet, Staszburg, Konigshofen, Els., #258394, June 15, 1912
..Hunting seat cane, which can be transformed into a tree stand, Ludwig Hambek, Zierdorf, Nied.- Osterr, #286577, June 18, 1914
..Cane stool, Rudolf Kohn, Marienbad, #315275, Nov. 16, 1917
..Cane with folding removable hunting seat, Erich Wahls, Brohm b. Friedland, Meckl, - Strelitz, #335384, Dec. 23, 1919
..Hollow cane which can be transformed into a three legged seat, Walter H. Thielemaan, Hamburg, #339271, Jan. 16, 1920
..Hunting seat cane consisting of one central and two side staffs, Herman Gradewalk, Magdeburg Buckau, #349690, May 8, 1920
..Crutch cane with attachable sitting device, Carl Hausmann, Glucksburg, Ostsee., #388883, Aug. 22, 1922
..Crutch cane with sitting device, Hugo Jellen, Carmerau b. Vossowska, O. -Schl. #393577. Dec. 12, 1922
..Cane stool, Crutch handle splits in two to make seat, Rudolf Dummler, Weimar, #42454, Oct. 4, 1924
..Cane or umbrella which is vertically divided and bolted together and can be changed to a sitting support, Ernst Buz, Sonnenberg, Thur. (Addition to Patent #462,433), #484920, Nov. 22, 1925
..Cane stool, Karl Kucera, Konigsberg, Schles, Czechoslovakia, #494905, Sept. 11, 1927
..Seat cane and for tracking, mountaineering, aiming and hunting, Kurt von Kaneke, Bad Doberan, Necklbg. and Carl Hermann, Eichhorn, Rostock, #481826, May 8, 1928
..Seat, umbrella, & Tripod cane, Edgar Mohry, Gleiwitz, #511591, June 14, 1928
..Seat cane or umbrella, Ernst Buz, Sonneberg, Thur. #46243 3, June 21, 1928
..Seat cane with bottom plate to prevent sinking into ground and with ball bearing swivel,

George Rothenberger, Obersontheim, Wurttbg. #468830, Nov. 8, 1928
..Stool cane, Otto Metzner, Chemnitz, #531638, April 5, 1929
..Hunting seat cane, Hermann Tambornino, Essen, #503016, Nov. 22, 1929
..Hunting seat cane whose handle splits in half to form a seat, Franz Bahr, Vienna, #547136, March 10, 1932
..Cane or umbrella seat, Hanz Schmitz, Aachen, #549748, April 14, 1932
..Cane or umbrella seat, Hans Schmitz, Aachen, #597,933, Addition to 549748, Aug. 16, 1932
..Cane or umbrella seat, Hans Schmitz, Aachen, #608916, Aug. 16, 19322
..Sitting cane, the sitting surface of which consists of webbing pulled out of the hollow staff and hangs between 2 spread parts of disassembled staff, Gustav Welp, Bielefeld -Sieker, #618340, May 13, 1934
..Seat cane, Sophie Noe geb. Neumeyer, Hannover, #629386, Oct. 28, 1934
..Seat cane, Sophie Noe geb. Neumeyer, Hannover, #645191, March 8, 1935
..Hunting seat cane and aiming cane, Herman Muller, Berlin -Baumschulenweg. #611516, March 14, 1935
..Seat cane, Heinrich Ottemeier, Lage, Lippe, #621994, Oct. 31, 1935
..Seat cane, Franz Hecker, Paderborn, #700599, July 18, 1936
..Hunting seat cane, Fritz Trautwein, Freiburg, Breisgau, #69 7278, July 6, 1938
..Hunting seat and aiming cane, Hermann Wandrey, Landsberg, Warthe, #690071, Nov. 10, 1938
..Hunting seat cane, whose seat can be folded and detached, Joseph Hillemeyer, Neuhaus, Kr. Paderborn, #700293, March 16, 1939
..Hunting seat cane with inner umbrella and folding seat, Karl Schrader and Dr. Hermann Lussenhop, Hamburg, #706 463, Sept. 16, 1939
..Cane, the handle of which folds out into a seat, Karl Siegel, Erda (Kr. Wetzlar) #811859, July 22, 1949
..Seat cane, Heinrich Steinhauer, Hennef/Sieg. #830 553, July 12, 1950
..Umbrella stool, Paul Klingbeil, Emden, # 89 80 70, July 28, 1951
..Cane support for sitting or standing, Georg Mann, Blaubeuren, #1771 167, May 31, 1958
..Seat cane, Dr. med. Karl Donges, Remscheid, #1777 973, Sept. 24, 1958
..Seat cane, Carsten Andersen, Sollerup uber Schleswig, #1785 714, Dec. 24, 1958
..One legged flexible seat cane with a rubber rod instead of a spiral spring, Heinz Hover, Runderoth - Ohl (Brz. Koln), #1808407, Oct. 10, 1959
..Seat cane (handle splits) with spring, Felix Sonnberger, Wurtzburg, #1968 255, June 29, 1967
..Seat cane - leather expandable seat pulls out of shaft & opens, Helmut Tkatz, Berlin, #1986 645, March 12, 1968
..Multipurpose cane -seat, umbrella, et., Frederich Walter Schmitz Garmisch - Parten Kirchen, #67 50499, Aug. 1, 1968
..Adjustable height seat cane for hunters, fishermen, etc., Hans Klug. Tauberbischofsheim, #6920 290 May 20, 1969
..Seat cane with light, stand, etc., Johannes Filippou, Hamburg, #6921683, May 30, 1969
..Folding seat cane for hunters, fishermen etc., Firma Wilhelm Meyer, Nurnberg, #69 365 565, Sept. 18, 1969
..Seat cane for hunters, fishermen, etc., Hans Klug, Tauberbischofsheim, #7333664, Sept. 17, 1973
..Cane with molded seat, Wolfgang Koppl, Nurnberg, #77 19675, June 23, 1977
..Seat cane for sport & hiking, Hans Klug, Tauberbischofsheim, #7736066, Nov. 25, 1977
..Seat cane, Heinrich Muller, Koln, #7900805,

Jan. 13, 1979
..Seat cane, Gunter Richter, Dortmund, & Hanno Bauer, Manheim, & Gerd Drespa. Dartmund, Aktenzeichen P 2748104,0, Ammeldung, Aug. 24, 1977, Offenlegungstag, March 1, 1979 115
..Strapped seat cane (Bipod), Joachim Mattulke, Garmisch -Partenkirchen, #7921021, July 23, 1979
..Emergency seat cane, Ernst Vogt -Spaltenstein, Effretikon, Zurich, (Switzerland) #7929513, Oct. 18, 1979
..Folding chair cane, Erwin Mittich, Munich, #7931450, Nov. 7, 1979
..Seat cane, Otto Behrendt, Haan, Akrenzeichen: #P 2931547.7, Ammeldetag: Aug. 3, 1979 Oftenlegungstag: Feb. 19, 1981

Shovel canes:

..Mountain cane which can be transformed into an ice pick or spade, Anton Schiebel, Wangen i. Allgau., #391028, July 1, 1922
..Shovel cane, Robert Ebert; Theodor Katz, Darmstadt, #7641222, Dec. 28, 1976 & Aug. 4, 1977

Smoking canes, match, lighters, pipes, Cigarettes, Humidors, etc.:

..Smoking pipe cane, August Ritter, Meerane, (Sachsen), #9762, Sept. 28, 1879
..Cigar & pipe cane, Louis Kronenberger, Hanau, #12603, July 3, 1880
..Cane & Tobacco pipe, F. Laesecke, Leipsig, #16999, June 30, 1881
..Umbrella useable as a walking stick, whose cane part serves as a container for a pipe which makes the handle, Carl Sondermann Niedersessmar, (Rheinpr.) #19710, April 28, 1882
..Umbrella which can be used as a cane & whose cane part serves as a container for a pipe, Carl Sondermann, Niedersessman, (Rhein Provinz) #23772, March 13, 1883
..Attachment on canes and umbrellas to hold, save or dispose of burning cigars, and cigarettes, Peter Schiffer, Crefeld, and Wilhelm Nisges, Osterrath, #292928, Oct. 9, 1915
..Cane smoking pipe, O. Sonnenbrodt, Pasewalk, #56567, April 19, 1890
..Tobacco pipe cane, H. Wimmel, Cassel, #76726, March 9, 1894
..Cane or umbrella handle to hold smoking paraphernalia, etc., Seb. Maier and Aug. Fischer, Schwab, Gmund, #111080, April 2, 1899
..Cane or umbrella handle as a smoking implement container, Seb. Maier and Aug. Fischer, Schwab, Gmund, #116221, Nov. 7, 1899
..Water Pipe cane, Sejed Ali Mohammed Khan, Temple (Grfsch, London) #130011, July 23, 1901
..Cane with cigar cutter beneath handle & in shaft, Alfred Volkmann, Hamburg, #267146, Feb. 8, 1913
..Cane containing handlamp, battery, cigar lighter, cigar cutter and container for the cut off pieces, August Muller, Berlin -Pankow, #285541, May 15, 1914
..Cane holding cigarettes in shaft & capable of being raised to and dispensed from top, Edouard Francois Michel Decobert, Paris, #511590, July 24, 1928
..Cane smoking pipe, Karl Fickenwirth and Frederich Kolbel, Lengenfeld i. Vgtl. #376044, Oct. 1, 1920
..Cigar or cigaret lighter cane, Aniceto R. Visitation, William Weigel and Louis G. Weigel, New York, #578025, Jan. 29, 1931

Sound Producing canes:

..Cane & umbrella knob with mechanical device -bell, R. Turck, Ludenscheid, #7049, Jan. 23, 1879
..Siren handle cane or umbrella, Max Blau, Berlin, #40773, Feb. 25, 1887

..Sound producing cane, Carl Amm, Forchheim (OFr.) #1789 700, March 6, 1959
..Interchangeable, Automatic light & alarm knob, (handle) for umbrellas & canes, Helmut Tkatz, Berlin, #66 01 622, March 12, 1968
..Cane with warning alarm system for day or night, Kurt Neumann, Watzenborn, steinberg, #70 03 368, Jan. 31, 1970

Spring canes:

..Spring cushioned cane, Bruno Ruthel, Burggrumbach, b. Wurzburg, #624246, Dec. 24, 1935

Table canes:

..Table cane, Otto Kuhl, Altona, #57128, Sept. 23, 1890
..Table cane, Rudolph Kroll, Zehlendorf bei Berlin, #63925, Feb. 14, 1892
..Cane which can be unfolded & spread into a table, seat, etc., Rudolf Kohn, Berlin, #453999, June 26, 1925
..Cane convertible to tripod for cameras, telescopes, tables, & with removable handle for same, Erich Gathwohl, Wesel, #   March 11, 1969

Telephone - hunting canes:

..Hunting seat cane containing a telephone instrument in its seat capable of making contact with over head wires, Joseph Strecker, Grottkau, #204490, March 18, 1908

Toiletry cane:

..Insert for canes to hold toiletry articles, etc., Paul Kampfe, Dresden, #67552, Sept. 22, 1892

Tool box canes:

..Cane containing file, screwdriver, wrench, chisel & other tools, Juan Lopez, Malaga, Spain, #381199, Oct. 6, 1922

Tripod or stand canes:

..Tripod cane capable of holding hats or other things, Johann Stoecker, Elberfeld, #62253, Aug 19, 1891
..Cane containing a tripod, Firma Rob. Tummler, Dobeln, S.A. #531637, March 18, 1930
..Cane convertible to tripod for cameras, telescopes, tables & with removable handle for same, Erich Gathwohl, Wesel, #   , March 11, 1969
..Seat cane with light, stand, etc., Johannes Filippou, Hamburg, #6921683, May 30, 1969
..Cane or umbrella camera stand, George Schwefess, Bielefeld, #74 32 707, Sept. 28, 1974
..Camera or telescope monopod cane, Albrecht Hagmayer, Ulm, #76 33 236, Oct. 23, 1976

Umbrella canes & cane umbrellas:

..Umbrella cane, Hugo Parnemann, Elberfeld, #8919, Sept. 12, 1879
..Umbrella which when closed becomes a cane, W. Loewenthal, Brieg (Reg. Bez. Breslau), #24756, Oct. 31, 1882
..Folding umbrella mechanism, which can be mounted on any cane, Carl Zimmermann, Dorotheendorf, O.S. & Oscar Gaertig, Zaborze, O.S. #136429, Feb. 23, 1902
..Umbrella which can be transformed into a simple cane by removing umbrella mechanism and corer, "Kronprinz" Aktiengesellschaft fur Metall industrie, Ohligs, #157158. April 3, 1903
..Travel device useable as a cane, umbrella, and stool, Karl Bachle, Wiesbaden, #170410, June 16, 1905

..Umbrella which can be transformed into a cane by a metal covering, Hans Denkmann, Helmstedt, #190807, Aug. 16, 1906
..Hunting cane opening into a fan-shaped umbrella, VonSchmeling, Potsdam, #216355, July 18, 1908
..Umbrella mechanism that can be mounted on a cane, Antonin Drahorad, Kittenberg, Bohmen, #232949, May 5, 1909
..Umbrella with hollow staff containing a cane, Alfred Alvers, Ahlen, I.W., #306024, Sept. 9, 1916
..Fastening device for umbrella mechanism, so it can be mounted on a cane, Lisbeth Orzegowski geb. Hoffman, Berlin, #397341, July 12, 1922
..Tourist umbrella, which can be disassembled into a tourist cane, ice pick, etc., and packed in a knapsack, Rudolf Franz ullmann, Vienna, #399970, July 26, 1926
..Cane convertable to a stand or an umbrella, Peter July, Oberehe, Post Dreis, Kn Daum, #538487, Oct. 29, 1931

..Cane with umbrella in shaft, Julius Richter, Zittau, #700266, Sept. 5, 1936
..Mountain cane with removeable umbrella, Suddeutsche Shirmfabrik, J. Becker, Munich, #6751914, July 26, 1968
..Multipurpose cane, Seat, umbrella, etc., Frederich Walter Schmitz Garmisch Partan Kirchen, #67 50499, Aug. 1, 1968

Weapon canes:

..Combination cane, dagger (in bottom) & Mountain cane, Michael Flurscheim, Eisenwerk, Gaggenau, #21619, Aug. 8, 1882
..Cudgel cane, cat o nine tails, Eisenwerke Gaggenau, Florscheim & Bergmann, Gaggenau (Baden) #34898, Oct. 2, 1885
..A weapon cane to catch and hold a fleeing person's legs, N. Heisdorf, Bad Ems, #194826, May 23, 1907

..Cane with knife or bayonet blade concealed in bottom of the stick (for army use), Julius Schroder, Celle, #306794, March 11, 1917
..Cane containing a knife or bayonet & (sawblade)-(for army use), Albert Mathe'e, G.m.b.H. Aachen, #306167, Sept. 18, 1917
..Multipurpose cane with flag, knife convertible to lance, or mountain climbing, etc., Chin-Tue Kuo, Taichung, Hsi Tun District Taiwan, #8130208, Oct. 16, 1981

Wheelbarrow canes:

..Wheelbarrow cane or luggage cart, Gottschalk Herzberger, Berlin, #72761, Jan. 31, 1893

Bibliography

Though canes were at one time very common and gadget canes are now considered rare, a surprising amount of material has been written about them. I enclose a most exhaustive up-to-date bibliography covering not only books, but periodicals which over the years I have compiled with the assistance of the late Theo Fossel, founder and former president of the British Stickmakers Guild.

The author acknowledges the contributions made herein by the late Theo Fossel, founder and former president of the British Stickmaker's Guild.

Early Lighting, a Pictorial Guide. Rushlite Club, 1972.
"Stick Dressing Exhibition." *Laing Art Gallery, Newcastle upon Tyne* (Dec. 1967).
Schirm Stock und Steiger. Fa. Steiger, Basel Switzerland (1987).
"Brollies, Bumbers, Blackthorns." *Gourmet* (March 1987).
"Canes, Walking Sticks and Poison Bottles." *Derbibooks, Inc.* (1974).
"Collecting Canes." *Rotarian* 71:60 (Oct. 1947).
"Curious Canes (Exhibit at the Cooper-Hewitt)." *American Craft* 43:36-7 (Aug./Sept. 1983).
"Curiosities of Walking Sticks." *Every Saturday* 11:119 (1871).
"La Canne, Artifice d'orfeverie precieuse." *Europa Star*. (Autumn 1980).
"In The Driftway." *The Nation* (June 24, 1934).
"Walking Sticks." *Chambers Edinburgh Journal* 39:12 (1862).
"Walking Sticks." *Chambers Edinburgh Journal* (May 1893): 330.
"Walking Stick Factory." *Chambers Edinburgh Journal* 48:81 (Feb. 11, 1871).
"Lincoln's Hickory Walking Stick." *Hobbies* 60:50 (May 1955).
"Old Walking Sticks." *Hobbies* 53:33 (Sep. 1948).
"Political Cane-Head Busts." *The Spinning Wheel* (Oct. 1953).
"Presidential Campaign Buttons, etc." *The Spinning Wheel* (Nov. 19, 1961).
"A Strange Wepon of a Century Ago." *Hobbies* (March 1937).
"Surgeon Urges Return of Walking Canes." *Science News Letter* 69:88 (Feb. 1956).
"Walking Cane's Return to Popularity Urged." *Science Digest* 39:49 (May 1956).
"Walking Hours." *Leisure Hour*. 2:525 (1853).
"The Lost Walking Stick." *London Magazine* 10:617.
"Los Domingos de ABC." *Una Collection de Bostones.* (Aug. 9, 1970). "Sticks, Historical & Contemporary Kentucky Canes." *The Kentucky Art & Craft Foundation*, 1988.
"Stick and Umbrella News." 1892 - 97.
"Bag, Portmanteau & Umbrella Trader." The Bag Trader Publishing Co., 1898.
"Shooting Sticks." *High-Gun Fieldsports, Ltd. Catalogue.* (1988)
"L'Uomo A Tre Gambe." *Antiquariato* (Summer 1980).
"In the Driftway." *Nation* 132:679 (June 24, 1931).
"Eighteenth Century Cane." *Antiques* 64:304 (Oct. 1953).
"Exhibition of Canes & Walking Sticks." *Cooper-Hewitt Newsletter* (Spring 1983).
"Hobby Hitching Post: Collecting Canes." *Rotarian* 71:60 (Oct. 1947).
"Hobbyhorse Hitching Post." *Rotarian* 55:67 (Oct. 1939).
"Walking-Sticks and How to Treat Them." *The Boys Own Paper* (1884).

"Assassination by Umbrella." *Chicago Tribune* (Oct. 1, 1978).
"Where There's Wood, There's A Crafty Way to Use It." *Choice Magazine* (April 1990).
"The Man Who Makes Shepherd Crooks." *Country Bazaar, Vol. 2 No. 9* (Spring 1984).
"Modern Stick Making." *Shooting Times* (Jul. 22 1982).
"Tsue (The Walking Stick)." *Fighters-Martial Arts Magazine* (May 1985).
"Fred Pricket: Master Ornamental Stick Maker." *Marshall Cavendish* (1981).
"The Jersey Giant Cabbage." *L'Etacq Woodrafts*. 1985.
Darstellung der Feldzuege d. Prinzen Eugen von Savoyen K.K. Kreigs- Archiv; Abt.f.Kriegsgeschichte (1876).
"Robbie Little and his Scottish Crooks." *Lands' End Catalogue* (Dec. 1990).
"Uses of the Scout Stave." *American Scout Association Monograph.*
"Why Does a Boy Scout Carry a Staff?" *The Scout Association* (1909).
"Umbrella Handles." *Cooper & Sons Ltd. Catalogue.*
"Catalogue of Walking Sticks." *Lintott & Sons Ltd. Catalogue.*
"The Work of Barry Saich, Stickmaker." *Craftsmans Cottages* (Winter 1990).
"Walking Sticks: Historic, Interesting and Unusual." *Spaulding & Co. Catalogue* (1900).
"Weapons in Walking Sticks." *Scientific American* 104:93 (Jan. 28, 1991).
"The Walking Stick Maker." London: Marshall Cavendish, 1986.
Elfenbein, Kunst. *Emil Vollmer Verl Wiesbaden* (1974).
"Treasures of Tutankhamun." *The British Museum Catalogue* (1972).
Two Dissertations on the Athenian Skirophoria. London: 1801.
"Notes & Queries" Oxford University Press.
Report of the Juries (Great Exhibition 1985). London: 1852.
Albridq. of Spec'ns rel. to Umbrellas, Parasols & Walking Sticks. London: 1871.
"The Umbrella." *Household Words* Vol. 6 (1853): 201-04.
"Final Report on the Census of Production for 1984." *HMSO Report* 1951.
"Catalogue of Fire-making Appliances." London: Bryant & May (1928).
"Tricks in Sticks." *Sports & Field.* Vol. 179 (March 1978); 53.
"The Trial of a Bus Stop Assassin." *The Sunday Times* London (Sept. 1978).
"Gentleman's Prop." *M.D.* (Feb. 1968): 236-45.
"Not Just a Stick: A Friend for Life." *The London Times* (Jul. 30, 1963).
"Walking Sticks & Fans." *Harper's New Monthly Magazine*. Vol 41 (July 1870): 221-24.

Bibliography of Francis H. Monek

Adburgham, Alison. *Gamages Christmas Bazaar 1913.* David & Charles, 1974.
Adburgham, Alison. *Shops & Shopping 1800 - 1914.* Allen & Unwin, 1964.
Adburgham, Alison. *Yesterday's Shopping: Army & Navy Stores Cat. 1907.* Devon: David & Charles, 1969.
Agnus, H. *Guides des Acheteurs.* 1896.
Aldred, Margaret. "Lament for the Walking Stick." *The Saturday Book* #124 (unknown): 199-201.
Allanson-Winn, R.G./Phillipps-Wolley, C. *Broadsword and Singlestick.* London: George Bell & Sons, 1905.
Allender, H.A. "Making Walking Canes in High School." *Industrial Arts & Vocational Education* 42 (Dec. 1953): 346-47.
Army & Navy Co-Operative Stores, Ltd. Catalogue. 1928.
Arnold, James. *Shell Book of Country Crafts.* London: John Baker, Ltd., 1968.

Arnow, Jan. *By Southern Hands: A Celebration of Craft Traditions in the South.* Birmingham, Alabama: Oxmoor House, 1987.
Ashley, G.O. "The Stick." *Outdoor Life Magazine* Vol. 119 (Feb. 1957): 66-7.
Auer, Michel & Lothrop. *Les Appareils Photographiques d'espionage.* Paris, 1978.
Austin, Robert. *Bamboo.* New York: Weatherhill, 1970.
Ayers, C.E. "My Stick Please." *The New Republic* Vol. 41 (Nov. 26, 1924).
Bacon, Reginald W. *The Juggler's Manual.* Newburyport, MA: Variety Arts Press, 1984.
Baden-Powell, Sir R. "Thumbsticks and Staves." *The Scout.* (Jan. 6, 1923).
Baden-Powell, Sir R. "How To Make Walking Sticks." *The Scout.* (Jan. 14, 1922).
Bahti, John. *South Western Indian Ceremonials.* KC Publications, Inc., 1990.
Baker, Cozy. *Through the Kaleidoscope.* Annapolis, Maryland: Beechcliff Books, 1985.
Bancroft-Hunt, Norman. *People of the Totem, The Indians of the Pacific Northwest.* Orbis Publ., 1979.
Bannerman, Francis. "Catalogue of Military Goods for Sale." (July 1907).
Banzhaf, Dr. D. "Dr. D.W. Banzhaf, Heilbronn" *Der Stocksammler.* (1978).
Banzhaf, Dr. Dieter. "Glaeserne Glueckbringer." *Kunst & Antiquitaeten Magazine.* (Mar/Apr 1981).
Bard, Julius. *Real Lexikon der Musik.* Berlin, 1913.
Barillet, _____. "Cannes a Systems Barillet." *Fabrique d'Armes Barillet.* Gervans, France.
Barton-Wright, E.W. "Self Defense with a Walking Stick." *Pearsons Magazine* (1901).
Bean, William B. "The Golden Headed Cane." 1969-70.
Beazley, J.D. "Narthez." *American Journal of Archeology* 37 (July 1933): 400-03.
Beihoff, Norbert J. *Ivory Sculpture Through the Ages - A Milwaukee Public Museum Publication* (1961).
Berry, Peter. "The Stickmaker." *Practical Woodworking.* (Jan. 1990).
Betensley, B. "Combined Cane and Stool." *Hobbies* 86 (1981): 126.
Betensley, B. "Old Patents Tell It Like It Was: Walking Canes." *Hobbies* 84 (1979): 126.
Bezzaz, Guy. "Le Monde Inconnu Des Cannes." *Le Louvre des Antiquaries.* (198_).
Bigham, Barbara. "Novelty Cameras." *Creative Crafts.* (May 1970): 16.
Binder, Pearl. *Muffs & Morals.* New York: Wm. Morrow & Co., 1938.
Bingham, K. "Carving Diamond Willow Canes." *Creative Crafts* 8 (1982): 49-50.
Bisp, Sandy. "Leaning on a Wooden Art." *The London Times.* (Oct. 13, 1990).
Blake, Joyce E. *Glasshouse Whimsies.* East Aurora, NY: 1984.
Block, Rudolph. *Catalogue of a Private Collection of Walking Sticks.*
Board of Trade. "Final Report on the Census of Production for 1948." *HMSO Report.* 1951.
Boehn, Max von. *Ornaments: Gloves, Walking Stocks, Parasols, etc.* New York: Benjamin Blom, Inc. (1970).
Boerner, Steve. "A Gift For a Prince." *Times* Rochester, New York (Sept. 26, 1984).
Bond, C. "Canes That Led a Double Life." *Smithsonian* 14 (May 1983): 156.
Boothroyd, A.E. *Fascinating Walkingsticks.* Bracknell: Salix Books, 1970.
Boothroyd, A.E. *Fascinating Walkingsticks* (Ed. 2) White Lion Publishers, 1973.
Boserup, *Boserup House of Canes & Walkingsticks Catalogue* (1987).
Boyce F.P. "Hobby Hitching Post: Collecting of Walking Sticks." *Rotarian* 87 (Sep. 1985): 62.
Bradley, Carolyn G. *Western World Costume: An Outline History.* New York: Appleton-Century Crofts, 1954.

Brigg, *Brigg Umbrellas and Walking Sticks*. London: Swaine, Adeney, Brigg & Sons, Ltd.

"The Stickmaker." *The British Stickmakers Guild* (1984).

Browning, Gertrude. "The Cane as Art and Artifact." *The Antique Journal* (Feb. 1973).

Brown, James & Sons. *Old Gun Catalogue* (1876).

Buchan, John. *The Magic Walking Stick*. Edinb.: Cannongate Publishing Ltd., 1985.

Buchner, Alexander. *Musical Instruments Through the Ages*. London: Spring Books, 1936.

Buck, A.M. *Victorian Costume & Costume Accessories*. Herbert Jenkins, 1961.

Burbridge, David. "Walking Wonders." *Country* Vol. 88 No. 11 (1988).

Burtscher, William J. *The Romance Behind Walking Canes*. Philadelphia: Dorrance & Co., 1945.

Campin, Francis. *The Practice of Hand-Turning*.

Carol, Sadtler. "The Shepherd's Art of Crooks and Cleeks." *Lands End Catalogue* (1989).

Carpenter, L. "The Snake Stick Just Took My Eye." *Foxfire* 18 No. 3 (Fall 1984).

Carpenter, C.E. "The Cultivation of Walking Canes." *Scientific American* 79:362 (Dec. 3, 1898).

Cazal, Rene Marie. *Assai Historique, Anecdotique Sur Le Parapluies*. Paris: L'ombrelle & la Canne, 1844.

Chalmers, J. "Walking Sticks Used by the Elderly." *British Medical Journal* 285 (1982): 57-8.

Chapuis, Alfred. *Hist. do la Boite A Musique & de la Musique Mecanique*. 1955.

Chamberlain, Essie. *Essays Old & New*. New York: Halcourt, Brace & Co., 1926.

Clark, Erland Fenn. *Truncheons, Their Romance & Reality*. 1925.

Clay and Court. "The History of the Microscope." (1932): 155.

Cochran, R. "Sticks." *Blair and Ketchum Country Journal 8* (Jan. 1981): 50-9.

Coe, Ralph T. *Sacred Circles*. London: The Arts Council, 1976.

Colbert, Paul. "Stick Dressing." *Countryside Monthly*. (July 1981).

Collier, John. *American Indian Ceremonial Dances*. New York: Bounty Books, 1972.

Conan Doyle, Arthur. *The Hound of the Baskervilles*. Grafton Books, 1902.

Cooper & Sons, Ltd. "Cooper & Sons, Ltd. Inc. Lintott & Sons Ltd. Catalogue." (1984).

Cooper, W. *A History of the Rod in All Countries*. Chato & Windus, 1874.

Coopers, "Cooper & Sons Ltd. Walking Stick Makers Through 6 Reigns."

Coradeschi, S. & Lamberti. *Bastoni*. Milan: Giorgio Mondatori, 1987.

Coriat, Isador H. "The Symbolism of the Gold Headed Cane." *American Medical History No. 6* (1974).

Cosner, Sharon. "Antique Walking Sticks and Canes." *Early American Life* (Dec. 1976).

Cowie, Keith. "K.C. Sales Leaflet." (1988).

Cox, Sandy. "King of the Stick Dressers." *Farmers Weekly* (Jan. 12 1979).

Craddock, Chris. "The Walking Stick Gun." *Shooting Times* (Oct. 11, 1984).

Craddock, Chris. "Guntalk — Readers' Queries." *Shooting Times* (June 19, 1986).

Craddock, Chris. "Walking-stick Gun." *Shooting Times* (Aug. 7, 1986).

Crawford, T.S. *A History of the Umbrella*. Devon: David & Charles, 1970.

Credland, Arthur. "The Blowpipe in Europe and the East." *The Journal of the Arms & Armour Society* (Dec. 1981).

Cromie, William James. *Single Stick Drill*. American Sports Publishing Co., 1919.

Crowell, I.H. *Horn Crafts*. 1945.

Culme, John. *Dictionary of London Gold & Silversmiths 1838-1914*. Suffolk: Antique Collectors Club, 1987.

Cunningham, Andrew C. "The Cane as a Weapon." *The Army & Navy Register* (1912).

Cunnington & Wille. *English Women's Clothing in the Present Century*. New York: Thomas Yoseloff, 1958.

Cunnington, C.W. & P. *Handbook of English Costume in the 18th Century*. London: Faber & Faber, 1963.

Curtis, E.S. *The North American Indian*. Mass.: Cambridge, 1908.

Curtis, Cecil-Ed. "Walking Stick Notes." *Cecil Curtis*.

Cuzacq, Rene. "Makhila et Agulhade." *Pyrenees*

D'Allemagne, Henry R. *Les Accessoires du Costume et du Mobilier*. Paris: Chez Schmit Libraire, 1928.

Daranatz. *Le Makhila*, 1923.

Davenport, Millia. *The Book of Costume*. New York: Crown Publishers, 1948.

Deacon, Ton. "A Stick to Beat All Others." *Trout and Salmon Magazine* (May 1990).

Deaver, George G. *Abnormal Gait Patterns*. New York: Inst. Rehabilitation Medicine, 196?.

Demura, Fumio. *Bo, Karate Weapon of Self-Defense*. California: Obera Publications, 1976.

DiPego, Pauline. "Raising Canes." *Modern Maturity* (Feb. - Mar. 1978).

Dick, Franziska. *Lituus and Galerus Wien 1973*. Vienna: Diss, 1973.

Dickie, Paul C. "The Subtle Art of Stick Dressing." *Heritage - The British Review* No. 30 (Dec. 1989).

Dike, Catherine. *Le Monde Inconnu des Cannes du 18e au 20e siecle*. Paris: Le Louvre, 1980.

Dike, Catherine. "Festival de Cannes." *Le Collectionneur Francais* (Oct. 1973).

Dike, Catherine. *Cane Curiosa*. Geneva: Catherine Dike, 1983.

Dike, Catherine. "A Horse Race." *Antique Collector's Club* (Dec. 1984).

Dike, Catherine. "Dual Purpose Walking Sticks." *Antique Collecting VIII* (Apr. 1974): 12.

Dike, Catherine. "From Weapon to Insignia." *The Australian Antique Collector* (Jan. - June 1985).

Dike, Catherine. "Prestigieuses ou inattendues, les cannes de collection." *L'Esampille 118* (Feb. 1980).

Dike, Catherine. "Silver & Gold Cane Handles in the US, 17th c. - Civil War." *Silver* 20:4 (Jul-Aug 1987).

Dike, Catherine. "Tiffany Silver & Gold Cane Handles 1950 - 1987." *Silver* 20:5 (Sep.- Oct 1987).

Dike, Catherine. "Gorham and Other Cane Handles." *Silver* 20:6 (Nov.-Dec. 1987).

Dike, Catherine. *Canes in the United States*. Ladue, MO: Cane Curiosa Press, 1994.

Dite, Tabor. "Stockflinten und Stockbuechsen." *Waffenjournal*. (Dec. 1975).

Donaldson, Gerald. *The Walking Book*. New York: Holt, Rinehart & Winston, 1979.

Douglas, John Murchie. *Blackthorn Lore and the Art of Making Walking Sticks*. Ayr: Alloway Publishing, 1984.

Duncan, John Shute. *Hints to Bearers of Walking Sticks & Umbrellas*. London: J. Murray, Fleet Street and Edinburgh: Harding St. James St. & A. Constables Co., 1808.

Dunphy, Robert J. "On Buying a Shillelagh in Shillelagh." *New York Times*.

Edings, Charles. "A Collection of Walking Sticks." *The Connoisseur* (1927).

Edings, Charles A. "Curious Walking Sticks in the Collection of _____." *The Connoisseur* 71:88-93 (Feb. 1927).

Edlin, Herbert L. *Woodland Crafts of Britian*. David and Charles: 1973.

Edmunds, Henry. "Blackthorn Bush to Walking Stick." *The Countryman* (1981).

Eggleston, Edward. *Mr. Blake's Walking-Stick*. 1870.

Elder, Peter. *The Art of Crookmaking*. 1987.

Elliott. *Carved Walking Sticks and Thumbsticks*.

Ellis, Anthony. "Collecting." *Sunday Observer London* (1990).

Emde. *Ernst Ludwig Emde - Catalog* (1983).

Escher, Martin R. "Stoecke mit Raffiniertem Innenleben." *Freizeit*.

Evans, Mary. *Costume Throughout the Ages*. Philadelphia: J.B. Linnicott Co. (1930).

Farnell, Jeremy. *Umbrellas & Parasols*. London: Batsford, 1985.

Farrelly, David. "The Book of the Bamboo." *Sierra Club Books* (1938).

Farrington, F. "Hand Me Down My Walking Canes." *Hobbies* 50:89 (March 1945).

Faveton, Pierre. *Les Cannes*. Paris: Cha. Massin, 1988.

Fedden, Robin. *Churchill at Chartwell Catalogue*. (1968).

Feild, Rachel. "What the Best Dressed Sticks are Wearing."

Fel, Edit. *Hungarian Peasant Art*. Budapest: Corvina, 1958.

Fenton, William Nelson. *The Roll Call of The Iroquois Chiefs*. Wash. DC: Smiths. Inst., 1950. Repr. NY: AMS Pr., 1980.

Fewins, Clive. "Handled with Care." *Country Times* (Sep. 1989).

Fewins, Clive. "Stick To It." *Weekend Telegraph*, London (Aug. 13, 1988).

Filepettini, et al. "Zauberriten und Symbole." *Bauer-Freilburg* (1979).

Finkenstaedt, H. & Th. "Stangsitzerheilige u. Grosse Kaerzen." *Weisshorn* (1968).

Finn, Mike. "Seitei Tanjo - The Power of the Stick." *Sticks Unlimited*.

Finn, Mike. "Seitei Jodo." All Japan Jodo Federation Video.

Fischer, H.G. "Notes on Sticks & Staves in Ancient Egypt." *Metropolitan Museum Journal* Vol. 1 (1977-78).

Fischer, Henry George. "Ancient Egypt in The Metropolitan Museum Journal." *Metropolitan Museum of Art, New York* (1980).

Flayderman, E.N. *Scrimshaw & Scrimshanders* New Milf. CN, 1972.

Fletcher, Nick. "Far From Sticks in the Mud." *Limited Edition* (Apr. 1989).

Forster, Lesley C. "By Hook or By Crook." *Country Life* (Aug. 26 1982)

Fossel, Theo. *Walking & Working Sticks*. The Apostle Press, 1986.

Fossel, Theo. *A Visit to Leonard Parkin*. 1985.

Fossel, Theo. "The Gentle Art of Stick Dressing." *Crafts and Leisure* (1983).

Fossel, Theo. *Shooting Handbook*. Northampton: Beacon Publishing.

Fossel, Theo. "These Sticks Were Made For Walking." *Woodworking International* (Nov. 1990).

Fossel, Theo. "Well-Dressed Walking Sticks." *Shooting Times* (Nov. 23, 1989).

Fossel, Theo. "Anniversary Walking Stick." *Practical Woodworking*. (Mar. 1987).

Fossel, Theo. "Chinning the Cosh." *Shooting Times* (Mar. 7, 1985).

Fournel, V. *Due role des Coups de Baton*. Paris: 1858.

Franklin, Alfred. *La Vie Prince d'autrefois*. Paris: E. Plom Nourret et cie, 1898.

Freedman, M. "Tuck It IN Your Walking Stick." *Saturday Evening Post* 222-87. (Apr. 29, 1950).

French, Harry J. *Umbrellas Past & Present*. London: Kendall's, 1923.

French, Mary. *A Victorian Village; Record of Quethiock Parish, Cornwall*. Falmouth: Glasney Press, 1977.

Frost, H. Gordon. *Blades and Barrels*. Texas: Walloon Press, 1972.

Futuro. "Future Patient Aids." *The Futuro Company Catalogue*.

Gardner, R.E. *Five Centuries of Gunsmiths, Swordsmiths and Armourers 1400-1900*. Columbus, Ohio: 1948.

Gastrock. "Gastrock Stoecke Catalogue." 1982.

German, Michael. "Strolling with Walking Sticks." 19??.

Gilliam, Laura E. et al. *The Dayton C. Miller Flute Collection*. Wash. D.C.: Library of Congress, 1972.

Ginsburg, Mirra. *One Trick Too Many*. New York: Dial Press, 1973.

Girard, Sylvie. *Cannes et Parapluies et Leurs Anecdotes*. Paris: MA Editions, 1986.

Girardin, Delphine de. *Le canne de Monsieur de Balzac*. Paris: 1853.

Girtin, Thomas. *Makers of Distinction*. Harvill Press: 1959.

Goodwin, Carol. "A Business to Lean On." *Record*, Ontario, Canada.

Gosset, Adelaide. *Scenes from a Shepherd's Life* (1911).

Goulding, Peter. "Swaine Adeney." *Shooting Times* (Oct. 28, 1982).

Gowan, Leo. "Making Antler Handled Sticks." *British Deer Society* (1987).

Graham, Winston. *The Walking Stick*. Garden City, NY: Doubleday, 1967.

Graham, Winston. *The Walking Stick*. London: Collins, 1967.

Graham, Samuel A. *The Walking Stick as a Forest Defoliator*. Ann Arbor: Univ. Michigan Press, 1937.

Grant, David. "Sticks from Stocks." *Shooting Times* (Jun. 7, 1948).

Hart, Edward. *Dalesman Books* (1972).

Grant, I.F. "Highland Folk Ways." *Routledge & Keegan Paul*.

Grasink, W. "Walking-Sticks From the Woods." *Profitable Hobbies* 12:28 (Feb. l956).

Green, D.M. "Canes or Walking Sticks." *Hobbies* 64:56-7 (Jan. 1960).

Greener, W.W. *The Gun & Its Development*. New York: Bonanza Books.

Greenberg, Joel. "Interesting Pistol Cane." *Monthly Bugle* (Sep. 1988).

Grider, Sylvia A. "Howard Taylor, Cane Maker and Handle Shaver." *Indiana Folklore 7*, No. 1 -2 (1974).

Hackley, Larry. "Sticks: Historical & Contemp. Kentucky Canes." *Kentucky Arts & Crafts Foundation* (1988).

Hall, Barbara A. *Hua, Kola* USA: Brown University, 1980.

Hardy, Thomas. *The Woodlanders*. Penguin English Library, 1887.

Harl, B.M. "MSS 1419, A & B" *British Museum Inventory*.

Harrell, D.T. "Walkers and Walking Sticks." *Hobbies* 56:64 (May, 1951).

Hart, Edward. *Walking Sticks* The Crowood Press: 1986.

Hart, Edward. "Stick Gathering." 19??

Hart, Edward. "Shepherds' Crooks." *Countryside Monthly*.

Hartley, Dorothy. *Made in England* (1977).

Hassan, Ali. *Stoecke u. Staebe im Phaeroischen Aegypten*. Munich: Deutscher Kunstverlag, 1976.

Hassan, Ali. "Stoecke u. Staebe im Phaeroischen Aegypten." *Muenchner Aegyptologische Studien No. 33* (1926).

Hattenroth, Fr. *Le Costume Paris*.

Hawthorn, Audrey. *Art of the Kwakiutl Indians (& Other N.W. Coast Tribes)*. The University of British Columbia.

Haythornthwaites, P. "Military Swagger Canes & Swagger Sticks." *Antique Arms & Militia*.

Haythornthwaites, P. *Army & Navy Stores Catalogue 1907*. Devon: David & Charles, 1969.

Heath, Veronica. "Sticks and Stones." *Countryside Monthly* (July 1981).

Herb, Karl. "Der Stab als Zeichen fuer Wuerde, Machut u. Autoritaet." *Salzburger Nachrichten* (Jan. 22, 1990).

Herzfeld, R. "Magie des Takstockes."

Hewitt, Charles. "Walking Stick Farm." *Picture Post* (Mar. 23, 1946).

Hill, Jack. *The Complete Book of Country Crafts*. David & Charles: 1979.

Hillaby, John. *A Journey Through Europe* (19??).

Hogg, Garry. *Country Crafts & Craftsmen*. London: Hutchinson, 1959.

Holliday, Robert C. *Walking-Stick Papers*. New York: George H. Doran Co., 1918.

Holiday, Robert C. "On Carrying a Cane." *Bookman* 48: 160-5 (Oct. 1918).

Holme, Charles. *Peasant Art in Australia & Hungary*. London: The Studio, 1911.

Hopkiss, E.J. *M. & M. Karolik Collection of 18th Century American Arts*. Boston: 1950.

Howell. "Natural Walking Sticks & Umbrella Sticks." *Henry Howell & Co. Catalogue*. 1890.

Hudson, W.H. *A Shepherd's Life; Impressions of the South*. London: Wilts, Downs Methuen & Co. Ltd., 1910.

Hudson, W.H. *A Shepherd's Life; Impressions of the South*. New York: AMS Press, 1968.

Hughes, Therle. *Small Antiques for the Collector*. Lutterworth: 1964.

Humphreys, John. "The Well Dressed Stick." *Shooting Times* (Apr. 6, 1989).

Humphreys, John. "With Hat and Stick." *Shooting Times* (Aug. 23, 1984)

Humphreys, John. "Sticks and the Flicks." *Shooting Times* (May 18, 1989).

Hutton, Alfred. *The Sword & The Centuries*. Rutland, VA: Charles E. Tuttle Co., 1973.

Ingraham, J.H. "An Essay on Canes." *American Monthly Magazine* 12:259, 1838.

J L H. *Umbrella Making & Repairing*. Liverpool: The Handbook Publ. Co., 1900.

Jackson, John R. "Walking Sticks." *Gardeners' Chronicle* (Jan. 27, 1877).

Jackson, John R. "Walking Sticks." *Good Words* 12:429 (1871).

Johnson, R.F. "Forerunner of the Shooting Stick." *Country Life* (Dec. 3, 1959).

Jones, J.A. "Sticks of Distinction." 137:116-18 *Forbes* (Feb. 24, 1986).

Jones, Peter. "Sticks & Crooks." *Country Magazine* (Oct. 1983).

Kaldenberg, F.J. *Manufacturers of Genuine Meerschaum Pipes & Amber Goods*. New York: Kaldenberg, 1889.

Kendall. *The House of Kendall*. London: Kendall & Sons Ltd., 1966.

Kennedy, J. "I'm Cane Crazy." *Hobbies* 60:60-1 (Sep. 1955).

Kind, Fa. *AKAH Lederwaren, Holster, Jagdzubehoer.* Germany: GmbH & Co. Gummersbach, annual.

Klever, Ulrich. *Stoecke*. Munich: Wilhelm Heyne Verlag, 1980.

Klever, Ulrich. *Spazierstoecke - Zierde, Werkzeug und Symbol*. Munich: Verlag Georg D.W. Callway, 1984.

Klever, Ulrich. "Spazier Stoecke." *Sammler Journal No. 3* (March 1974).

Klever, Ulrich. "Die Stockindustrie began im Biedermeier." *Sammler Journal* (July 1979).

Klever, Ulrich. "Das Wichtigste ist meist die Kruecke." *Sammler Journal* (June 1977).

Klinkenberg, Jeff. "The Cane Man." *St. Petersburg Times* (Feb. 1, 1987).

Klinkhart, Wilhelm Stauder & Bierman Braunschweig. *Alte Muskenstrumente*, 1973.

Kocher, G. "Richter und Stabuebergabe im Verfahren der Weistuemer." *Leykam* (1971).

Koehler, M. "Spazierstoecke waren oft mehr als nur Spazierstoecke." *Sammler Journal* (1974).

Kopp, Ernst Ott. "Allerlei Spazierstoecke." *Bibliothek d. Unterh.u.d. Wissens* No. 12 (1898).

Kovac, Eva. *Romanesque Goldsmiths' Art*. Budapest: Corvina Press, 1974.

Kuchler, Hans. *Wanderstoecke*. Roven: Olten, 1982.

Langel, Rene. "La canne revele ses secrets." 19??

Lauffer, Ott. "Der Laufende Bote." 1954.

Lester, Cath M. & Kerr, R.N. *Historic Costume*. Peoria, IL: Charles A. Bennet Co., 1967.

Lester, Cath. M./Oerke, Bess V. *Accessories of Dress*. Peoria, IL: Charles A. Bennet Co., 1954/67.

Lindboom, Gerhard. *Spears & Staffs with Two or More Points in Africa*. Thule: Tryckeri AB, 1937.

Lorz, Kurt. "Das Hirtenmuseum in Hersbruck." *Sammler Journal* (July 1976).

Lovat, The Lord. "Baron Simon Joseph Fraser Lovat." Portrait c. 1908.

Love, Dane. "Stick-Dresser's Day." *The Countryman*, Burford, Oxfordshire (Summer 1987).

Luard, Elisabeth. "Rounding the Horn." *Country Times Leicester* (July 1989).

Lucos, E.V. *Luck of the Year*. London: Methuen & Co., 1923.

Lucos, E.V. *Fireside and Sunshine*. Freeport, NY: Books for Libraries Press, 1968.

Ludgale, Mrs. Howard. "The Evolution of the Stick." 6:28 (May 1897).

MacManus, Seumas. *The Bewitched Fiddle & Other Irish Tales*. New York: Doubleday & McLure Co., 1900.

Macmichael, William. *The Gold-Headed Cane*. The Royal College of Physicians, 1968.

Macmichael, William. *The Gold-Headed Cane*. Paul B. Hoeber, Inc., 1915.

Mann, Sir James. "European Arms and Armour." *The Wallace Collection*. Book 2 (1915).

Manners, J.E. *Country Crafts in Pictures*. Devon: David & Charles, 1976.

Manners, J.E. *Country Crafts Today*. Devon: David & Charles, 1974.

Manners, John. *Crafts of the Highlands & Islands*. Devon: David & Charles, 1978.

Marchal, Charles. *Essai Historique*. Paris: Typogr. Lacrampe et Cie, 1844.

Margerand, M.J. "La Canne." *Carnet de la Sabretache 402* (1941).

Marinas, Amante P. *Arnis Lanata*. Burbank, CA: Unique Publications, 1984.

Marcuse, Sibyl. *Musical Instruments - A Comprehensive Dictionary*. Doubleday, 1964.

Markham, Leonard. "Cane & Able." *Woodworker* (1988).

Martin, Ray. "British Canemaker is in the Stick of Things." *The Cambridge Times*, Ontario, Canada (Oct. 29, 1986).

Masaaki, Hatsumi & Chambers, Quintin. *Stick Fighting*. Palo Alto, CA & Tokyo: 19??

Mase-Spencer, Alphonse. *Historie des Cannes* (before 1927).

Massingham, H.J. *Shepherd's Country*. London: Chapman & Hall, Ltd., 1938.

Matzenauer. *Erste Wiener Peitschen-Stock-Manufaktur*. Jos. Matzenauer, Wien: pre-1918.

Mayes, Herbert R. "The Walking Stick." *Diversion* (Nov. 1983).

McClellan, E. *Historic Dress in America*. Phil.: George W Jacobs, 1904/1910.

McIlroy, A.J. "Villagers beaten by Walking Stick Makers." *The Daily Telegraph,* London (1991).

McKay, James A. *Rural Crafts in Scotland*. 1976.

Merriden, Howard. "Walking Stick Wonderland." *Pearson's Magazine*. Vol. 4 (Nov. 1897): 533.

Meyer, George H. *American Folk Art Canes, Personal Sculpture*. 1992.

Michaelson, P. "Walking Sticks used by the Elderly." *British Medical Journal* 185:58 (1982).

Miles, C. "Sticks and Stones." *Hobbies* 141:2 78:141 (July 1973).

Milnee, A.A. *Not That It Matters*. New York: E.P. Dutton & Co., 1920.

Milton, Roger. *The English Ceremonial Book*. David & Charles, Newton Abbot, 1972.

Mitton, Mervin. *The Policeman's Lot*. Quiller Press Ltd., 1985.

Moeck, Herman. *Spazierstockinstrumente*. Celle, 19??

Moeller, Ernst v. *Die Rechtssitte des Stabbrechens* Weiman: H. Bohlaus, Hachf., 1900.

Mogridge, George. *Family Walking Sticks*. London, 1865.

Monek, Francis H. *List of US Cane Patents up to ca. 1980*.

Monek, Francis H. *List of British Walking Stick Patents up to ca. 1980*.

Monek, Francis H. *List of German Cane Patents*.

Monek, Francis H. *Canes: Staffs of Many Lives; Encyclopedia of Collectibles Vol. 3*. Alexandria, VA: Time-Life Books, 1978.

Monek, Francis H. "The Pleasures and Surprises of Collecting Canes and Walking Sticks." *Der Stocksammler* (1992).

Monek, Francis H. "Gun Canes." *The Cane Collectors Chronicle* Vol. 4, No. 4 (Oct. 1993).

Monek, Francis H. "The Rate Anemometer Cane." *Der Stocksammler* (Dec. 1987).

Morgan, David W. *Whips and Whipmaking*. Cambridge, MD: Cornell Maritime Press, 1972.

Moseman. *Moseman's Illustrated Guide - Horse Furnishing Goods*. New York: Arco Publ., 1892/1976.

Moser, O. *Ein Meisterstab der Zimmerleute*. Wien: Museum f. Volkskunde, 1981.

Mosoriak, Roy. *The Curious History of Music Boxes*. Lightner Pub. Co., 1943.

Mouillesseaux, Harold R. "The Search for Doctor Lambert's Cane Rifle." *The Gun Report*. (Dec. 1975).

Moxon, Stanley. *Umbrella Frames 1848-1948* Samuel Fox, 1948.

Mulley, Graham P., M.D. "Walking Sticks - Everyday Aids & Appliances." *British Medical Journal* Vol. 296 (Feb. 13, 1988).

Munk, William. *The Golden-Headed Cane*. London: Longmans, Green & Co. (1884).

Mutz, Mag J. *Reiten Fahren Gehen*. Vienna, Austria: Galerie Palais Starhemberg, 1987.

Neillands, Robin. *Walking through France*. Collins, 1988.

Neillands, Robin. "Walking Sticks Galore." *The Rambler* (Spring 1991).

Nelson, Edna DeuPree. "Walking out with the Walking Stick." *Antiques* 32:3, 128ff (Sep. 1937).

Nemec, H. *Zauberzeichen.* Schrol, 1976.

Niederer, Jean. "Dressing Up Walking Sticks." *Exchange,* Waterloo, Canada Vol. 6, No. 3 (1988).

Norwood, John. *Craftsmen at Work.* London: John Baker, 1977.

Oblin-Briere, Mireille. *La Canne Blanche.* Tulouse: Private, 1981.

Parker, Dr. South. *The Giant Cabbage of the Channel Islands.* Jersey, C.I.: The Toucan Press, 1970.

Paul, J.S. "Fashionable Cane for a Lady." *Workbench* 34:55 (July 1978).

Payne, Blanche. *History of Costume.* New York: Harper & Row, 1965.

Peel, J H B. "Give Them Some Stick." *The Daily Telegraph, London.*

Peterson, Harold L. *Encyclopedia of Firearms.* London: The Connoisseur, 1964.

Petrel. "A Bit of Stick." *Shooting Times* (1984).

Peumery, S.E. "Les Templiers." *Historia* No. 385 (19??)

Philp, Peter. "There a Run on Walking Sticks." *Unknown* (1988).

Pilkington, William. "Self Defense for All Ages Pt. 1." *Survival Weaponry & Techniques* (July 1986).

Pilkington, William. "Self Defense for All Ages Pt. 2." *Survival Weaponry & Techniques* (Aug 1986).

Pinto, Edward H. *Treen and Other Wooden Bygones.* London: Bell & Sons, Ltd., 1969.

Pollet, Sylvester. *Entering The Walking Stick Business.* Brunswick, ME: Blackberry, 1982.

Polonec, Andrej. *Tvarovane a Zdobene Palice Catalogue.* 1977.

Poese, Bill. "Hand Me Down My Walking Cane." *The Antique Trader.* (Dec. 17, 1974).

Proteus. "The Changing Year." *The Field.* (Sept. 26, 1979).

Raj, J. David Manuel. *Silambam: Technique and Evaluation.* Madras: Higginbothams, 1971.

Ray, Charles. "The Story of the Umbrella." *Pearsons Magazine* (1898).

Réal, Anthony. *The Story of the Stick in all Ages and Lands.* New York: J.W. Bouton, 1875.

Reale, Paul J. "Presidential Canes." *The Antique Trader* (1977).

Redford, R.A. "Man and His Walking Stick." *The Gentleman's Magazine* (1898).

Reeder, Cliff. "My Friendship Cane." *Chip Chats* Vol. 38, No. 1 (Jan. 1991).

Rees, David Morgan. *Yorkshire Craftsmen at Work.* Dalesman Books, 1981: 30-31, 76-77.

Richardson, Robert G. *La Canne a pomme d'or.* London: Abbottempo, 1969.

Ritchie, C.I.A. *Bone and Horn Carving.* New York: 1975.

Ritz, J.M. *Stock und Stab.* Deutschen Landesv f. Heimatschutz - Jahrb., 1937.

Roe, Frederick W. *Early Essayists 1923.* Freeport, NY: Books for Libraries Press, 1971.

Rouse, Parke Jr. "Southern Almanac: Mr. Peanut." *Southern Magazine* (Aug. 1987).

Sangster, William. *Umbrellas and their History.* London, 1855.

Sarry, Maurice. "Le canne: arme de defence." (1978).

Sauer. *Stsoecke kauft man bei Sauer.* Germany: A.K. Sauer GmbH & Co., unknown.

Schiffer, P., N. & H. *The Brass Book.* Schiffer Publishing, 1978.

Schmidt, L. "Horn." *Volkskunde in Niederoesterreich.* 1966.

Schroeder, Joseph J. Jr. *Arms of the World 1911.* Chicago: Follett Publishing Co., unknown.

Schlumberger, Eveline. "Cannes a coup, Cannes a reverse..." *Connaissance des Artes,* No. 339 (May 1980).

Scoggins, Charles E. *The Walking Sticks.* Indianapolis: The Bobbs-Merril Co., 1930.

Sela, Francisco. *El Baston en la Defence Personal.* 194?.

Selfridge, Oliver *Sticks.* Boston: Houghton Mifflin, 1967.

Serven, James E. *The Collecting of Guns.* Stockpole Company, 1974.

Seymour, John. *The Forgotten Arts.* The National Trust, 1984: 139.

Shearston, Trevor. *Sticks That Kill.* New York: St. Lucia, Qld., 1983.

Silverman, J.H. "Praising Canes." *Town and Country* (May 1980).

Smith, W.H.B. *Gas, Air & Spring Guns of the World.* Harrisburg, Pennsylvania: MSP Company, 1957.

Smith, J.J. "Stalking Skills." *Survival Weaponry & Techniques* (Feb. 1987).

Snowmann, A. Kenneth. *Farberge 1846-1920.* London: Debrett's Peerage Ltd., 1977.

Snyder, Jeffrey B. *Canes: From the Seventeenth to the Twentieth Century.* Atglen, Pennsylvania: Schiffer Publishing Ltd., 1993.

Soble, Ronald L. "The Not-Exactly-Humble Walking Stick." *San Francisco Chronicle* (Jan. 9, 1987).

Soble, Ronald L. "Cane Fancy Is Walk of Life for Hobbyists." *Los Angeles Times.* (Dec. 30, 1986).

Sortais, F.L. "Load Off My Feet: Shooting Stick." *Harvest Years.* 8:48 (1968).

St. Aubyn, Fiona. *Ivory.* London: Thames & Hudson, 1987: 142, 274.

Stanley, Albert A. *Catalogue of the Stearns Collection of Musical Instr.* New York, 1916.

Stein, Kurt. *Canes & Walking Sticks.* York, PA: G. Schumway Publisher, 1974.

Stein, Kurt. *Swordcanes.* Man at Arms.

Stephano, Peter. "In Praise of Walking Sticks." *Wood Magazine* Des Moines, Iowa (Feb. 1990).

Stephano, Peter. "On-The-Job Classes." *Better Homes & Gardens* (Dec. 1989).

Stevenson, W. *The Trees of Commerce.* London: W. Rider & Son, 1894/1920.

Stewart, Henry M. "Lewis and Clark and the American Air Gun School of 1800." *Monthly Bugle* (Feb. 1977).

Stewart, Henry M., Jr. "The Air Gun in Antiquity." *Air Gun Magazine* (unknown).

Stone, J.W. Jr. "Walking Sticks in a Southern Collection." *Antiques* 111:338 (Feb. 1977).

Stoner, E. "Novel Walking Sticks." *Profitable Hobbies* 9:33 (Sep. 1953).

Strenge, F.H. "You Can Bend Wood at Home." *Popular Science* Vol. 167 (Sept. 1955): 22.

Summerhays, Jill. "Cane Trivia." *Phoenix (The Stroke Recovery Association)* (1985).

Surtees, R.S. *Mr. Sponge's Sporting Tour.* London: Bradbury & Evans, 1853/1981.

Swaine, Adeney. *Swaine Adeney Brigg Catalogue.* 1988.

Tegner, Bruce. *Stick Fighting.* Ventura, CA: Thor Publ. Co., 1982.

Thaler, Mike. *The Staff.* NY: Joseph Schindelman, 1971.

Thiel, E. *Geschichte des Kostuems.* Berlin, 1968.

Thonet. *Thonet Bros Catalogue.* Vienna: Thonet, 1927.

Tibodeau, Michelle. "A Cane Scrutiny." *Traditional Homes* (Spring 1989).

Tobey, James A. "The Magic Wand of Medicine." *Hygeia* (Apr. 1930).

Tressle, Robert. *The Ragged Trousered Philanthropist.* unknown.

Tulip, Norman. *The Art of Stickdressing.* Newcastle: Frank Graham, 1978.

Tyson, Stuart L. "The Caduceus." *Science Monthly* Vol. 34 (June 1932).

US Bureau of Census. "Census of Manufacturers 1931." *US Govt. Printing Office Report* (1933).

Underwood, Peter. *Ghosts in Cornwall.* Cornwall: Bossiney Books 1983.

Untersteiner, Eva. "Der Stock - Buerdezeichen, Wuerdezeichen Catalogue." (1983).

Vance, J.M. "Something to Lean On." *Audobon* 88:68-72 (Nov. 1986).

Vince, John. *Old Farm Tools.* Aylesbury Bucks: Shire Publications, 1974.

Waele, Ferdinand. *The Magic Staff or Rod in Graeco-Italian Antiquity.* Gent: Drukkerij Erasmus, 1927.

Wagner, Mary. "Stuck on Sticks." *Farmers Weekly* (Sep. 5, 1986).

Wall, John. "Carving Canes." *Insight* (Feb. 9, 1987).

Walters, F.G. "Man & His Walking Stick." *The Gentleman's Magazine* Vol 61: 567 (1898).

Warr, Gordon. "People and Places: Theo Fossel." *Practical Woodworking* (1983).

War Office. *Manual of Instruction for Single Stick Drill.* London: Harrison & Sons, 1887.

Warwick E./Pitz, H./Wyckoff, A. *Early American Dress.* New York: Benjamin Bloom 1965.

Walters, John M. Jr. "Uncle Tom's Therapeutic Walking Stick." *Florida Wildlife* (Jan-Feb 1984).

Webb, Wilfred Mark. *The Heritage of Dress.* The Times Book Club, 1912.

Wesley, L. *Air-Guns and Air-Pistols.* Cassell, London: A.S. Barnes & Co., 1955.

Wilcox, Ruth Turner. *The Mode in Costume.* New York: Charles Scribner's Sons, 1947.

Wills, Barclay. *The Downland Shepherds.* Book Club Ass./Alan Sutton Publ., 1989.

Winant, Lewis. *Firearms Curiosa.* New York: Bonanza Books, 1955 (1961).

Winter, H.J.J. "A Shepherd's Time-Stick, Ngari Inscribed." *Revista intern. de Storia d. scienza* VI:4 (1964).

Winternitz, Emanuel. *Musical Instruments of the Western World.* New York: McGraw Hill, 1967.

Wolff, Elden G. *Air Guns (Publications in History No. 1.* Milwaukee Public Museum, 1958.

Wong, James. *Hung Chia, Double End Staff.* Stockton, CA: Koinonia Productions, 1982.

Wyand, John. "Showing Off." *Country Living* (May 1986).

Wyllie, Margaret. "Hooked on Crooks." *The Craftsman Magazine,* Driffield, E. Yorks (1990).

Yahroes, Herbert. "Wood Detective." *Saturday Evening Post* #220 (1947).

Yates, Peter. "A Countryman's Sticks." *Shooting Times* (Apr. 7, 1988).

Yolen, Jane. *The Seeing Stick.* New York: Thos. Y. Crowell Co., 1979.

Zern, E. "Staff of Life: Wading Staff." *Field and Stream* 83:136-8, 1978.

Prices of Canes at Two Auctions

This is a very variable and uncertain subject. I have purchased canes for $10.00 when others would ask over $1,000.00 for the same or a similar stick. Sincerely, I once paid $600.00 to a dealer for a rare gadget cane and about two months later found and bought the identical cane for $50.00

One cane, a whalebone fist-handed scrimshaw, of which I have several, sold at auction in October of 1994 for $44,000.00!! I have a letter from a large and reputable antiques house in Philadelphia offering a presidential cane of which I have many, for - believe it or not - $65,000.00!

The value of canes seems to go up and down depending on such variable factors as weather keeping people from an auction, the financial need of the seller, the ability of the purchaser to pay, etc. Many price guides I have read are way out of line on the value of canes, due to the limited number of knowledgeable people in this field.

Rather than be confronted hereafter with an alleged misappraisal, I feel that the only fair way for me to evaluate a stick is to educate the prospective purchaser with what similar sticks sold for - not on a one by one confrontation, but by the prices obtained at an auction attended only by cane collectors.

Such an auction is given periodically by a dealer who deals in and auctions only canes. He contacts collectors world wide and sells to and solicits from them their canes for sale in his auctions. His firm is Henry & Nancy Taron, Tradewinds Auctions, 24 Magnolia Avenue, Manchester-By-The-Sea, MA 01944 (508) 768-3327; the only "sole cane-auction house" in America.

Their brochure of an upcoming auction - again only of canes - is very beautiful, and expertly and finely displays every stick with a most exact and detailed description. Their appraisal of each stick is listed under each picture and very fairly states the probable low and high bid on each item. Subsequently, after the auction, a final sale sheet is mailed to each purchaser of the brochure.

As the brochure is mailed out many weeks before the auction, prospective buyers can leisurely examine the canes pictures, read the descriptions, ponder the appraisal values, and then either attend the auction or mail in a bid. The sale price is consequently a well weighed and contemplated figure.

I have found this auction house to be most fair and have noted that their high and low appraisals invariably are proven correct by the final sale price.

As I believe this is the fairest way of appraising a cane, I have included in this book two brochures plus final sales prices on two of their most recent auctions.

You too can read and study the pictures, the descriptions, the appraisals and final sales prices and then mentally compare this with any stick you have or will later find and wish to purchase.

What could be a fairer method of determining the value of a walking stick?

The auction price estimates and results for each auction are listed separately; the Saturday, October 23, 1993 auction results are listed first, followed by the May 20, 1994 results. The results are listed in the following order: auction lot number, description of the cane handle in that lot, description of the shaft material, probable country of origin, the height of the cane, the approximate date of the cane's manufacture, the low and high estimates for each cane, and finally the actual auction price received for each cane (without the added ten percent). The values are in U.S. dollars.

October 23, 1993 auction at Samoset Resort, Rockport, Maine, conducted during the first American International Cane Collectors Conference.

1. Large silver knob handle, single bark malacca, Continental 34 1/2" c. 1850 $500-800 $250
2. Sterling 2 1/2" handle, coconut wood shaft 35 3/4" $200-400 $100
3. Sterling 5" long handle, partridge wood shaft, American 34 3/4" c. 1880 $200-400 $200
4. Large 4" silver knob handle, sandlewood shaft, Continental 33" c. 1880 $500-800 $200
5. Art Deco, sterling & ebony handle, mahoganized hardwood shaft, American 36" c. 1920s $200-400 $325
6. Chinese export silver handle, full bark malacca shaft 37" c. 1880 $300-500 $325
7. 7" long 800 silver handle, snakewood shaft, Continental 36" c. 1870 $600-900 $325
8. Parade master's, 3 1/4" large English smooth sterling handle, malacca shaft, sterling eyelets 35 1/2" $500-700 $350
9. Meissen porcelain man handle, pattern #269, 19th c. remake, malacca shaft 36" c. 1860 $1500-2000 $2000
10. Whale ivory scrimshaw captains cane, fist w/ baton handle, mahogany shaft 38" c. 1850 $1100-1500 $1200
11. Nautical, 1 3/4" fluted whale ivory handle, whalebone diamond sawtooth carved shaft, English 35" c. 1830 $600-900 $500
12. Nautical, 2 3/4" carved, fluted, baleen inlaid handle, shaft fluted, matches handle, English 34" c. 1840 $700-1000 $1300
13. Nautical, ivory handle (carved) depicts Greek Andromeda myth, whalebone shaft, American 34" c. 1850 $2600-3600 $2700
14. Nautical, 3 1/4" polished bone knob/walrus cap handle w/ bone ring, hemp shaft in sailor's knots, American 33" c. 1850 $900-1300 $1100
15. Civil War Union, burnished copper handle w/ eagle & flag, coconut wood shaft, American 35" Pat. 1862 $400-700 $600

16. American political cast pewter elephant handle, ebonized hardwood shaft 34 1/2" c. 1880 $200-400 $350
17. Silver handle w/ dog & snake, American 37 3/4" c. 1890 $200-400 $350
18. Flick stick, ivory knob, 3 1/2" spike, malacca shaft w/ eyelet, Continental 32 3/4" c. 1830 $500-700 $800
19. Ivory tau Masonic handle, malacca shaft, English 36" c. 1890 $400-600 $350
20. Ladies cane, all ivory, high relief decoration, Continental 32 1/2" c. 1860 $1200-1500 $600
21. Japanese staghorn monkey grappling snake handle, bamboo shaft, American made 36" c. 1880 $600-900 $475
22. Ivory knob, flexible elephant tail shaft 34" c. 1830 $700-1000 $550
23. Folk art schoolmaster's, wood knob handle and shaft, carved #s & letters, American 36" c. 1770s $3500-4500 Passed
24. Ivory lion handle, mahoganized hardwood shaft, English 34" c. 1900 $500-700 $325
25. Folk art, wood knob, carved & painted wood shaft, American 34" c. 1850 $1300-1800 $500
26. Folk art, one piece soft wood, painted & carved pig faces, Native American 34" c. 1900 $700-1000 $500
27. L handle wood carved monkey, hardwood shaft, English 37" c. 1880 $500-700 $500
28. Ivory duck handle, hazelwood shaft 35" c. 1890 $600-800 $900
29. Solid 18K gold presentation knob handle, snakewood shaft, American 33 3/4" 1865 $800-1200 $750
30. Skull w/ 8 emeralds, ruby eyes, polished bone handle, mahoganized hardwood shaft, English 37" c. 1890 $2000-3000 $3000
31. Gun cane, brass dog handle, faux tortoiseshell shaft, floating firing pin 38 1/2" c. 1850s $1500-2500 $2200
32. Gun cane, rosewood L handle, breech loader, painted metal shaft, English c. 1890 $1200-1800 $1000

33. Blow gun rifle, metal cap over mouthpiece, cartridge gun, brass barrel under stepped malacca shaft, French c. 1870 $1500-2000 Passed
34. Sword cane, gold filled knob handle, 25" blade, whalebone 5" collar, bamboo shaft 36" c. 1870 $500-800 $550
35. Underhammer percussion gun cane, signed, American c. 1825 $1500-2000 $1900
36. Breech loading gun cane, black horn crook handle, walnut covered shaft c. 1870 $1200-2000 $800
37. Sword cane, marked Toledo blade, snakewood shaft, American 35 1/4" c. 1890 $800-1200 $450
38. 5 cane makers samples of exotic wood shafts, carved w/ wood names, American 30" c. 1890 $800-1200 $450
39. African chieftan folk art, well carved wood handle and shaft 34 1/2" c. 1850s $1600-2200 $1700
40. Tortoiseshell & sterling silver blackmoor cane (handle fashioned as man's head, silver hair), French 36" c. 1880 $1200-1600 $1700
41. Wood gray parrot head handle, ebonized shaft, English 34 1/2" c. 1880 $400-600 $300
42. Folk art, tau handle, well carved hardwood shaft w/ Masonic symbols, etc., American 36" $1500-2500 $2400
43. Ivory carved Scotty dog handle, ebonized hardwood shaft, English 35 1/4" c. 1890 $500-700 $500
44. Silver pique, 3" ivory handle w/ "95" date inlaid, malacca shaft 37" 1695 $900-1200 $1100
45. Porcelain 4 1/4" tau hanlde, ebonized shaft, Continental 35 1/4" c. 1890 $600-900 $450
46. Folk art, spaniel wood handle, carved wood shaft, American 35" c. 1860 $600-800 $400
47. Folk art (poss. missionary), faces w/ headdresses handle, carved snakes shaft, all wood 36" c. 1840 $800-1000 $450
48. Folk art hardwood, root crook handle, carved snake shaft, American 36" c. 1870 $600-800 $200
49. Folk art hardwood, man's head handle, relief carved shaft, American 43" 1897 $600-800 $200

50. Rare field microscope gadget, signed, black walnut & brass, American c.1850s-1890s $1500-2500 $3100
51. Ivory ball handle, Japanese shibiyama decor, inlaid jade, coral, mother of pearl, signed, single bark malacca shaft, American 34 1/4" c. 1880 $1200-1500 $800
52. Mushroom shaped rhino horn knob, 14K gold receptacle & collar, inscribed, full bark malacca shaft, American 35 1/2" early 20th c. $1100-1300 Passed
53. Sterling silver encased root handle, silver snake, medlar shaft, American 36" c. 1870 $1200-1500 $1350
54. Relic cane, wood from Confederate gun boat, carved & hemp decorated, American c. 1911 $2000-3000 $1700
55. Walnut & glass cane case, fans open, 5 sections, 120 canes held, American 32" wide, 28" deep $2500-3000 $4400
56. Sterling Tiffany & Co. decorated, signed handle, mahoganized hardwood shaft 33" c. 1890 $800-1200 $1300
57. Rare bronze bearded man cane handle mold c. 1870 $500-800 $400
58. Japanese 4 3/4" carved handle, rosewood shaft, American 37" c. 1880 $1000-1400 $550
59. "Faces of man" ivory ball (4 faces), briarwood shaft, Continental 36" c. 1890 $900-1200 $1000
60. Very rare violin cane, beechwood, nickle rings, fitted bow, German c. 1850 $9000-12000 $9000
61. Perched eagle 6" carved handle, ebonized shaft, English 34" c. 1870 $400-600 $400
62. Lapis Lazuli ball top cane, bamboo shaft, gold plated presentation collar, English 36" c. 1870 $400-600 $300
63. Automata gadget cane, horses head, moving ears & mouth, segmented horn shaft 36 3/4" c. 1890 $800-1200 $1050
64. Sterling silver folding Masonic ball handle, ebonized shaft, English 35" c. 1900-1925 $2000-2500 $3600
65. Unusual carved Japanese grotesque faces ball handle, partridge handle, American 35" c. 1890 $1200-1500 $1100
66. Nautical cane, shepherd's crook baleen top, 18K gold end cap, baleen shaft, American 35 1/8" c. 1840s $900-1200 $500
67. "Six Gods" gold gilt cast brass handle, rosewood shaft, Continental 34 1/4" c. 1880 $400-600 $650
68. Historical relic cane, "Jason" shipwreck, turned knob, inscribed 34" c. 1890s $700-1000 $600
69. Lady's enameled handle, silver mounts & polished rose quartz, thin malacca shaft 35 1/2" c. 1900 $300-400 $600
70. Rare 18th c. boxwood handle with nude, stepped malacca shaft, German 36" c. 1740 $1400-1800 Passed
71. Folk art doctor's cane from medical school, all wood w/ incised & inked designs, American 35" 1883-1886 $2500-3500 $2600
72. Folk art historical relic cane, carved wood shaft from Fayetteville Arsenal, N.C., American 38 3/4" c. 1863 $400-600 $500
73. Ivory ball handle in silver cup sword cane, 13" quadrafoil blade, malacca shaft 34" c. 1860 $400-600 $600
74. Sword cane, crook wood handle, stepped hardwood shaft, "Toledo" marked blade 35" c. 1890 $700-900 $700
75. Horn glove holder cane, hand holding ball handle, malacca shaft 33 1/2" c. 1870 $200-400 $350
76. Rhino horn crook handle, 14K gold collar, rosewood shaft 35 1/4" c. 1900 $400-600 $300
77. Green aventuring handle, tropical hardwood shaft, Continental 36" c. 1870 $500-800 $600
78. Ivory setter handle, solid silver collar, coconut wood shaft, American 36" c. 1880 $800-1000 $1500
79. L carved ivory handle w/ sleeping nude, mahogany shaft, Continental 36" c. 1890 $1200-1500 Passed

80. Folk art all walnut wood cane depicting bearded man with bible 36" c. 1850s $1500-2000 Passed
81. L ivory handle doctor's cane with skull and cross-bones motif, natural wood shaft, American 33" c. 1860 $700-900 $800
82. Political, William Jennings Bryan cast pewter handle, hardwood shaft, American 35 1/4" c. 1896 $200-400 $275
83. Folk art, carved wood man's head handle, wood shaft, German 34" c. 1880 $200-400 $100
84. Folk art carved black man's head with skull cap, one piece dark stained oak down shaft, American 35 1/2" c. 1880 $300-500 $150
85. Political cane, William McKinley pewter & gold gilt (rare) handle, maple shaft, American 36" 1896 $300-400 $275
86. Folk art, carved black man handle, pink lips, white teeth, one piece hardwood through shaft 35 1/2" c. 1890 $300-500 $400
87. Grotesque man's head handle carved from root, rosewood shaft, Continental 35 1/4" c. 1890 $400-600 $475
88. Knobkerrie weapon, helmetted man silver plated handle, mahogany shaft 33" c. 1890 $300-500 $250
89. Brass railroad watch handle w/ key, ebonized hardwood shaft c. 1900-1925 $600-900 $600
90. Historical cane, sterling silver handle w/ 1904 Panamanian coin inset, presentation from Col. George W. Goethals $800-1200 $550
91. Folk art, carved drum, bag & snake 33 3/4" $400-600 $200
92. Wood turk's head knot ball handle, wood cane, black paint, American 37 1/2" c. 1860 $400-600 $300
93. Folk art, one piece wood cane, knot and fluting handle, simulated thorn shaft 36" c. 1860 $700-900 $275
94. Gambler's cane, hollow ivory ball handle w/ bone dice under glass, stepped partridgewood shaft 35" c. 1900 $350-550 $575
95. L ivory handle, crouching hound carved, ebony shaft 36" c. 1880 $600-800 $500
96. Elephant ivory handle, relief carved horse and setter, solid gold collar, single bark malacca shaft 35" c. 1860s $1000-1300 $500
97. Odd ivory monkey face w/ black ebony robe, bamboo shaft c. 1870 $600-900 $375
98. L ivory handle, carved alligator, snakewood shaft, American 34 1/2" c. 1880 $800-1200 $550
99. L whale ivory handle, scrimshaw whaling decor, malacca shaft, American 35 1/4" c. 1850 $1500-2000 $650
100. Solid 18K gold knob handle, gold continues down ebony shaft, American 36" c. 1850 $900-1200 $2700
101. Relic cane from sidewheeler steamboat "New Orleans", inscribed & imbedded spike at handle, American 34" c. 1880s $1200-1800 $550
102. Relic cane from Commodore Perry's flagship "Lawrence" 33 1/2" c. 1830s $1500-2000 $750
103. Crook ivory handle, simulates bamboo, stepped partridge shaft, American 36" c. 1890 $500-700 $850
104. Ivory L handle carved as bamboo, inlaid silver simulating whorl, stepped hardwood shaft, American 35 1/4" c. 1890 $500-700 $425
105. Ebony pug handle 5 1/4" long, sterling collar, medlar shaft, American 34 1/4" c. 1880 $500-700 $750
106. Folk art polychrome decor snake & frog, all wood, American 34 1/8" c. 1840 $800-1200 $250
107. Confederate folk art hardwood, carved & black painted snake, American 33" 1861 $300-500 $100
108. Folk art polychrome cane, snakes, carved simulated thorns shaft, American 38 1/2" c. 1870 $700-1000 $350
109. Chieftan's cane, tropical wood ball knob, 3 twining snakes shaft, South Seas or African 35" c. 1900 $400-600 $375
110. Ivory pique handle w/ inlaid silver "97", malacca shaft, English 41 1/2" 1697 $800-1200 $900

111. Ivory bust of 15th c. man, mounted 19th c. hardwood shaft 33 1/2" c. 1890 $600-800 $500
112. L ivory eagles claw & egg handle 34" c. 1890 $500-700 $500
113. Ivory half crook handle, relief carved hunting equipment, dark malacca shaft, American 36" c. 1870 $700-900 $500
114. 4" straight carved ivory perched bird handle, whangee bamboo shaft 37" c. 1890 $600-800 $375
115. Carved ivory L handle w/ owners name carved through center, rosewood shaft 36" c. 1890 $400-600 $275
116. Ivory carved dog L handle, hardwood shaft, American 34" c. 1890 $500-700 $625
117. Horn handle carved as elephant w/ ivory tusks, slim bamboo shaft 36" c. 1890 $400-600 $400
118. Stepped partridge wood crook handle w/ sterling whippet at end w/ London hallmarks 36" $600-800 $375
119. Ivory Japanese L handle carved w/ monkeys on arbor, mahoganized hardwood shaft, American 35 3/4" c. 1880 $600-800 $700
120. Folk art wood knob handle, carved twist, moon, man's face, branch & leaves, maple shaft, American 35 1/4" c. 1880 $300-400 $375
121. Wood ball handle incised w/ initials, hardwood shaft incised w/ 2 figures (flappers), American 34" $400-600 $150
122. Chinese foo dog wood handle & shaft, gold eyelets 34 1/4" c. 1840 $400-600 $200
123. One piece carved wood half crook sleeping bear handle, hardwood shaft, Continental 33 1/2" c. 1880 $400-600 $150
124. Folk art natural hickory stick, applied knob handle, relief carved animals, American 37" c. 1900 $400-600 $200
125. Major Frank E. Harris' Philippines cane, silver handle, ebony shaft 35" 1913 $900-1200 $550
126. French ebony, ivory & rosewood aristocrat's cane, leather carrying case. Silver disk, family crest, 3 pieces rosewood shaft w/ ivory & ebony separators 35 1/4" c. 1900 $700-900 $500
127. Silver tau handle w/ relief pointer, Art Nouveau style, American 36" c. 1880 $500-800 $475
128. Folk art whale & Jonah handle in wood, shaft poker burn decorated 37" c. 1860 $600-900 $475
129. Horn L handle, carved crouching hound, briar shaft, English 36" c. 1870 $400-600 $275
130. Staghorn Japanese handle, carved monkey & snake, square bamboo shaft, American 34 3/4" c. 1890 $400-600 $275
131. Staghorn L handle, Japanese w/ monkey & snake, squared bamboo shaft, American 35 1/2" c. 1890 $400-600 $275
132. Ebony hand holding mother-of-pearl baton handle, mahogany shaft, silver eyelets, American 33" c. 1840 $400-600 $350
133. Knob handle on malacca cane, presentation cane w/ inscribed band 35" $400-600 $225
134. Folk art, heeled boot handle, relief carved animals on shaft, European 35" c. 1850s $600-900 $350
135. Silver skull handle, hinged movable jaw, ebonized shaft, Continental 35" c. 1890 $800-1200 $750
136. Folk art stylized snarling dog handle, heavy shaft w/ poker burning decor, French 33 1/2" c. 1700s $700-1000 $350
137. All rhino horn slim cane w/ L handle, braided silver collar 33" c. 1860 $400-600 $500
138. Folk art Odd Fellows carved wood cane w/ 3 1/2" stepped bone handle, American 36" 1914 $500-700 $200
139. Hammered silver putter handle sporting cane, bamboo shaft, English 35 1/2" c. 1900 $600-800 $450
140. Glass whimsey cane, L handle, twisted shaft, 3 stripes, milk glass core, American 38 1/4" c. 1880 $300-500 $500

141. Ivory crook handle w/ carved elephant head end, ebonized hardwood shaft, English 35" c. 1880 $500-700 $200
142. Oak & glass cane case, round, holds 39 canes, American 21" x 43" c. 1880 $1500-2000 $1600
143. L handle elephant ivory w/ carved rings & rope garlands, gold collar presentation, full bark malacca shaft c. 1880s $800-1000 $550
144. Walrus ivory L handle (4" long) w/ bear's head & paws, malacca shaft 34" c. 1890 $500-700 $300
145. Elephant ivory handle (3") carved as Egyptian lady, rosewood shaft 37" $500-700 $250
146. Elephant ivory handle relief carved hound (4 3/4"), briar shaft 31" c. 1890 $600-800 $325
147. Sterling Y handle fashioned dowsing twig, ivory inset, ebony shaft, American 33 3/4" c. 1890 $600-800 $450
148. Staghorn L handle relief carved running stag, medlar shaft, German 34" c. 1880 $400-600 $175
149. Horn crook handle, silver plated owl end piece, compressed paper shaft over metal rod, English 35 1/2" c. 1890 $300-500 $225
150. All horn cane w/ 2" knob & decorative rings over metal rod, American 35 1/2" c. 1890 $200-400 $225
151. Staghorn 4" turned handle, hand carved spiral rosewood shaft 34" c. 1880 $300-500 $250
152. Sterling silver college cane molded as staghorn handle marked Rutgers '01, heavy ebony shaft 35" $200-400 $175
153. Unusual leather, brass & bone cane with twist c. 1900 $200-400 $450
154. Black horn & walrus ivory segmented cane over metal rod, American 37 1/4" c. 1890 $200-400 $350
155. Polychrome folk art carved wood cane, ball handle, American 37" c. 1870 $700-900 $200
156. Folk art cane, one piece oak, crude carved snake & man, American 35 1/2" c. 1860 $300-500 $125
157. Folk art, one piece cane carved w/ long knob handle, carved decor, fraternal society cane, American 40" c. 1890 $500-700 $100
158. Solid tortoiseshell crook handle, stepped partridgewood shaft c. 1890 $300-500 $425
159. Lady's cane, 8 1/2" elephant ivory carved handle, rare purple heart wood shaft, Continental 35 1/2" c. 1890 $400-600 $400
160. 7" straight ivory carved handle of robed woman, 19th c. bamboo shaft, shallow relief monkeys, Japanese & signed 39 1/2" $700-900 $425
161. Elephant ivory hound, thin malacca shaft, lady's cane c. 1880 $200-400 $275
162. Tau porcelain lady's cane, rosewood shaft 31" c. 1890 $250-350 $250
163. Ivory L handle fashioned as horse's leg w/ gold filled hoof, natural ash shaft, American 34" 19th c. $400-600 $400
164. Staghorn cane w/ 14K gold mounts, mahogany shaft 35 1/4" c. 1910 $300-500 $300
165. Horn horse head 4 1/2" handle, palisander shaft, American 36" c. 1890 $350-550 $200
166. Ivory ball turned on rose lathe for spiral decor, gold plated collar, malacca shaft, plain eyelets, Continental 33 1/2" c. 1840 $350-550 $375
167. Ivory shepherd's crook handle, snakewood shaft, English 36" c. 1890 $800-1000 $400
168. Wooden one piece cane, large pondering monkey handle, Oriental 34 1/2" c. 1880 $400-600 $200
169. Whimsical pewter man's round face w/ housefly, ebonized hardwood shaft, German 35" c. 1890 $400-600 $225
170. Carved one piece knobby root handle as bearded man, American 36" c. 1855 $700-1000 $275
171. T handle carved ebony early whale concept, thick soft wood shaft 42 1/2" c. 1850-1900 $600-800 $325
172. Wild boar's tusk relief carved w/ woman, natural hardwood shaft, Continental 36 1/2" c. 1870 $400-600 $300

173. Polished boar's tusk, gold filled collar, malacca shaft, American 35 1/2" c. 1880 $400-600 $300
174. Carved oriental boy's head Kachina nut handle, bamboo shaft 35 1/2" c. 1890 $200-400 $200
175. Walrus ivory L handle carved hound, malacca shaft, American 35 1/4" c. 1860 $500-700 $325
176. Folk art root handled cane carved dog, rabbit & bear, soft wood shaft, American 36" c. 1870 $500-800 $350
177. Folding seat cane, removable nickel plated cap allows split walnut shaft to separate as tripod & hold cloth seat, American 35" c. 1880 $300-500 $325
178. Wild boar's tusk, relief carved reclining semi-nude woman, hardwood shaft, English 36 1/2" c. 1890 $800-1200 $600
179. Carved ivory Victorian lady's leg w/ boot, lace garter, malacca shaft, English 35" 1874 $700-900 $1250
180. Carved man's head w/ tricornered hat handle, mahogany shaft, English c. 1890 $800-1200 $450
181. Japanese carved handle w/ 4 monkeys climbing, signed, ebony shaft, gold filled collar, English 40 1/2" c. 1890 $1000-1300 $500
182. Black horn poodle handle, ebonized mahogany shaft, simulated thorns, English 38" c. 1900 $600-800 $350
183. 2 polished whale's teeth mounted in T shape handle, whalebone shaft 36" c. 1860 $800-1000 $825
184. Large carved ivory skull, ebonized shaft, English 35" 1868 $800-1000 $575
185. Ivory carved Chinese kneeling woman w/ rose, rosewood shaft, ivory eyelets, English 36 1/2" c. 1890 $900-1300 $400
186. L ivory hound handle, malacca shaft, English 36" c. 1890 $600-800 $375
187. Ivory L handle w/ carved boar & hound, ebony shaft, English 36" 1917 $1000-1400 $850
188. Macabre wooden handle of robed skeleton as death w/ throne of skulls & snakes, briar shaft, Continental 37" c. 1880 $600-800 $375
189. Japanese carved ivory handle w/ frog & lotus leaves (netsuke quality), signed, ebony shaft, English c. 1890 $700-900 $1600
190. Rhino horn phallus handle, snakewood shaft, Continental 36" c. 1900 $800-1200 $1000
191. Important Americana, tortoiseshell handle embossed w/ bust G. Washington & Seal of U.S., mahogany shaft (w/ partial replacement) 37 1/2" $600-900 $550

May 20, 1994 auction at Kings Grant Inn, Danvers, Massachusetts

1. Silver (8" on handle) overlaid wooden cane, hardwood shaft 35 1/4" c. 1900 $100-300 $150
2. Chestnut shooting stick gadget cane, German 35 1/2" c. 1900 $200-400 $200
3. Shagreen (coral colored) crook handle, malacca shaft, American 35" c. 1920 $100-300 $200
4. Rhino horn pistol handled cane, 800 silver eyelets, malacca shaft, German 37 1/2" c. 1890 $100-300 $250
5. Wooden dog head glove holder, rosewood & cherry shaft 36 1/2" c. 1890 $300-500 $375
6. Tool container cane, 4 metal tools w/in screw top cap, yew shaft, English 36" c. 1890 $300-500 $350
7. Tortoise shell crook handle, gold plated end cap, stepped partridge shaft, American 33 1/4" c. 1890 $300-500 $300
8. Relic cane from WWI airplane propeller, pistol grip handle, silver plaque 35 1/2" $400-600 $300
9. Corkscrew cane w/ carved ivory reclining lion handle, malacca shaft, English 35" c. 1890 $700-1000 $700
10. Pique cane dated 1700, 3" ivory handle w/ eyelets, malacca shaft, English 37" 1700 $900-1300 $450

11. Ivory tiger handle, realistic, snakewood shaft, French 35 1/2" c. 1900-1925 $600-800 $800
12. Plain silver Tiffany & Co. handle, shaft from Washington Elm in Cambridge, MA 35 1/2" $400-600 $425
13. Masonic cane w/ elephant ivory ball handle, carved black walnut shaft, American folk art 35 1/4" c. 1890 $600-800 $575
14. Elephant ivory L handle, doctor's cane, reindeer relif carved, narrow malacca shaft, American 35 1/2" 1865 $400-600 $300
15. Ivory handle w/ sterling mounts, rosewood shaft, American 36" c. 1890 $400-600 $775
16. Anglo-Egyptian segmented ivory cane w/ Egyptian Pharoah handle, onyx simulated thorns in shaft 34 1/2" c. 1900 $500-700 $375
17. Silver capped (London hallmark) knobby natural wood shaft, bronze crabs & ants in branch stubs 36" c. 1880s $300-500 $300
18. Elephant ivory knob handle w/ baleen dot inlay, silver collar, snakewood shaft, American 32 3/4" c. 1840 $400-600 $575
19. Spectroscope cane, examine optical spectra, sterling cap, marked w/ maker & seller, hallmarked 1929, malacca shaft 35 1/2" $500-700 $425
20. Rare "going ashore" cane, 10" heavy narwhal tusk handle, hardwood shaft (heavy), English 39 3/4" c. 1830 $1200-2000 $1850
21. Solid gold "race track tout's" pencil cane, 9K gold knob, single bark malacca shaft 35 1/2" 1920 $600-800 $525
22. Elephant ivory "trio of horses" handle, malacca shaft, American 36" 1893 $800-1200 $1100
23. Nautical cane, whale turks head knot handle, baleen separators, white whalebone shaft, American 36" c. 1850 $500-800 $600
24. Well carved 3" ivory handle w/ 3 nude maidens & swan, single bark malacca shaft, Continental 36" c. 1860 $2400-3000 $3500
25. Cold painted Vienna bronze fox handle, walnut shaft 36 1/2" c. 1880 $500-800 $1700
26. Ivory & 14K gold American Banker's decorative cane handle, presentation, stepped partridge shaft 34" $800-1200 $1350
27. Ivory handle carved w/ dog chasing cat & nipping tail, rosewood shaft, English 38 1/2" c. 1870 $800-1000 $800
28. Scrimshaw whales tooth cane, southern American wood shaft c. 1875 $400-600 $150
29. Ivory horse head handle, narrow, stepped malacca shaft, American 34 3/4" c. 1860 $400-600 $375
30. Rare narwal tusk cane w/ silver end cap, American 38 3/4" c. 1850 $3000-4000 $3800
31. Ivory & brass spyglass cane (3 1/4" long as handle), rosewood shaft 36 1/2" c. 1920 $500-800 $625
32. Lapis Lazuli all handle, ebony shaft, English 35 1/2" $400-700 $350
33. Lady's powder puff cane, silver plated handle (flat), opens to mirror & puff, hardwood shaft, American 38 1/2" c. 1900-1925 $400-600 $525
34. Carved wooden blackmoor handle on dark wood shaft (one piece) 36" c. 1880 $600-800 $425
35. Rare ivory monkey automata cane (eyes roll, tongue sticks out), malacca shaft, Continental 36" c. 1890 $2800-3600 Passed
36. Sterling half crook handle, Art Nouveau motif of oak leaves & bark, acorns & twigs, thick ebony shaft, Continental c. 1880 $400-600 $300
37. Harmonica cane, walnut w/ ebony cap & ebony separator, English 36" c. 1900-1925 $400-600 $1000
38. Historical cane from "U.S.S. Constitution" w/ short ivory knob, coin silver cap & eyelets, oak shaft, American 33 3/4" c. 1830 $800-1200 $1400
39. Ivory Japanese carved ball handle, owl & 14 rats battling, snakewood shaft, American 36 3/4" c. 1890 $1100-1400 $1250
40. Rare sailor's knobkerrie weapon, woven baleen over lead ball handle, flexible malacca shaft 34 1/2" c. 1850 $300-500 $500
41. Nautical cane, whale ivory fist w/ cuff handle, shaft 40 segments alternating ivory & Koa wood, eyelets 34 1/2" c. 1850 $1500-2500 $2200

42. Sword cane, silver top & collar, 26 1/2" long Toledo marked sword, mahoganized malacca shaft 34" c. 1900 $400-600 $350
43. Ivory carved horse's leg & hoof, silver collar w/ relief horse's head, French 36 1/2" c. 1890 $600-900 $375
44. Gadget cane, ebony handle & sterling mounts, contains matchsafe w/in unscrewing handle, ebonized hardwood shaft, England 35 3/4" c. 1920s $300-500 $375
45. Race track tout's pencil cane, pencil within crook of handle, bamboo shaft, 12K gold mounts, England 38" c. 1905 $600-800 $425
46. Nautical cane, turned whale ivory knob, mahogany shaft w/ inlaid satinwood & mother of pearl diamonds & dots, English 35 1/4" c. 1830 $600-800 $350
47. Ivory crook handle, solid gold 1" collar, snakewood shaft, English 36" c. 1930s $600-800 $375
48. Sword cane w/ parrot handle, double edged steel blade 27 1/4" long, Continental 35 3/4" c. 1920 $400-600 $550
49. Siren cane, filigree decoration, ash shaft c. 1890 $400-600 $425
50. Rare pie shaped 50 cane case, 43" x 39", walnut wood & glass, American c. 1860 $1500-2000 $1950
51. L ivory carved bearded man handle, silver collar w/ raised fox, malacca shaft, Continental 35 1/4" c. 1880 $500-700 $275
52. Ivory parrot handle, rosewood shaft, American 35 3/4" c. 1890 $500-700 $300
53. Horse measuring cane, knobby wood handle, bamboo shaft, brass measuring arm, English 37" c. 1870 $500-800 $600
54. Ivory L handle w/A. Lincoln bust scrimshaw inked, malacca shaft, American 1865 $700-900 $1100
55. Nautical cane, polished whale tooth, 3 baleen separators, polished whalebone shaft, American 35 1/4" c. 1850 $500-800 $450
56. Polished whale ivory nautical cane, handle belaying pin shaped, ebony shaft, American 34 1/4" c. 1870 $500-800 $500
57. Japanese ivory Shibayama cane, brown ceramic cap, inlay birds, etc. in abalone, jade, mother of pearl, & ivory, ebony shaft, Japanese 36 3/4" c. 1890 $700-1000 $750
58. Nautical cane, carved elephant ivory ball in hand handle, whalebone shaft, American 35 1/4" c. 1860 $500-800 $600
59. Solid silver handle presentation cane, inscribed, ebony shaft 36" 1884 $400-600 $900
60. Utility knife gadget cane, 7 1/2" long blade, poker burned & stepped shaft, simulating bamboo, French 34 3/4" c. 1890 $400-600 $275
61. Large 4 1/2" carved ivory handle carved w/ The Legend of Saint Hubertus, single bark malacca shaft, ivory eyelets, German 36 1/4" c. 1820 $2000-3000 $2750
62. Polished staghorn dog head whistle cane, malacca shaft, English 33" c. 1880 $300-500 $325
63. Walrus ivory carved elephant head 4" handle, mahogany shaft 35 1/8" c. 1880 $400-600 $400
64. Solid silver handle w/ vine & flower decor, satinwood shaft, Far Eastern 39" 1890 $300-500 $300
65. Ivory handle cane assoc. w/ Ringling Bros. history, carved 3 different dogs heads, stepped partridge shaft 35 1/2" c. 1890 $1200-1500 $1100
66. 2" jade handle, 1 1/2" gold mount, zebra wood shaft 35 1/2" c. 1890 $200-400 $275
67. Lady's cane, 3 1/2" mother-of-pearl handle w/ daisies, ebonized hardwood shaft, English 36 1/2" c. 1910 $200-400 $325
68. Watch cane handle w/ flip up lid, rosewood shaft, French 35 1/2" c. 1925 $700-1000 $1000
69. Solid 9K gold decorative knob handle, malacca shaft, England 34 1/4" 1890 $500-700 $275
70. Automata (gadget), wooden parrot head, eyes roll & beak opens w/ push button, ash shaft, English 36" c. 1890 $1500-2000 Passed

71. Elephant ivory well carved ball-in-fist handle (2"x2"), rosewood shaft 34 3/4" 1919 $600-800 $500
72. Elephant ivory well carved parrot 4 1/2" handle, rosewood shaft 38" c. 1890 $600-800 $1100
73. Flask cane, copper mounts, top unscrews & reveals 2 1/4" footed drinking glass, 6" down shaft unscrews to reveal 13 1/2" slender glass flask w/ metal & cork stopper, congo wood shaft, Austrian 36 1/4" c. 1900 $400-600 $550
74. Whimsical wooden carved man handle, stepped hardwood shaft, English 37" c. 1900 $200-400 $125
75. Sterling snuff-box handle w/ erotic view inside lid. Lid snaps open to reveal snuff compartment, ebonized hardwood shaft, English 35 1/4" 1880 $2500-3500 $3500
76. Folk art, hickory, dunce w/ broad nose & pout as handle, American 37 1/2" c. 1880 $300-500 $150
77. Horn crook handle w/ bulldog at end w/ composition ears, malacca shaft, German 36" c. 1900 $200-400 $275
78. Brass ball handle w/ compass (under unscrewing top cap), ebonized hardwood shaft, English 33 1/2" c. 1880 $400-600 $400
79. Elephant ivory segmented cane, 3" knob handle, simulated thorns w/ black dots (onyx?), Anglo-Egyptian 35" c. 1890 $600-900 $400
80. Walrus ivory mermaid masthead handle (5 1/2"), ebony shaft, American 34 1/4" c. 1860 $800-1200 $600
81. Walrus ivory male lion eating twisting snake (4 3/4") handle, hardwood shaft 35 1/2" c. 1890 $300-500 $325
82. Reveling monk (gambling & drinking) ivory handle, mahogany shaft, German 34" $2000-2500 $2400
83. Sterling 2 1/4" knob w/ swirls & C scrolls, snakewood shaft 36" $200-400 $225
84. Poacher's percussion gun w/ ebony L handle, overhammer trigger w/ pull ring, metal shaft, removable ferrule, Continental 33 1/2" c. 1880 $1000-1500 $1500
85. Rare gadget, beheading handle w/ bearded man handle, unscrews & knife removed from snakewood shaft, knife inserted behind head, beheads but man escapes unharmed! American 35 1/2" c. 1900 $2400-3000 $2800
86. Ivory L handle Masonic, relief carved square & compass w/ G, American 34 1/4" c. 1895 $300-500 $475
87. Masonic ceremonial sword cane, etched Masonic symbols, hand guard & blade stored w/in shaft, encased leather shaft, English c. 1890 $1000-1500 $1100
88. Round 1 1/4" agate handle, solid gold collar, brown painted hardwood shaft, English 36 1/2" c. 1900 $200-400 $175
89. Rhino horn whippet handle, briar shaft, American 34 1/8" c. 1880 $300-500 $325
90. Ape head automata crook handle w/ ivory ears, push button under jaw, sticks out red tongue, hardwood shaft, English 35 1/4" c. 1880 $900-1200 $900
91. Lady's Japanese cloisonne crook handled (9") cane, smooth partridge shaft, American 38 1/4" c. 1900 $500-700 $650
92. Folk art carved diamond willow, Western motif, completely carved shaft, knob handle, American 38 1/4" c. 1910 $700-1100 $400
93. Faceted bloodstone handle, solid gold collar, rosewood shaft 35 3/4" c. 1890 $500-700 $1000
94. Ivory & silver L handle, overlaid 3 sterling 4 leaf clovers, mahogany shaft, American 35 1/2" c. 1890 $300-500 $275
95. Pique pomander handle, unscrewing perforated cap w/ pocket inside for medicinal herbs, silver collar & eyelets, malacca shaft, English 39 1/2" c. 1730 $1200-1500 Passed
96. Elephant ivory (5") twisted handle w/ carved hand lady's cane, ebonized hardwood shaft, English 33 1/3" c. 1880 $300-500 $325

97. Elephant carved in ivory ball handle, hardwood shaft, American 35 1/2" c. 1880 $800-1000 $500
98. Silver eagle weighted knobkerrie weapon handle, eagle holds apple in beak, hardwood shaft, Continental 34 1/4" c. 1880 $400-600 $675
99. Well carved elephant ivory Shakespeare bust (3") handle, heavy rosewood handle, English c. 1870 $1300-1800 $1200
100. Glove holder, 4 segment rhino horn w/ stylized bird handle, handle pistol grip shape w/ central hole for gloves, Chinese 36" c. 1890 $400-600 $425
101. Elephant ivory straight handle carved w/ 2 oriental dragons, lady's cane w/ exotic hardwood shaft, Chinese 35" c. 1890 $400-600 $400
102. Superb KPM Berlin large porcelain veiled lady (painted) handle, rosewood shaft 39" c. 1850s $1200-1700 $1000
103. Nautical cane, whale ivory turk's head knot handle, octo-carved piece of whalebone below w/ inked whales and names on each, natural wood shaft 36 1/2" c. 1860 $400-600 $400
104. Solid oak cane case w/ glass front & top, holds 49 canes, 50" tall, 21 1/4" wide, 20" deep, American c. 1880 $800-1200 $1200
105. Carved ivory upright lion (3 1/2") handle, ebony shaft, English 37" c. 1890 $500-700 $300
106. Sterling rabbit handle, gilded gold, ebonized hardwood shaft, English 34" 1919 $400-600 $575
107. Carved ivory ram's head handle, single bark malacca shaft, English 37 1/2" c. 1880 $1200-1700 $1700
108. Rare T handle Meissen porcelain spotted hound handle (3" long), mahogany shaft 36" late 18th c. handle $1200-1700 $1350
109. Carved elephant ivory lion & 2 dogs battling constricting snake, malacca shaft 34" 1890 hallmark $1600-2200 $1800
110. L ivory horses head handle, ebonized shaft, gold gilt collar, English 36" c. 1890 $500-800 $375
111. Carved boxwood bearded man handle, single piece of wood handle & shaft, German 35" c. 1880 $400-600 $200
112. Damascene metal-work egg shaped knob handle, cedar shaft, Middle Eastern 35" c. 1900 $200-400 $175
113. Carved elephant ivory acrobats 4 1/2" straigh handle, malacca shaft, German c. 1880 $1200-1500 $600
114. Walrus ivory whaling scene L handle w/ relief carved rope & harpoon, heavy mahogany shaft, English 34 1/4" c. 1890 $500-800 $250
115. Carved wood see no evil monkey 2" high handle, stepped hardwood shaft, English c. 1900 $200-400 $175
116. Large carved elephant ivory 3 dogs attacking mountain lion 5" handle, heavy ebony shaft 37 1/2" 1919 hallmark $1500-2000 $2000
117. Ivory L animal paw handled short sword, diamond shaped 12" blade, smooth partridge shaft 35 1/2" c. 1880 $700-900 $950
118. Transverse cane, ivory handle, silver mounts, 13" flute, rosewood shaft, Continental 36" c. 1900s $500-700 $800
119. Spyglass w/ nickel handle, ebonized malacca shaft, American 34" 1880 pat. $300-500 $575
120. Carved elephant ivory Irishman w/ cap 2" handle, rosewood shaft 37 1/2" 1912 hallmark $600-800 $325
121. Large elephant ivory carved bulldog handle (2"), gold collar inscribed, malacca shaft, English 34 3/4" $600-800 $400
122. Elephant ivory Disraeli bust 2" high handle, 1" sterling collar, presentation cane, rosewood shaft w/ simulated thorns 36 1/2" $900-1300 $1700
123. Polished carnelian pistol grip handle, gold plated collar, rosewood shaft, English c. 1880 $400-600 $200
124. Carved wooden Oriental man, freely moving ball in mouth, wood shaft poker burned & relief carved, ball rattles when shaken, Thailand 37" c. 1900 $200-400 $125

125. Macabre carved ivory T 2 skulls facing outward w/ 2 snakes at abutted backs of skulls at center of T, briar shaft, Continental   33 1/4"   c. 1880 $1000-1500 $1800

126. Large carved detailed ivory cat handle, rosewood shaft, English   c. 1890 $1100-1600 $1800

127. Automata wooden bison, push button in back & tongue sticks out, mahoganized hardwood shaft, English 37 1/2" c. 1890 $1300-1800   Passed

128. Carved elephant ivory Elizabethan lady w/ ruff collar handle (2"), malacca shaft, English 34 1/2"   c. 1890 $600-800 $350

129. Carved elephant ivory Friar Tuck head handle, malacca shaft   34 1/4"   1912 hallmark $600-800 $400

130. Silver w/ solid gold overlay handle, heavy lignum shaft, French   35 1/4"   c. 1900 $500-700 $375

131. L horn handle w/ sterling mounts, studs & eyelets, ebonized shaft, American   36"   c. 1890 $200-400 $175

132. Underhammer percussion gun cane, firing mechanism hidden for poaching, crook handle, muzzle loader   36"   c. 1840 $1200-1600 $1400

133. Carved ivory fox & grapes pistol grip handle (5"), 14K solid gold collar, thin malacca shaft, German 34" c. 1880 $500-700 $275

134. Rhino horn erotic phallic (L shaped) handle, gold collar, tropical exotic wood shaft, French c. 1890 $800-1200 $800

135. Carved elephant ivory round faced man w/ tricornered hat handle, malacca shaft   35 1/4" $500-700 $350

136. Carved elephant ivory Roman man handle, heavy rosewood shaft 35 1/4" $700-900 $325

137. Carved elephant ivory bison handle, rosewood shaft, American 34 1/2" c. 1880 $600-800 $800

138. Macabre carved ivory skull handle, gold gilt collar, ebony shaft, English   33 3/4"   c. 1890 $600-800 $275

139. Carved elephant ivory whippet L handle, malacca shaft, English   33"   c. 1890 $500-700 $350

140. Polished staghorn Japanese whimsical "treed" elephant by turtle motif handle (5 1/3"), ebonized hardwood shaft 38"   c. 1895 $400-600 $475

141. Elephant ivory 12 segment cane, L handle w/ thumb rest, 2 black horn separators, Anglo-Egyptian 33 3/4"   c. 1900 $400-600 $375

142. L walrus ivory hound handle, ebonized malacca shaft, 14K gold collar, American   34 1/2" c. 1860 $300-500 $325

143. Whimsical ivory terrier w/ long jockey cap (4" long) handle, hardwood shaft, English 34 1/4" c. 1890 $400-600 $425

144. Ebony handle, breech loading gun cane, underhammer trigger, metal shaft, Continental 34 3/4"   c. 1880 $1000-1500 $1100

145. Umbrella cane, crook dark malacca handle, 14K solid gold collar, light wooden shaft, umbrella hidden w/in, German   35 1/4"   c. 1900 $300-500 $200

146. Golf driver mahogany handle, golf head inlaid w/ lead & ebony heel, oak shaft, English 35 1/2" c. 1900 $500-700 $375

147. Large staghorn L handle overlaid w/ sterling simulated staghorn & snake, briar shaft, American 35 1/2"   c. 1880s $400-600 $400

148. Christopher Columbus souvenir cane, pewter bust handle, marked 1893 Columbus, Chicago, Souvenir, hardwood shaft   34 1/3" $300-500 $225

149. Carved ivory eagle head handle, ebonized hardwood shaft, English   37"   c. 1880 $300-500 $250

150. Tau sterling Art Nouveau handle, snakewood shaft, American 35 1/4"   c. 1890 $500-700 $350

151. Silver & 2 inlaid panels of ivory, curved L handle, medlar shaft, American   33"   c. 1880 $200-400 $175

152. Carved ivory L huchbacked jester reclining on pillow handle, medlar shaft, American   35 3/4" c. 1870 $500-700 $475

153. Large, heavy going-a-shore cane, 7" polished whale tooth handle, thick exotic tropical wood shaft, American   38"   c. 1860 $600-800 $300

154. Nautical scrimshaw half-crook whale ivory handle w/ incised bird's head, whalebone shaft, carved c. 1860 $600-800 $1200

155. Ivory & sterling mounts tau handle (4 3/4" long), stepped partridge shaft, American   36" c. 1890 $300-500 $275

156. 2 Dartmouth College senior canes, father & son, (one w/ Indian head handle), signed by seniors down wood shaft $500-800 $325

157. Nautical cane, round turned whale ivory handle w/ 1848 Liberty dime inlaid in top, whalebone shaft, American   38 1/4" $600-900 $850

158. Nautical cane, L horn handle, 7 horn spacers, narrow shark spine shaft, American   33 1/4" c. 1860 $200-400 $250

159. China Trade silver knob handle, decorated scenes, tropical mahogany shaft, American   37" c. 1850 $300-500 $275

160. Large rhino horn crook handle, stepped partridge wood shaft, American   34 3/4"   c. 1890 $200-400 $125

161. Decorative cane, ivory w/ silver overlay handle, stepped partridge shaft, American   35" $300-500 $200

162. Polished staghorn skull cane, mahogany shaft 37" $400-600 $400

163. Ebony L handle w/ ivory bear endcap, malacca shaft, Continental   35 1/2"   c. 1880 $300-500 $125

164. Faceted crystal ball-knob handle, bamboo shaft, French   36"   c. 1890 $200-400 $150

165. Large silver pistol handle w/ overlay bee & flowers, ash shaft, American   35"   c. 1870 $200-400 $325

166. Silver hound head handle, thick bamboo shaft, Continental   34 1/2"   c. 1900 $200-400 $225

167. Pistol ash handle w/ ivory overlay of wolf killing deer, ash shaft, German   35"   c. 1890 $300-500 $100

168. Ivory lion's paw handle, baleen shaft, silver collar, American   35"   c. 1850 $300-500 $200

169. Chinese rosewood opium pipe, elaborately carved T handle w/ fish (mouth for opium), carved 7 Immortals shaft   35"   early 1900s $400-600 $1400

170. Early short sword (13" blade) cane in bamboo, English   33 3/4"   c. 1830 $300-500 $150

171. Solid silver crook handle etched w/ niello highlights, ebony shaft 36"   c. 1890 $200-400 $250

172. Silver plated dog w/ hat, shirt & bow tie handle, malacca shaft, English   35 1/4"   c. 1900 $200-400 $200

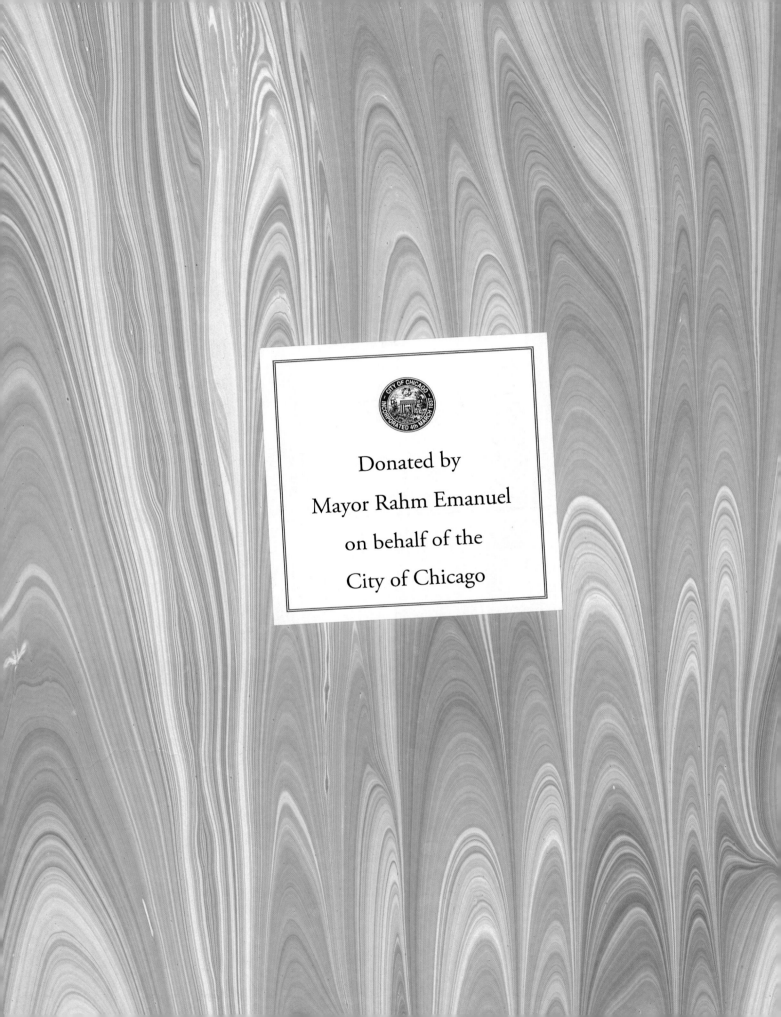